Study Guide for the

# Core Curriculum for Oncology Nursing

Study Guide for the

# Core Curriculum for Oncology Nursing

*6th Edition*

**Suzanne M. Mahon, DNSc, RN, AOCN®, AGN-BC**
Professor, Internal Medicine
Division of Hematology/Oncology
Saint Louis University;
Professor, Adult Nursing
Saint Louis University School of Nursing
St. Louis, Missouri

**Rose Bell, PhD, ARNP-C, AOCNP®**
Director
Professional Practice
Education and Research, Nursing
Roswell Park Comprehensive Cancer Center;
Adjunct Assistant Clinical Professor, Nursing
University of New York at Buffalo
Buffalo, New York

ELSEVIER

Elsevier
3251 Riverport Lane
St. Louis, Missouri 63043

STUDY GUIDE FOR THE CORE CURRICULUM
FOR ONCOLOGY NURSING, SIXTH EDITION

ISBN: 978-0-323-59546-9

---

**Notice**

Practitioners and researchers must always rely on their own experience and knowledge in evaluating and using any information, methods, compounds or experiments described herein. Because of rapid advances in the medical sciences, in particular, independent verification of diagnoses and drug dosages should be made. To the fullest extent of the law, no responsibility is assumed by Elsevier, authors, editors or contributors for any injury and/or damage to persons or property as a matter of products liability, negligence or otherwise, or from any use or operation of any methods, products, instructions, or ideas contained in the material herein.

---

Previous editions copyrighted 2018, 2016, 2005, 1998, 1992, and 1987 by Oncology Society

*Executive Content Strategist:* Lee Henderson
*Senior Content Development Specialist:* Heather Bays
*Publishing Services Manager:* Deepthi Unni
*Project Manager:* Srividhya Vidhyashankar

Printed in United States of America

Last digit is the print number: 9  8  7  6  5  4  3  2  1

Working together
to grow libraries in
developing countries

www.elsevier.com • www.bookaid.org

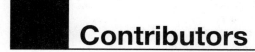

# Contributors

**Diane Bartella, MSN, RN, OCN®**
Clinical Educator, Nursing Education
Roswell Park Comprehensive Cancer Center
Buffalo, New York

**Susan Weiss Behrend, MSN, RN, AOCN®**
Clinical Nurse Specialist, Nursing
Fox Chase Cancer Center
Philadelphia, Pennsylvania

**Christine Boley, MSN, RN, ACNP-BC**
Oncology Nurse Practitioner, Medical Oncology
Providence St. John's
Santa Monica, California

**Jeannine Brant, PhD, APRN, AOCN®, FAAN**
Oncology Clinical Nurse Specialist and Nurse Scientist
Nursing, Billings Clinic
Billings, Montana;
Assistant Affiliate Professor
College of Nursing
Montana State University
Bozeman, Montana

**Christa Braun-Inglis, MS, APRN-Rx, FNP-BC, AOCNP®**
Nurse Practitioner, Oncology
University of Hawaii Cancer Center
Honolulu, Hawaii;
Assistant Researcher, Clinical Trials Office
University of Hawaii Cancer Center
Honolulu, Hawaii;
Clinical Faculty
School of Nursing
University of Hawaii at Manoa
Honolulu, Hawaii

**Dawn Camp Sorrell, MSN, FNP, AOCN®**
Oncology Nurse Practitioner
Oncology
Children's of Alabama
Birmingham, Alabama

**Ellen Carr, MSN, AOCN®**
Nurse Case Manager
Multispecialty Clinic
Moores Cancer Center
La Jolla, California

**Suzanne Carroll, MSN, BSN, AAS, OCN®**
Clinical Nurse Manager
Leukemia
Roswell Park, Buffalo, New York

**Jill Cooper, BSEd, BSN, MSN**
Nurse Practitioner
Briskin Clinical Research Center, City of Hope
Duarte, California

**Diane Cope, PhD, ARNP, BC, AOCNP®**
Oncology Nurse Practitioner, Nursing
Florida Cancer Specialists and Research Institute
Fort Myers, Florida

**Stacie Corcoran, MSN, RN**
Program Director, Adult Cancer Survivorship
Department of Medicine
Memorial Sloan Kettering Cancer Center
New York

**Patti Davis, BSN**
Manager of Nursing Operations
Infusion Center
Medical Oncology and Radiation Oncology
Frontier Cancer Center
Billings, Montana

**Elizabeth Delaney, DNP, CNS, FNP-BC, OCN®, ACHPN**
Nurse Practitioner
Medical Oncology
Dayton Physicians Network
Dayton, Ohio;
Assistant Professor
School of Nursing
Cedarville University
Cedarville, Ohio

**Katrina Duncan, MSN, BSN**
Nurse Practitioner
Hematology/HSCT
City of Hope Medical Center
Duarte, California

**Julia Eggert, Phd, GNP BC, AGN-BC, AOCN®, FAAN**
Professor Emerita
School of Nursing
Clemson University
Clemson, South Carolina;
Advanced Practice Nurse Genetics Counselor
Oncology Services
Bon Secours St. Francis Hospital System
Greenville, South Carolina

**Denise L. Falardeau, MSN, AGPCNP-BC, AOCNP®**
Nurse Practitioner
Medical Oncology
City of Hope National Medical Center
Duarte, California

**Elizabeth Freitas, PhD, MS, BSN**
Clinical Nurse Specialist
Pain and Palliative Care
The Queen's Medical Center
Honolulu, Hawaii

**Jaya Mini Gill, MD, BSN, RN**
Clinical Trials Supervisor
Neuro-Oncology
Providence Saint John's Health Center/John Wayne
Cancer Institute
Santa Monica, California

**Cathy Glennon, RN, MHS, OCN®, NE-BC**
Director, Patient and Community Education
Nursing, Cancer Center
University of Kansas Cancer Center
Westwood, Kansas

**Catherine Jansen, PhD**
Oncology Clinical Nurse Specialist
Department of Oncology and Hematology
The Permanente Medical Group
San Francisco, California;
Clinical Professor
Physiological Nursing
University of California
San Francisco, California

**Marcelle Kaplan, MS, RN, CNS**
Oncology Nursing Consultant, Writer, Editor
Test Developer, Independent Contractor
Merrick, New York

**Brenda Keith, MN, RN, AOCNS®**
Sr. Oncology Clinical Coordinator III, Genentech
South San Francisco, California

**Santosh Kesari, MD, PhD**
Chair and Professor
Translational Neurosciences and Neurotherapeutics
John Wayne Cancer Institute
Santa Monica, California

**Hana Kim, PhD, MS, CP**
Staff Psychologist
Comprehensive Pain Center
Minneapolis VA HCS
Minneapolis, Minnesota

**Erin Kopp, BSN, MSN, ACNP-BC**
Nurse Practitioner
Department of Hematology
City of Hope
Duarte, California

**Tricia Montgomery, BSN, RN**
Clinical Coordinator, Research
Cancer Research, Tumor Registry
Oncology Social Work Billings Clinic
Billings, Montana

**Patricia W. Nishimoto, BSN, MPH, DNS**
Adult Oncology Clinical Nurse Specialist
Department of Medicine
Tripler Army Medical Center
Honolulu, Hawaii

**Janis Marie Petree, RN, MSN, FNP, AOCNP®**
Nurse Practitioner
Medical Oncology
Infusion Treatment Center
Redwood City
Stanford Healthcare
Redwood City, California

**Cynthia Samborski, AAS, BS, MSN, MHA**
Clinical Research Educator
Clinical Research Services
Roswell Park Comprehensive Cancer Center
Buffalo, New York

**May San, MSN, FNP-C**
Department of Hematology and Hematopoietic
Transplantation
City of Hope National Medical Center
Duarte, California;
Clinical Adjunct Faculty
School of Nursing
Azusa, California

**Marlon Garzo Saria, PhD, RN, AOCNS®, FAAN**
Oncology Clinical Nurse Specialist
Professional Development
Providence Saint John's Health Center
Santa Monica, California;
Clinical Nurse, Nurse Corps
United States Air Force
March Air Reserve Base, California;
Director and Assistant Professor
Translational Neurosciences and Neurotherapeutics
Pacific Neuroscience Institute
Santa Monica, California

**Shama Shrestha, BSN, RN, OCN®**
Nurse Case Manager
Palliative Care
University of California in San Diego
Moores Cancer Center
La Jolla, California

**Mady C. Stovall, MSN, ANP-BC**
PhD Student
School of Nursing
Oregon Health & Science University
Portland, Oregon

**Joseph D. Tariman, PhD**
Assistant Professor, Co-Director for the DNP Program
Department of Nursing
DePaul University
Chicago, Illinois;
Nurse Practitioner
Section of Hematology-Oncology
Northwest Oncology and Hematology
Hoffman Estates, Illinois

**Tia Wheatley, DNP, RN, AOCNS®, BMTCN**
Oncology Clinical Nurse Specialist
Professional Practice and Education
City of Hope National Medical Center
Duarte, California

**Barbara J. Wilson, MS, RN, AOCN®, ACNS-BC**
Director Oncology Professional Practice
Cancer Network, WellStar Health System
Marietta, Georgia

# Preface

This Study Guide is a companion text to the *Core Curriculum for Oncology Nursing*, Sixth Edition. Each chapter in this new edition has a corresponding chapter in that text, reflecting content updates in the practice of oncology nursing since the previous edition. Among the changes, you will notice totally new chapters with content that is critical to our work. Question content, formats, focus, and distribution have been revised to match those of the 2018 OCN® examination test blueprint, to reflect important changes in cancer treatment and related nursing care, and to reflect the latest research evidence.

In general, certification helps assure and validate that a nurse has met rigorous requirements for both experience and knowledge in oncology nursing. Specifically, attaining an OCN® credential is a formal recognition of specialized knowledge in oncology nursing. Knowledge in both the science of oncology and in how to best care for patients and families affected by a diagnosis of malignancy is continually evolving. Oncology nurses are continually challenged to keep up with these changes and apply state-of-the-art knowledge to clinical practice. Certification tests this nursing knowledge.

Written by nurses working in the specialty of oncology and contributors to the ONS *Core Curriculum*, and edited by oncology nursing experts selected by ONS, this revised study guide is the only question-and-answer review book for the OCN® examination developed in collaboration with ONS, providing a tool for nurses to not only assess their knowledge, but to expand their knowledge base as well with the goal of providing excellent clinical care. Questions reflect content that oncology nurses need to understand and apply to provide safe and effective care. The rationale for each question provides information not only on why an answer is correct but also why the other options were either not correct or not the best choice. Reviewing the rationale provides an additional educational opportunity to expand oncology knowledge on not only the content in the question, but related knowledge. To ensure accuracy and consistency between the two books, chapters have been written by authors who contributed to the ONS Core Curriculum, as well as subject matter experts in the field, and edited by experts chosen by ONS. An answer key with detailed rationales is provided for review and remediation.

Persons utilizing this text are encouraged to spend time studying and reflecting on the information in the rationale section and when indicated consult the *Core Curriculum for Oncology Nursing* for additional information.

# Contents

**PART SEVEN:   PROFESSIONAL PRACTICE**

# 1 Epidemiology, Prevention, and Health Promotion

1. Cancer epidemiology is defined as the study of the:
   A. rates of cancer occurrence in a population
   B. number of deaths from cancer in a given time period
   C. distribution and determinants of cancer in a population
   D. most common types of new cancer cases diagnosed each year

2. Which of the following types of cancers have an increasing annual incidence trend in the United States?
   A. breast and ovary
   B. lung and prostate
   C. stomach and larynx
   D. kidney and pancreas

3. There are 15.5 million patients with cancer living as survivors in the United States. A statistical breakdown of cancer survivors reveals:
   A. Almost 60% of survivors are age 65 years or older.
   B. African Americans have higher relative survival rates than whites.
   C. The greatest increase in five-year survival rates is for cases of lung cancer.
   D. Relative survival rates decreased for patients with chronic myeloid leukemia.

4. Which of these findings is accurate about disparities in cancer epidemiology among different ethnic groups in the United States?
   A. Asians/Pacific Islanders have the highest incidence and death rates of all groups for kidney cancer.
   B. African American men are more than twice as likely as white men to die from prostate cancer.
   C. White women have higher mortality rates for breast cancer than African American women.
   D. Hispanic/Latina women have the lowest incidence rate for cervical cancer but the highest death rate.

5. Tobacco cessation is an important focus of education about cancer prevention in the United States because:
   A. Smokeless tobacco products are an approved alternative to cigarettes.
   B. Adults with a college degree are most likely to use tobacco products.
   C. Tobacco use is the greatest modifiable risk factor for cancer.
   D. Smoking prevalence has increased in the past ten years.

6. Maintaining a healthy weight is considered to be an important strategy in efforts to promote general health in the United States. Overweight populations and people who are obese continue to be one of the largest concerns in promoting general health because:
   A. Obesity and being overweight are responsible for 50% of cancer deaths
   B. Obesity and being overweight are linked to cancers of the gastrointestinal system
   C. Obesity and being overweight are associated with increased risk for cancers of the lung
   D. The highest prevalence of obese and overweight people is in non-Hispanic white women

7. For which of the following groups is the vaccination for chemoprevention of the human papilloma virus (HPV) recommended?
   A. Vaccination is recommended for female children only
   B. Vaccination is recommended for all sexually active adult men and women over the age 26 years
   C. Vaccination is recommended to be given to girls between the ages of 15 and 18 as a single dose
   D. to begin in children aged 11 or 12 years as a two-dose series

8. The Federal Drug Administration (FDA) has approved drug treatments to reduce the risk of breast cancer in the general population. These drugs include which one of the following?
   A. raloxifene
   B. diethylstilbestrol
   C. anabolic steroids
   D. menotropins

9. Ms. P. is a 40-year-old woman, who has identified herself as a smoker, and who is undergoing a preventive cancer risk assessment. A thorough medical history and physical examination is being conducted, and she is being assessed for motivation for preventative behavior as per the health belief model. Which of the following questions should she be asked during the motivation for preventative behavior assessment?

A. "Do you currently have any medical conditions and what medications for those medical conditions are you currently taking?"

B. "Have you or anyone in your immediate family ever been diagnosed with cancer?"

C. "Have you ever undergone treatments for cancer such as chemotherapy, radiation therapy, or immunotherapy?"

D. "How difficult do you think it will be to decrease your risk for cancer by quitting your smoking habit?"

10. According to statistics from the American Cancer Society, several factors contribute to cancer mortality in the United States. Factors such as age, gender, geography, and socioeconomic status play a role in cancer deaths. Regarding socioeconomic status, which of the following is true regarding the cancer mortality in poorer populations?

A. High socioeconomic status is associated with increased risk of lung cancer, cervical cancer, stomach cancer, and cancer of the head and neck.

B. The use of alcohol has increased among poorer populations, leading to a higher rate of cancer mortality.

C. A higher rate of advanced disease is found at diagnosis among poorer populations and those who live in rural regions than in the rest of the U.S. population.

D. Low SES is associated with increased risk of breast, prostate, and colon cancers.

11. As of 2016, the U.S. Food and Drug Administration (FDA) classified Electronic nicotine delivery systems (ENDS), also known as *e-cigarettes,* as a tobacco product, bringing them under FDA regulation. Of the following, which statement is true regarding the use of ENDS?

A. As of 2016, more than 2 million middle and high school age students were identified as e-cigarette users, with a variety of appealing flavors cited as the primary reason for use.

B. As of 2016, the U.S. Food and Drug Administration (FDA) has approved e-cigarettes as a cessation aid.

C. Electronic cigarettes are battery-operated devices in which the inhaled vapor is produced from cartridges that contain flavoring and other chemicals, but has not been found to contain any nicotine, like in traditional tobacco products.

D. Use of e-cigarettes has so far not been linked to leading non-smokers and children to begin smoking.

# 2 Screening and Early Detection

1. A new fecal occult blood test screening designed to correctly identify individuals with colon cancer is an example of the test's:
   A. reliability
   B. negative predictive value
   C. sensitivity
   D. specificity

2. A 44-year-old patient with colorectal cancer asks about screening for his son. His nurse advises him that the recommended screening guidelines for prevention includes which of the following?
   A. 50 years of age, or 10 years before the youngest case in the immediate family.
   B. 40 years of age, or 10 years before the youngest case in the immediate family.
   C. 60 years of age, or 10 years before the youngest case in the immediate family.
   D. Colonoscopy every 10 years and every 6 years after the age of 55 years.

3. A 27-year-old female comes in for her routine cervical cancer screening. Which screening test is recommended for her age group?
   A. Pap test every 3 years.
   B. Human papillomavirus (HPV) test with Pap test every 5 years.
   C. HPV test with Pap test every 3 years.
   D. Screening would not be recommended if she has been vaccinated.

4. A patient with cervical cancer asks whether an HPV vaccine would be recommended for her. The nurse responds based on her understanding that HPV vaccine is a method of:
   A. primary prevention
   B. secondary prevention
   C. tertiary prevention
   D. quaternary prevention

5. In women 45 years of age and older with an average risk of breast cancer, which of the following are included in the recommended screening guidelines?
   A. Clinical breast exam every 6-12 months.
   B. Prophylactic surgery (e.g. bilateral salpingo-oophorectomy).
   C. Annual breast MRI.
   D. Annual mammography.

6. A 27-year-old woman who was treated with chemotherapy and thoracic radiation for childhood Hodgkin disease asks about her breast screening guidelines. Based on her history, the screening guidelines should include:
   A. clinical breast exam every 12 months
   B. mammogram every other year
   C. annual mammogram
   D. bilateral salpingo-oophorectomy

7. A 45-year-old healthy African American male with a significant family history of prostate cancer asks whether he should be screened for prostate cancer. Which one of the following is the best response to give?
   A. Screening is not recommended until age 50 years.
   B. It would be beneficial to begin screening.
   C. Screening should only be done in men with comorbidities.
   D. Screening should only be done in men who are healthy with little to no comorbidities.

8. A 62-year-old woman with a 22-pack-year smoking history asks if she should be screened for lung cancer. According to the National Comprehensive Cancer Network (NCCN), what would you recommend?
   A. Lung cancer screening is not recommended.
   B. Low-dose computed tomography (LDCT) is recommended.
   C. Sputum cytology with or without chest x-ray is recommended.
   D. Chest radiography is recommended every 5 years.

9. Cancer screening tests are:
   A. always safe and not harmful if only done annually.
   B. diagnostic tests to find out what is the cause of certain symptoms.
   C. designed to detect early disease or risk factors for a disease in healthy individuals.
   D. offer a cure which may otherwise not be found if it were not done.

10. The percentage of persons who screen positive and actually have the disease is referred to as:
    A. positive predictive value
    B. negative predictive value
    C. sensitivity
    D. specificity

11. *BRCA1* and *BRCA2* mutations are:
    A. responsible for approximately 50% of hereditary breast cancers
    B. are not common enough to recommend testing for the general population
    C. responsible for approximately 20-25% of hereditary lung cancers
    D. indicative of a developing cancer if the mutation is found

12. Which one of the following is an important component to discuss when performing an assessment on a patient to determine if cancer screening is recommended?
    A. current medications
    B. family history
    C. sleep pattern and exercise
    D. allergies

13. When reviewing cancer-related symptoms, which one of the following would be considered suspicious for cancer?
    A. Fatigue, malaise, recent weight gain or weight loss.
    B. Increased blood pressure.
    C. Increased urination, thirst, and perspiration.
    D. Stiffness in joints.

14. A 55-year-old male has a prostate-specific antigen (PSA) blood test with a value of 2.46 ng/mL. What are the National Comprehensive Cancer Network (NCCN) guidelines for this PSA value?
    A. Repeat digital rectal exam (DRE).
    B. Repeat PSA testing in 6-12 months.
    C. Repeat PSA testing at 1-2 year intervals.
    D. Repeat PSA testing at 2-4 year intervals.

15. J. L. is a 45-year-old African American female who calls to make a mammography appointment. She is asymptomatic without a personal history of breast cancer or breast implants. She will be scheduled for which one of the following types of mammograms?
    A. breast tomosynthesis
    B. screening mammogram
    C. 2D mammogram
    D. diagnostic mammogram

16. A 35-year-old woman is very worried about her risk for developing breast cancer. Her mother was diagnosed with breast cancer at age 34 and her sister was recently diagnosed with breast cancer at age 39. When she was 30 years old she had a benign fibroadenoma removed from her breast. Her first menstrual period was at age 11 and her first birth was at age 28. The nurse uses which model to calculate her estimated risk for developing breast cancer in the next five years and over a lifetime:
    A. PREMM model
    B. BRCAPRO model
    C. Gail model
    D. Penn II model

17. An ideal screening testing would be which one of the following?
    A. be administered annually
    B. be available in the hospital setting
    C. have a low negative predictive value
    D. be cost-effective

18. The nurse is conducting a cancer risk assessment on a 26-year-old female. The components of the patient's history should include which one of the following?
    A. assessment of pain and stiffness in bones and joints
    B. assessment of the cranial nerves
    C. assessment of daily exercise habits
    D. assessment of all skin surfaces

# 3 Survivorship

1. In relation to cancer survivorship, the term survivor refers to which one of the following?
   A. anyone with a cancer diagnosis, as well as their family and significant others
   B. someone who is greater than 5 years from a cancer diagnosis
   C. anyone who is given the diagnosis of an early-stage cancer
   D. a parent or child who also has a cancer diagnosis

2. An important component of survivorship care that the oncology nurse must understand regarding long-term and late effects is that:
   A. Long-term effects are those that begin at least one year after treatment completion.
   B. The first year after treatment is the most critical for treatment sequelae development.
   C. Late effects may manifest months or years later depending on treatment exposures.
   D. Adolescent and young adult (AYA) survivors are at lower risk for significant late effects.

3. Which one of the following statements is *inaccurate* when considering social concerns of cancer survivors:
   A. Relationships that have been altered, or even ended, after treatment may cause feelings of isolation and depression in cancer survivors.
   B. The Americans with Disabilities Act (ADA) only applies to cancer survivors with limb prosthetics.
   C. Survivors experience a higher rate of unemployment than their non-survivor counterparts, causing personal stress and possible financial hardship during search for employment.
   D. Transition back to "life after cancer" can be difficult for survivors at any age.

4. T.R. is a 35-year-old female patient, who was treated for Hodgkin lymphoma at the age of 25, and received mantle field radiation. Which one of the following should be reviewed by the health care team with the patient regarding her screening?
   A. Screening for second malignancy is not needed until age >50 years old.
   B. Annual mammogram, breast MRI or both are recommended.
   C. A PET scan is indicated to screen for second malignancies.
   D. Factors such as lifestyle behaviors need not be addressed.

5. J. C. is a 47-year old male patient, and a prostate cancer survivor of three years. He arrives at his 3-year post-treatment follow-up with his healthcare team. After the appointment is complete, and he is about to leave, J. C. asks if he is allowed to schedule a follow-up appointment with his local urologist. The oncology nurse's response is based on which one of the following?
   A. J.C. no longer needs follow-up care for this diagnosis if he is showing no new signs or symptoms or evidence of recurrence.
   B. A survivorship care plan might be useful to his local provider, and can be shared with the provider if the provider requests it.
   C. A local provider can assume care with a coordinated transition of care, with recommendations for disease surveillance, potential late treatment effects, and health promotion.
   D. His post-treatment care can only be provided by cancer specialists and the oncology nurse advises that J.C. must continue his care with the clinic he has been visiting for at least the next 10 years.

6. Which one of the following is not a standard that is included in conducting a patient history?
   A. Actual or potential insurance coverage limitations.
   B. Genetic history and test results, if available.
   C. Adherence to cancer screening recommendations.
   D. Assessment of health behaviors.

7. Which one of the following statements best describes psychosocial considerations for cancer survivors?
   A. Screening tools to assess anxiety or depression are of limited value and should be avoided.
   B. Frequent changes in occupation or living arrangements should generally be viewed as positive signs of adaptation.
   C. Symptoms such as anxiety and depression may be indicative of post-treatment issues such as pain, fatigue, and insomnia.
   D. Personal questions can be difficult for both the patient and the healthcare provider, and may detract from more important aspects of the visit.

8. A nurse's work healthcare setting is interested in partnering with a nearby rehabilitation center. When asked for feedback, the nurse would most likely share which one of the following opinions?
   A. "Advances in treatment leave most cancer survivors with few or no post-treatment limitations, and it is doubtful this collaboration will be beneficial for our institution."
   B. "Since the benefits of rehabilitation are not well known to providers and survivors, the program may not be widely utilized and the decision to partner with a rehabilitation center would have a negative impact."
   C. "Rehabilitation is very time consuming, and can negatively impact time and productivity at work, so the decision to partner with a rehabilitation center would not be worthwhile for our institution."
   D. "Utilizing such a service may help to decrease the severity of actual and potential post-treatment impairment, so the decision to partner with a rehabilitation center would be worthwhile."

9. Mr. S is a 75-year-old colon cancer survivor. Previously, he had led an active lifestyle, participating in a regular exercise routine, and had been an avid golfer and was even in a bowling league. He states his intention to restart exercising again. His oncology nurse advises which one of the following?
   A. If he maintains a healthy body mass index (BMI), light-intensity exercise once a week can be beneficial.
   B. If he wants to begin exercising again, 150 minutes of moderate-intensity or 75 minutes of vigorous-intensity exercise per week is recommended.
   C. When preparing to exercise or recovering from exercise, be warned that stretching can often lead to strained muscles, and she recommends replacing a stretching regimen with a warm bath.
   D. Rest, rather than exercising, is recommended for the first-year post treatment to promote continued healing, especially for patients > 60 years of age.

10. As part of preventative and ongoing treatment and follow-up, oncology nurses frequently counsel patients on healthy weight management with the understanding that which one of the following is true?
    A. Fast foods are acceptable in moderation once goal weight is achieved.
    B. Portion control is only relevant for weight loss, not ongoing weight maintenance.
    C. Routine weight checks can be discouraging, and should be avoided.
    D. A plant-based diet contributes to achieving and maintaining healthy weight.

11. A cancer survivorship care plan does not include which one of the following?
    A. potential long-term effects associated with treatment
    B. recommended health promotion behaviors and maintenance activities
    C. recommended cancer screening for high-risk siblings
    D. summary of treatment, including all chemotherapy, radiation therapy, hormone therapy, and surgery

12. When caring for AYA survivors, the oncology nurse understands that which one of the following is true?
    A. A younger age at diagnosis places survivors at lower risk for physical and psychosocial sequalae.
    B. Younger survivors generally have greater access to insurance coverage based on their age and limited healthcare needs.
    C. Limited financial resources may result in prioritization of expenses such as paying rent instead of filling medication prescriptions.
    D. Cognitive impairment does not typically impact ability to manage high school or college courses.

13. An institution is preparing to launch a new survivorship program. An oncology nurse is assigned to prepare for the launch and, during her preparation, she correctly recognizes that:
    A. General counseling topics such as sun protection and safe sex need not be incorporated in the visits.
    B. Immunization recommendations for both children and adults should be included.
    C. Sun protection recommendations should be addressed only with AYA patients who have received total body irradiation.
    D. Information on safe amounts of tobacco or vaping products should be included.

14. In preparing for survivorship care delivery over the next decade, oncology nurses recognize that:
    A. The number of cancer survivors is expected to remain stable for the next 8-10 years.
    B. The population of cancer survivors are expected to increase by more than 5 million by the year 2026.
    C. Cancer diagnoses are expected to decrease significantly in patients who are 64 years and older.
    D. The expected increase in the oncology workforce will continue to meet the needs of survivors.

15. R. J. is a 30-year-old patient, who has a 10-year history of osteosarcoma. R. J. arrives for a follow up appointment with symptoms of new onset dyspnea and lower extremity edema. When considering the next steps, the oncology nurse correctly recognizes which one of the following?
    A. These symptoms are not related to RJ's disease and treatment.
    B. The patient is too young to consider cardiac etiology, unless there is a strong family history.
    C. Close monitoring of these symptoms over the coming months is recommended.
    D. The patient should be referred to a cardiologist for further evaluation.

16. T. L. is a 40-year-old patient, who has a history of testicular cancer. He calls in to the clinic to state that he had been doing well up until this past week. He is now dreading his survivorship appointment and reports feeling increasingly anxious about his upcoming visit. Hearing his concerns, the nurse taking his call correctly understands that which one of the following is true?
    A. The patient should be referred to psychiatry for evaluation prior to his visit.
    B. These symptoms he is reporting are common around the time of scans and appointments, and she encourages him to keep his appointment.
    C. Postponing the visit will help him to overcome these feelings.
    D. Anxiety and fear of recurrence in survivors actually help to promote vigilance and compliance with follow up recommendations.

# 4 Hospice and Palliative Care

1. Which one of the following statements below best describes the concept of palliative care? Palliative care:
   A. focuses on improving the quality of life for the patient
   B. focuses on treating the cancer with the fewest number of and severe side effects
   C. is delivered by a specialized physician rather than delivered by a healthcare team
   D. provides care to the dying patient at end of life

2. The palliative care treatment team is comprised of interdisciplinary palliative team members. Initially, which one of the following sets of three team members should be included on the team?
   A. family, pastor, friends
   B. pain management specialist, chaplain, social worker
   C. pharmacist, physical therapist, occupational therapist
   D. significant other, integrative practitioner, nurse

3. In order for a patient to access Medicare hospice benefits, the patient must have an estimated life expectancy of less than:
   A. 3 months
   B. 4 months
   C. 6 months
   D. 12 months

4. According to the position statements published by the Oncology Nursing Society and the American Society of Clinical Oncology, palliative care should be considered early during the course of illness for any individual with metastatic cancer and/or a high symptom burden. Which one of the following is considered as a main advantage of early palliative care consultation?
   A. decreased burden of care for the primary care team
   B. Cost savings for patients admitted with advanced cancer
   C. chemotherapy administration is increased
   D. extended disease-free survival

5. Tertiary palliative care refers to which one of the following?
   A. care provided by rural palliative care team
   B. basic palliative care principles carried out by a home health nurse
   C. advance care planning in the terminal setting
   D. care provided in a cancer center with Joint Commission Palliative care certification

6. Although rural communities may not have tertiary palliative care readily, available providers in these settings can connect to a variety of services via which one of the following?
   A. home health aids
   B. telehealth connectivity systems
   C. social work services
   D. the local emergency services

7. Certification of prognosis must be provided for hospice care by which one of the following combination of staff members?
   A. referring physician and social work supervisor
   B. Pastor and hospice medical director
   C. referring physician and hospice medical director
   D. hospice medical director and insurance adjuster

8. Both as a philosophy of care and as a regulated insurance benefit, hospice care is a model of high-quality, compassionate care. When a patient signs up for hospice care, they are agreeing to which one of the following?
   A. chemotherapy if the doctor thinks it is an option
   B. transferring care to a different oncologist
   C. cessation of aggressive therapy
   D. intubation for respiratory distress

9. Physicians are often overly optimistic when anticipating life expectancy for patients with terminal or advanced disease, and usually overestimate survival time of their patients by a factor of which one of the following?
   A. four
   B. three
   C. five
   D. two

10. Unfortunately, it is common for hospice care referrals to occur quite late in the trajectory of a patient's illness. The median number of days a patient lives while on hospice care, according to 2018 data by the National Hospice and Palliative Care Association, is which one of the following?
    A. 25
    B. 30
    C. 7
    D. 17

11. Unlike other areas of clinical practice, it may be appropriate in a hospice setting for team member to do which one of the following?
    A. conduct a physical examination on the caregiver or family member
    B. evaluate the patient once at the beginning of hospice assessment
    C. assess patient and family member or support providers separately
    D. talk to family members without the knowledge of the patient

12. From the United Kingdom to the United States, the hospice movement began with pioneers such as Dr. Florence Wald and Dame Cicely Saunders leading the way for the care of the terminally ill. The roots of the modern hospice movement can be traced to which one of the following time periods?
    A. 1960's in England
    B. 1970's in Scotland
    C. 1980's in the United States
    D. 1960's in Connecticut

13. The process of dying can be a traumatic and painful experience for any family dealing with the illness and associated suffering of a loved one, even a loved one who is elderly or has been experiencing the trajectory of a long illness. Which one of the following is responsible for assisting the family through the dying process and grieving period?
    A. It is the responsibility of extended family members only.
    B. It is the responsibility of the psychotherapist of the patient.
    C. It is the responsibility of the RN who attends to the patient at home.
    D. It is the responsibility of the whole interdisciplinary hospice team.

14. The tool that was developed and adopted by the National Hospice and Palliative Care Organization in 2007 to assess the sociocultural needs of the patient is is called which one of the following?
    A. NCCN
    B. SWAT
    C. ECOG
    D. EQOL

15. Distress is a common psychosocial symptom, not only in patients, but also for the families, loved ones, and caregivers involved. More physical and emotional distress, as well as more prolonged caregiver grief, is experienced by patients who die in which one of the following manners?
    A. Dies unexpectedly
    B. Dies alone
    C. Dies at home
    D. Dies in the hospital

16. Terminal secretions – also commonly referred to as a "death rattle" – occur when the dying patient is too weak to clear or swallow pharyngeal secretions. Which of the following is one of the least invasive ways to manage terminal secretions in dying patients?
    A. anti-cholinergic drugs
    B. elevation of the head of the bed
    C. suctioning
    D. cool wash cloths

17. According to the National Comprehensive Cancer Network (NCCN) Distress Screening tool, a patient who scores a "4" or below should be referred to which one of the following services or members of the healthcare team?
    A. psychiatrist
    B. support group
    C. primary oncologist
    D. clergy person

18. Mr. S. is an 80-year old male, who has been admitted into hospice care with an advanced form of cancer. He has been in hospice care for less than 24 hours, but his health is rapidly declining, and after an evaluation from the hospice team, it is determined that his death is eminent. Which one of the following signs could the hospice team have considered as a sign of eminent death?
    A. rapid breathing
    B. restless movements
    C. Cheyne-Stoke breathing
    D. bounding pulse

19. Mrs. L. is an 83-year old female, who has been admitted into hospice care, and based on her declining condition, the recommendation is to place her on artificial nutrition and hydration (ANH). Which of the following statements is false regarding the effects of ANH on a dying patient?
    A. May increase the risk of aspiration and its complications.
    B. Artificial nutrition given via tube feedings is associated with increased infection, and fluid overload.
    C. ANH is known to reduce the sensation of thirst or dry mouth.
    D. According to a Cochrane review, no clinical difference on quality of life was found in artificial hydration versus a placebo.

20. Shared Decision Making and goals of care are known to be essential elements of palliative care practice. Which one of the following is NOT an element of shared decision making or goals of care?
    A. The plans are based on the wishes and beliefs of both patients and caregivers.
    B. The plans are flexible, and the goals may change over the course of an illness.
    C. Plans are elicited in an intentional and structured way.
    D. Plans are meant to map out advance care planning.

21. G. T. is a 48-year-old mother of two with metastatic breast cancer, which has metastasized to her pancreas. She has recently begun palliative care. She has been suffering from periods of extreme pain, to the point of being debilitating. After consulting with the patient and the patient's family, her palliative care team has decided to place her on a regimen of pain medication. Which one of the following statements best illustrates a standard of palliative care?
    A. G.T.'s palliative care team respected her autonomy as a patient, as well as her family's wishes, and developed a treatment plan to aggressively treat her cancer.
    B. G.T.'s palliative care team dealt with her psychosocial and spiritual distress.
    C. G.T.'s palliative care team began end-of-life care
    D. G.T.'s palliative care team respected her autonomy as a patient, as well as her family's wishes, and initiated a plan to ease the pain caused by her cancer.

# 5 Navigation Across the Cancer Continuum

1. Harold Freeman, in 1990, developed the first patient navigation program for underserved patients in the Harlem neighborhood of New York City. The goal of the first patient navigation program was to reduce mortality in women with which one of the following types of cancer?
   - A. Breast
   - B. Cervical
   - C. Colon
   - D. Melanoma

2. Which one of the following is a goal of a patient navigation service?
   - A. Identify and resolve barriers to care.
   - B. Care for patients at end of life.
   - C. Supply medical advice by phone.
   - D. Provide telehealth services.

3. In 2012, a role delineation study (RDS) was conducted by the Oncology Nursing Society (ONS) to clearly define the role of the nurse navigator. This study led to the development of which one of the following?
   - A. The study led to changes to breast screening guidelines.
   - B. The study led to improved guidelines for the use of personal protective equipment.
   - C. The study led to improved staffing ratios on inpatient bone marrow transplant (BMT) units.
   - D. The study led to the development of the oncology nurse navigator (ONN) core competencies.

4. According to the Cancer Care Continuum Model, a trained nonprofessional or volunteer who provides individualized assistance to patients, families, and caregivers to help overcome health care system barriers and facilitate timely access to quality health and psychosocial care is which one of the following types of navigators?
   - A. Lay
   - B. Novice
   - C. Expert
   - D. Community clinic

5. The first navigation program in 1990 started by Harold Freeman in the Harlem neighborhood of New York City focusing on an underserved population of women with breast cancer demonstrated an increase in five-year cancer survival rates from which one of the following ranges?
   - A. 10% to 17%
   - B. 25% to 49%
   - C. 39% to 70%
   - D. 75% to 92%

6. The Academy of Oncology Nurse and Patient Navigators (AONN+) was incorporated in which one of the following years?
   - A. 1990
   - B. 2000
   - C. 2009
   - D. 2018

7. In 2015, the American College of Surgeons (ACOS) Commission on Cancer issued updated program standards that states which one of the following?
   - A. The program standards amendedmended the administration guidelines for outpatient chemotherapy
   - B. The program standards required organizations to be accredited by the Joint Commission
   - C. The program standards increased adherence rules for "time out" procedures prior to surgery
   - D. The program standards required patient navigation to become a facility's standard to gain and maintain certification

8. Data compiled from the Patient Navigation Research Program (PNRP) revealed that a delay in diagnosis has been correlated withwhich one of the following conditions?
   - A. Unemployment
   - B. Coverage from disability insurance
   - C. Adequate social support
   - D. Higher education levels

9. Sue is collecting and organizing information for a report that she must compile to show the value of the new navigation program that her department is considering implementing. A key part of her report is to show the value of an individual oncology nurse navigator (ONN). As Sue is developing her report, which one of the following methods should be utilized to calculate and measure the value of an ONN?
   - A. Improved staffing ratios in inpatient oncology units.
   - B. Increased length of stay for patient comfort.
   - C. Provider, patient, and family satisfaction scores.
   - D. Improved drug costs.

10. As part of their role, nurse navigators assess the level of psychosocial distress in patients with cancer as a barrier of care. Which one of the following represents the best time for a nurse navigator to access psychosocial distress in a patient?
    A. at each clinic visit
    B. during the end stage of disease
    C. when a psychologist is present during a clinic visit
    D. when patients have a remote psychiatric diagnosis

11. The most appropriate way to overcome the limitations that determine the effectiveness of nurse navigator programs would be to include data from which one of the following prospective studies?
    A. gather data from lung cancer patients
    B. provide navigation services focused on newly diagnosed patients
    C. standardize instruments to gather data and measure outcomes
    D. gather data from large metropolitan cities

12. Ms. J is a 74-year-old woman who is currently receiving immunotherapy. She calls that her car has broken down and she is unable to attend the treatment appointment. She is unsure how long it be will be until her car is repaired and she is concerned about transportation to her future treatment appointments. Ms. J's car trouble is an example of which one of the following types of barriers to care that nurse navigators must try to mitigate for their patients with cancer?
    A. Transportation
    B. Cultural
    C. Language
    D. Family support

13. J. S. is a 42-year old female, who has been diagnosed with breast cancer. She calls stating that she just lost her job and is now unemployed. With mounting medical bills and no income coming-in, she'll have no choice but to file for bankruptcy and, from now on, she will no longer be able to afford her medications. After hearing her story, her nurse navigator knows that which one of the following resource(s) may be available for her?
    A. transition to hospice care because of her financial barriers
    B. charity care and medication assistance programs
    C. receiving donated medications from other patients
    D. the treating facility's staff members will pay for her medications

14. Navigators can receive navigator-specific certification via which one of the following?
    A. ACOS
    B. ONS
    C. OCN
    D. AONN+

15. Which type of navigation model of care is defined by having a holistic, patient-centered focus, supporting patient's autonomous decision-making, and encouraging patient participation?
    A. Transitional care
    B. Planetree
    C. ONN care
    D. Survivorship

16. Which one of the following types of navigators requires professional backgrounds (i.e., medical assistants), educational degrees higher than bachelor's degree, but does not necessarily need to be clinically focused?
    A. Nurse navigators
    B. Lay patient navigators
    C. Social work/counselors
    D. Allied health patient navigators

17. The Oncology Nurse Navigation (ONN) competency categories for nurse navigators lists four competency categories for navigation. Which one of the following is NOT part of the coordination of care category?
    A. Identifies potential and realized barriers to care (e.g., transportation, child care, elder care, housing, language, culture, literacy, role disparity, psychosocial, employment, financial, insurance) and facilitates referrals as appropriate to mitigate barriers.
    B. The ONN provides appropriate and timely education to patients, families, and caregivers to facilitate understanding and support informed decision making.
    C. Applies knowledge of clinical guidelines (e.g., National Comprehensive Cancer Network, American Joint Committee on Cancer) and specialty resources (e.g., ONS Putting Evidence into Practice resources) throughout the cancer continuum.
    D. Facilitates timely scheduling of appointments, diagnostic testing, and procedures to expedite the plan of care and to promote continuity of care.

18. According to the Cancer Care Continuum Model from the Institute of Medicine, at which one of the following stages of the continuum does care planning begin?
    A. Care planning begins at the treatment stage.
    B. Care planning begins at the diagnosis stage.
    C. Care planning begins at the screening stage.
    D. Care planning begins at the survivorship stage.

# 6 Communication and Shared Decision-Making

1. What is the definition of Shared Decision Making (SDM) according to Charles, Gafni, and Whelan's breakthrough paper in 1997 on the SDM?
   A. A theoretical model of care delivery designed to lower healthcare costs.
   B. An *a priori* model lacking structural validation in actual practice.
   C. A theoretical care delivery model that involves collaboration of the patient and clinician.
   D. A model of local care delivery within regions of the state.

2. In 2014, the Agency for Healthcare Research and Quality (AHRQ) developed five steps for SDM. Which one of the following clinician's statements exemplifies the first of the five steps?
   A. "Do you already know which treatment you want to choose?"
   B. "Share with me what you are taking away from our discussion of treatment options."
   C. "There are two treatments we should discuss, I would like to explore your thoughts for treatment."
   D. "When reviewing the treatment options, are there any worries that immediately come to mind?"

3. Which one of the following key elements of SDM has the lowest likelihood of being actualized during SDM implementation?
   A. Sharing of information between family and patient.
   B. Collaborative approach between services.
   C. Consensus building between the treatment team.
   D. Explicit mutual agreement on treatment decision between patient and treatment team.

4. SDM has demonstrated short- and long-term benefit and has become a preferred model of care delivery by lawmakers and policymakers. Which one of the following statements by the patient reflects an immediate, short-term benefit of SDM?
   A. "My quality of life is I think good to very good on the treatment I was prescribed."
   B. "I have been taking my oral chemotherapy regularly."
   C. "My confidence in my provider really improved after receiving the information that I needed."
   D. "I have been in remission for over 4 years now without any episode of cancer recurrence."

5. In a study among oncology nurses on their perceived barriers to SDM, which one of the following statements on SDM is correct?
   A. There is no nursing scope of practice limitation for SDM and nursing practice.
   B. Oncology nurses have more than adequate time for SDM.
   C. Oncology nurses reported lack of resources for education and training on SDM.
   D. All nursing leaders embrace and support SDM as a standard of care.

6. Which of the following is not a significant influence in an older adult's cancer treatment decisions:
   A. Convenience of therapy
   B. Trust with the physician
   C. Provider recommendations
   D. Access to patient decision aids

7. The most frequently used instrument to measure the degree of patient role preferences in the cancer setting is the:
   A. OPTION tool
   B. Pattern of Treatment Decision Making questionnaire (Control Preferences Scale)
   C. Decisional Conflict Scale
   D. Satisfaction with Decision Scale

8. The oncology nurse must anticipate that the top patient priority after a cancer diagnosis would include information on:
   A. treatment options and timing
   B. self-care and family support
   C. cancer diagnosis and disease
   D. prognosis and financial options

9. Which one of the following has the least significant impact on the quality communications between the clinician and the patient?
   A. Locus of control.
   B. Informed decision-making style.
   C. Socio-emotional approach.
   D. Empathy.

**13**

10. Which one of the following statements reflects the complex role of variables within the context of uncertainty?
    A. I will reinforce to the patient that she should make her decision on treatment after a discussion of options with her oncologist.
    B. The patient has been given education based on National Comprehensive Cancer Network (NCCN) guidelines.
    C. The patient lives on her own and her support comes from her neighbor, who has a full-time job.
    D. I didn't tell the patient my concern regarding the possibility of her developing brain metastasis. I know that her mom is currently in hospice care and I didn't want to add even more stress to her life.

11. In the 1970s, the shared model of care began to become popular in health care, especially in cancer care settings, as more patients wished to have a larger say in how their care was determined. Which one of the following is NOT a major factor in the emergence of Shared Decision Making as the dominant model of care in modern health care?
    A. An increased desire from consumers to take more control, have more autonomy, and being a more active participant in their own health care.
    B. The signing into law of the Patient Protection and Affordable Care Act (PPACA), often shortened to the Affordable Care Act (ACA), in 2010.
    C. An explosion of cancer treatment choices and options for patients to consider.
    D. An increase in health care consumerism in Australia, Canada, Europe, and the United States.

12. An oncology nurse's role in Shared Decision Making can be complex and take on many different aspects. A single mother of three, Mrs. S, a 52-year old female, who has been newly diagnosed with breast cancer, meets with her nurse to discuss the diagnosis and next steps. The nurses shares brochures and pamphlets with the patient on her type of cancer and the cancer treatments available. The institution where the nurse works has produced these educational materials for nurses to utilize when meeting with new patients. These materials describe some of the possible tests and treatments and outline what patients can expect next to happen. During their conversation, Mrs. S expresses her concern over, not only the diagnosis, but how she will be treated during the continuum of care, and shares her deep worries over caring for her teenage children. Which of the following best represents the manifestation of a nursing role during Shared Decision Making.
    A. Patient education and psychosocial support
    B. Psychosocial support and advocacy
    C. Patient education and patient needs assessment
    D. Patient education and outcome evaluation

# 7 | Carcinogenesis

1. L.S. is a 49-year-old female with pancreatic cancer. During the course of her diagnosis and treatment, L.S. asks the oncology nurses in her care about the cause of her cancer. The oncology nurse responds to the question from L.S. with the understanding that the gene mutation frequently affecting this condition is caused by which one of the following:
   A. a missense gene mutation
   B. a chromosome translocation
   C. a proto-oncogene mutation
   D. an insertion mutation

2. According to 2018 statistics from the American Cancer Society, colorectal cancer is the third leading cause of cancer-related deaths in men and in women, and the second most common cause of cancer deaths when men and women are combined. Mr. P. is a 55-year-old man who is has been diagnosed with metastatic colon cancer. The nurse caring for Mr. P. is aware that the signaling pathway that may be playing a role in his metastases is:
   A. vascular endothelial growth factor
   B. epidermal growth factor receptor
   C. medial growth factor
   D. nerve growth factor

3. A new oncology nurse is reviewing a patient's medical record and requests help in understanding the process of carcinogenesis. A seasoned nurse explains that the process is due to which one of the following?
   A. clonal evolution
   B. convergent evolution
   C. coevolution
   D. perseverance

4. R.J. is a 70-year old male whose lung metastases have spread to other regions of his body. He asks the nurse attending to him how the spread of his lung metastases has occurred. The nurse explains to R.J. that the process involves feeding the tumor with oxygen and nutrients that, therefore, allows the tumor to enlarge. The process the nurse has described to her patient is called which one of the following?
   A. carcinogenesis
   B. glycolysis
   C. pathogenesis
   D. angiogenesis

5. An oncology nurse is caring for a newly diagnosed patient with osteosarcoma who has "skip metastasis". The nurse is aware that this occurs when
   A. cells bypass one organ and metastasize in another
   B. cells bypass the first node and reach more distant sites
   C. cells spread into nearby capillary beds or pulmonary arteriovenous shunts
   D. tumor cells embed into distant arteries

6. The primary tumor that most frequently metastasizes to the brain is which one of the following?
   A. non–small cell lung cancer
   B. prostate cancer
   C. liver cancer
   D. colorectal cancer

7. Which one of the following is a key association and cause of cancer?
   A. Three servings of fresh fruits and vegetables weekly
   B. White meat in daily diet
   C. Too much fiber in daily diet
   D. Sun exposure and indoor tanning parlors

8. A tumor is formed from a single precursor cell with genetic alterations that undergoes clonal expansion. Clonal evolution is the process of cells within a tumor accumulating genetic changes over time that are different from one cell to the next. Thus, a tumor may be heterogeneous and consist of cells that arose from the same mother cell that are genotypically different from one another. In this model, which is the <u>third</u> phase in the process of cell mutation?
   A. Acquisition of cancer hallmarks
   B. Acquisition of genomic instability
   C. Initiating mutation
   D. Further genetic mutation

9. Which one of the following is a definition of carcinogenesis?
   A. The creation of new blood vessels from existing ones to provide nutrients and remove waste products.
   B. The transference of normal cells into cancer cells through a complex and dynamic process that starts with mutations in regulatory cells and is promoted by genomic instability, inflammation, and interactions within the tumor microenvironment.
   C. The process which causes epithelial cells to lose cell polarity and cell–cell adhesion and have invasive properties so that they can become mesenchymal cells.
   D. A mechanism that may change the activity of a gene without changing the sequence of DNA.

# 8 Immunology

1. Recent surveillance imaging has revealed that an oncology patient, who is currently in remission, has developed new lesions. The phase of tumor suppression mechanism most likely to be implicated in this new development can be classified as which one of the following?
   A. elimination
   B. equilibrium
   C. escape
   D. progression

2. The concept of immune surveillance occurs:
   A. when innate and adaptive immunity destroy clinically unmeasurable tumors
   B. when a rare cancer clone requires resistance to innate immunity but is stabilized by the adaptive immune system
   C. when tumors enter the equilibrium phase of the proposed tumor suppression mechanism
   D. as a result of receiving multiple, sequential chemotherapeutic agents

3. Adaptive immunity differs from innate immunity in that adaptive immunity:
   A. creates memory cells for a longer lived immune response
   B. uses humoral immunity through T-cell activation
   C. uses feedback inhibition mechanisms to control tissue damage due to inflammatory response
   D. uses nonspecific processes for immune defense

4. An example of how tumor cells can evade the adaptive immune system would include which one of the following?
   A. becoming resistant to chemotherapy through drug activation
   B. promotion of T-cell exhaustion by upregulating checkpoint molecules
   C. the innate immune system keeping the disease in check
   D. increasing antigens that are recognized by the adaptive immune system

5. An example of humoral immunity is:
   A. during antigen presentation to naïve T cells by antigen-producing cells (APCs)
   B. T lymphocyte activation
   C. the destruction of foreign particles by neutrophils
   D. the production of plasma cells

6. Cytokines function to do which one of the following?
   A. assist with cell signaling during immune responses
   B. recognize, ingest, and kill microbes
   C. produce antibodies against antigens after exposure
   D. supply tissue nourishment, improve oxygenation, and modulate blood viscosity

7. Organ and tissue components of the immune system include primary lymphoid organs and secondary lymphoid organs and tissues. Secondary lymphoid tissues are sites where antigens are captured and processed in the body. Which one of the following is an example of both primary and secondary lymphoid tissue?
   A. Spleen
   B. Lymph nodes
   C. Bone marrow
   D. Thymus

8. Lymphoid stem cell lineage has several types of lymphocytes that play a key role in immune responses. Which one of the following cells migrate to the thymus gland for maturation and are integral to immune surveillance and response?
   A. NK cells
   B. Cytotoxic T cells
   C. T cells
   D. B cells

9. Which one of the following is the most abundant granulocyte?
   A. Neutrophils
   B. Basophils
   C. Eosinophils
   D. Macrophages

# 9 Precision Medicine

1. Which of the following information is more important in the application of precision medicine in a patient with a cholangiocarcinoma?
   A. 11.5 x 10.0 x 9.5 cm right hepatic lobe mass
   B. high positive expression of programmed death-ligand 1 (>50%)
   C. tolerated adjuvant therapy with leucovorin, fluorouracil, and oxaliplatin (FOLFOX)
   D. alanine aminotransferase 80 U/L, aspartate aminotransferase 123 U/L, total bilirubin 2.9 mg/dL

2. Cancer prediction tools include the following criteria, EXCEPT:
   A. demographics
   B. medical history
   C. family history
   D. tumor stage

3. K.T. is a 29-year old female patient, who has been newly diagnosed with breast cancer. K.T. has asked her oncology nurse why the oncologist would require the result of the biomarker test to determine the treatment plan. Which of the teach-back responses indicates that the patient did not fully understand her oncology nurse's explanation?
   A. The results will tell us if I need surgery.
   B. The results can predict if the treatment will work for me.
   C. My doctor will use the results to find out if I will need chemotherapy after surgery.
   D. The results can be used to measure how aggressive my cancer is.

4. The use of ER/PR/Her-2/Neu status to guide decisions on the use of adjuvant systemic chemotherapy is an example of:
   A. use of a cancer-risk assessment tool to confirm suspected familial cancer syndromes.
   B. dose determination based on genomics.
   C. use of biomarkers to guide treatment decisions.
   D. use of testing to determine eligibility for a clinical trial.

5. The field of pharmacogenomics has revolutionized cancer care because it:
   A. increased rates of non-adherence to therapy.
   B. lowered the cost of cancer treatment.
   C. increased enrollment in clinical trials.
   D. increased the safety and efficacy of cancer drugs.

6. The use of targeted therapies is common within oncology practice and involves the use of genetic and genomic information of the cancer tissue to guide selection of an appropriate targeted drug therapy. One of the benefits of using targeted therapies is:
   A. less severe adverse reactions.
   B. not classified as hazardous drugs.
   C. spare normal cells.
   D. only available in oral formulation.

7. K.T., a 29-year old female patient with breast cancer, has requested information on genetic and molecular testing. Her oncology nurse knows that her patient will need more information when she is heard saying:
   A. Please expedite the results. I need them in 2 days for my second opinion.
   B. I understand that my results may have implications to the rest of my family.
   C. I will need to inquire if my health insurance will cover the costs related to genetic and molecular testing.
   D. There are known risks to my privacy and confidentiality.

8. Which of the following is a definition of gene amplification?
   A. Loss of all or part of a gene found in cancer and other genetic diseases.
   B. Heritable change that does not alter the DNA sequence but changes gene expression.
   C. Increase in the number of copies of a gene that may cause cancer cell growth or resistance to anti-cancer drugs.
   D. Increase in the copies of a protein made from a gene that may play a role in cancer development.

9. Which of the following is a definition of gene deletion?
   A. Heritable change that does not alter the DNA sequence but changes gene expression.
   B. Loss of all or part of a gene found in cancer and other genetic diseases.
   C. Increase in the copies of a protein made from a gene that may play a role in cancer development.
   D. Increase in the number of copies of a gene that may cause cancer cell growth or resistance to anti-cancer drugs.

10. Which is the following is an example of pharmacokinetics?
    A. Examination of how a drug will affect an individual patient
    B. Examination of how an individual patient will affect a drug
    C. Study of how a patient's genomes affect responses to certain types of medications
    D. Study of heredity and the variation of inherited characteristics

11. When administering precision medicine treatments, the healthcare team must be aware of ethical considerations of the patient. Which one of the following is an ethical concern?
    A. After beginning treatment of a targeted therapy, the patient develops an unexpected adverse event, leading to life-threatening complications that neither the patient nor the patient's family had expected.
    B. Though the patient has been educated on the topic, the side effects of a particular treatment have severely comprised the patient's quality of life.
    C. The cost of the treatments is such that the patient experiences financial toxicity and must stop treatment while deciding how to pay the price of drugs.
    D. The patient is concerned about data security and fear government intrusion that may affect health care coverage.

**19**

# 10 Genetic Risk Factors

1. Application of the Central Dogma of molecular biology to oncology nursing practice is important because:
   A. canines have the same DNA nucleotides as humans.
   B. it explains the production of protein for all body functions.
   C. DNA and RNA contain identical nucleic acids for genetic information important in genetic testing in hereditary risk.
   D. RNA to DNA to protein explains the chain of events for protein production.

2. A patient with history of exposures to an environmental carcinogen has come to a class on environmental risk and epigenetics. The audience asks "why/how" that matters. The nurse responds with the understanding that:
   A. epigenetics causes pieces of the DNA sequence to be "chopped out".
   B. only epigenetic changes associated with aging, drug use, and addiction cause cancer.
   C. most cancers are the result of inherited DNA and RNA mutations in single cells over the lifetime of an individual.
   D. changing the histone structure of DNA by allowing transcription and preventing transcription can alter the protein product outcome.

3. The oncology nurse is caring for a 29-year-old female patient newly diagnosed with bilateral breast cancer. Which of the following would raise suspicion for hereditary breast and ovarian cancer (HBOC) syndrome?
   A. Maternal aunt and paternal uncle with a history of brain cancer at unknown ages.
   B. Mother was diagnosed with ovarian cancer at age 33 years.
   C. Brother was diagnosed with testicular cancer at age 25 years after he served in the military during Vietnam.
   D. 4-year-old nephew diagnosed with leukemia.

4. A new oncology nurse asks how to determine if a cell is somatic or germline. You explain that:
   A. Germline cells will have single nucleotide polymorphisms (SNPs) associated with a mutation.
   B. A somatic cell acquires mutations during the monthly reproductive cycle of the body.
   C. Germline mutations occur in reproductive cells of a person with an inherited cancer predisposition.
   D. Somatic cells accumulate mutations prior to conception while *in utero*.

5. Which of the following statements explains the derivation of a cancerous tumor?
   A. Genetic mutations in genes that control cell growth and proliferation are commonly associated with the development of cancer.
   B. Proto-oncogenes are frequently associated with the proliferation and development of malignancies.
   C. Passenger mutations are essential to cancers caused by driver mutations.
   D. Mutations in a DNA repair gene are not associated with environmental carcinogens or inheritance.

6. A patient is being seen in the high-risk cancer clinic because there are features suggestive of a risk for hereditary cancer. These features could include:
   A. passage of a trait to future generations on only one allele of a chromosome.
   B. no known germline deleterious mutation in a cancer susceptibility gene.
   C. autosomal dominant designation of a cancer.
   D. a unique variety of cancer types in multiple generations.

7. Pedigree construction that identifies a family at high risk for inherited cancer should include:
   A. at least four generations of cancer information for both lineages.
   B. the use of squares to designate females and circles to designate males.
   C. race, ethnicity, and age of individuals, but only if there is cancer in the generation.
   D. history of treatments that may have reduced risk of cancer.

8. A negative genetic testing result with "known family genetic mutation" should include the following caveat:
   A. the technique used has limited sensitivity.
   B. the family may be affected by a mutation in another gene.
   C. family history from the other parent influences the risk of developing cancer.
   D. the cancer in the family may not be caused by a germline genetic mutation.

9. A "variant of unknown significance" (VUS) has which of the following characteristics:
   A. It is identified when a cancer risk has been established.
   B. A VUS identifies a genetic change in which the association with cancer risk cannot be established.
   C. Once identified, a VUS maintains that label forever.
   D. A VUS is an uncommon genetic finding.

10. A patient with a family history of breast cancer has had genetic testing with "23 and Me" and reports her result was "negative". Which of the following information should be discussed with her?
    A. This tests for *BRCA1/2* genetic testing only and includes three mutations.
    B. Breast cancer predisposition testing from this test is not United States Food and Drug Administration approved.
    C. Direct-to-consumer testing is approved for use in diagnosis and treatment of breast cancer.
    D. All direct-to-consumer testing is the same.

11. Which mutation-identifying technique will determine the number of mutations in chromosomes?
    A. cytogenetics
    B. Sanger sequencing
    C. genome-wide association studies (GWAS)
    D. microarray

12. A germline mutation occurs in the gametes and:
    A. is present only in first generation.
    B. is present in non-reproductive cells.
    C. can include a *de novo* mutation.
    D. includes every cell in the body.

13. Which of the following may be a psychological consequence to the patient that receives genetic testing results that reveal substantially increased risk for developing cancer or another primary lesion?
    A. Depression yet a sense of relief
    B. Transmitter guilt
    C. Heightened anxiety
    D. Survivor guilt

14. Which of the following groups are not included in the Genetic Non-Discrimination Act (GINA)?
    A. Native Americans
    B. African Americans
    C. Jewish Americans
    D. Southern Baptist Association

15. Which of the following provisions of informed consent for genetic testing is not included when consented for testing?
    A. Purpose of the test
    B. Motivation for testing
    C. Impact of test result on healthcare decision making
    D. Longevity of life after testing

16. Which of the following diseases does not increase the risk for a primary brain tumor?
    A. Huntington disease
    B. Neurofibromatosis type 1
    C. Li-Fraumeni syndrome
    D. von Hippel-Lindau disease

17. The small arm of the chromosome is labeled as
    A. o
    B. p
    C. q
    D. s

18. The protein coding section of a gene is referred to as
    A. Exon
    B. Codon
    C. Intron
    D. Autosome

19. Which of the following hereditary cancer syndromes is inherited in an autosomal recessive fashion?
    A. Hereditary retinoblastoma
    B. MUYTH associated polyposis
    C. Hereditary diffuse gastric cancer
    D. Multiple endocrine neoplasia type 1

20. Mutations in the MSH2 gene are associated with cancers of the
    A. lung
    B. ovary
    C. sarcoma
    D. thyroid

# 11 Clinical Trials

1. A clinical trial study where participants are not assigned to a specific intervention and health care outcomes are assessed is described as which one of the following?
   A. experimental
   B. interventional
   C. expanded access
   D. observational

2. Individuals from the general population who are enrolled in a clinical trial study to evaluate a new technique for early detection of skin cancer are in which type of the following clinical trials?
   A. Screening
   B. Diagnostic
   C. Quality of life
   D. Prevention

3. Which one of the following is a characteristic of an expanded access protocol?
   A. An investigational drug is used outside of a designated clinical trial.
   B. Provides a means to use a therapy off label.
   C. Patient must have early-stage cancer.
   D. Requires United States Food and Drug Administration approval within 72 hours of use.

4. A "3+3" Phase I trial to determine maximum tolerated dose is an example of which type of clinical trial design?
   A. Factorial
   B. Parallel
   C. Adaptive
   D. Basket

5. The individual with primary responsibility to ensure the ethical conduct of the research study is which one of the following?
   A. study coordinator
   B. principal investigator
   C. statistician
   D. data manager

6. The code of ethics and conduct that focuses primarily on beneficence, respect for persons, and justice is known as which one of the following?
   A. Nuremberg Code
   B. Declaration of Helsinki
   C. Common Rule
   D. Belmont Report

7. A common inclusion criteria for eligibility used broadly in oncology clinical trials is termed as which one of the following?
   A. geographic area of residence
   B. performance status
   C. no prior research participation
   D. number of children

8. The approximate number of subjects needed for a Phase I study is which one of the following?
   A. 10-12
   B. 20-100
   C. 80-300
   D. 500-1000

9. The clinical trial endpoint of "time from randomization until death" is known as which one of the following terms?
   A. disease-free survival
   B. objective response rate
   C. overall survival
   D. time to progression

10. Which one of the following depicts a factorial design? Randomization to treatment:
    A. A or B.
    B. A→outcome→B.
    C. A, B, A and B.
    D. A, B, A and B, placebo.

11. A clinical trial study where subjects who have no reported outcomes or conditions are followed and compared, based on exposure, is described as which one of the following?
    A. experimental
    B. outcomes research
    C. cohort studies
    D. observational

12. A clinical trial study which explores the results of health care practices and interventions, includes patient-based outcomes, as well as the study of populations, databases, and the delivery of healthcare is described as which one of the following?
    A. interventional
    B. outcomes research
    C. cohort studies
    D. experimental

13. J. L. is a 49-year male with lung cancer who has recently enrolled into a clinical trial. The clinical trial explores new drug therapies to minimize toxicities related to cancer and cancer treatments. The clinical trial is an example of which one of the following?
    A. screening
    B. prevention
    C. quality of life
    D. therapeutic

# 12 Bone and Soft Tissue Cancers

1. Primary tumors that have been known to spread to the bone include which one of the following?
   A. prostate
   B. brain
   C. leukemia
   D. melanoma

2. Ewing family tumors (EFT) are associated with:
   A. distant metastasis
   B. adolescence
   C. age over 65 years
   D. hormonal therapy

3. A.R. is a 60-year-old woman who arrives at an office visit complaining of bone pain. She explains to her nurse how she is feeling and what the sensation is like. Typically, patients describe bone pain as which one of the following?
   A. prickly
   B. intermittent
   C. aching
   D. sharp

4. T. K. is a 43-year-old male patient. During a physical assessment, the nurse notes a palpable mass in the area of a patient's fibia. A key part of assessment and documentation would be to include a(n):
   A. needle aspiration
   B. incision and drainage
   C. comparison to the unaffected side
   D. evaluation of complete blood count results

5. The goal for the surgical treatment of bone/soft tissue malignancies includes which one of the following?
   A. amputation
   B. altered function
   C. survival
   D. removing the blood supply

6. Post-reconstruction management of a bone or soft tissue tumor includes a focus on which one of the following?
   A. thrombocytopenia
   B. pruritis
   C. cytokine response
   D. infection

7. Adjuvant radiotherapy can be a component of treatment in soft tissue tumors:
   A. only before surgery.
   B. when the tumor has metastasized.
   C. as the primary standard of care.
   D. after the tumor has been debulked.

8. After amputation, the patient may experience phantom limb pain:
   A. for 1-2 weeks after surgery.
   B. postoperatively, starting 8 weeks or more after surgery.
   C. chronically.
   D. intermittently when standing.

9. A sarcoma of the blood vessels is characterized as which one of the following?
   A. Kaposi sarcoma
   B. liposarcoma
   C. rhabdomyosarcoma
   D. leiomyosarcoma

10. Chondrosarcoma is best characterized as:
    A. originating in the lymph nodes.
    B. originating in osteoid tissue.
    C. a pediatric disease.
    D. occurring in middle age (50-60 years old).

11. R. J. is a 42-year-old male who is complaining of abdominal pain and has mentioned that his stools have been tarry with a foul smell. His nurse should conduct a physical examination with the suspicion that R.J. might be suffering from which one of the following?
    A. Chondrosarcoma
    B. Kaposi sarcoma
    C. Soft Tissue sarcoma
    D. Osteosarcoma

12. According to the American Cancer Society and the National Cancer Institute, which one of the following is a risk factor for developing a soft tissue cancer?
    A. Exposure to radiation
    B. Damaged immune system
    C. Food allergies
    D. Exposure to certain viruses

13. Based on statistics reported by the National Cancer Institute (NCI) in 2018, between 1975 and 2010, childhood osteosarcoma mortality decreased by more than which one of the following percentages?
    A. 56 percent
    B. 66 percent
    C. 50 percent
    D. 40 percent

# 13 Breast Cancer

1. The two most important risk factors that make a person more susceptible to breast cancer include age and which one of the following?
   A. gender
   B. race
   C. reproductive/hormonal factors
   D. pregnancy

2. Which one of the following factors makes a patient more likely to have a genetic abnormality based on family history of breast cancer?
   A. History of multiple breast surgeries
   B. First-degree relative with breast cancer
   C. Age of menopause or menarche prior to diagnosis
   D. Nulliparity

3. Which one of the following patients should undergo genetic testing for mutation?
   A. A 60-year-old male with breast cancer.
   B. An 80-year-old female with grade 1, estrogen receptor (ER)-positive, progestogen receptor (PR)-positive breast cancer.
   C. A 55-year-old female with ductal carcinoma *in situ* (DCIS).
   D. A 60-year-old female who is post-menopausal with no family history.

4. An approved agent that could be utilized for the primary prevention of breast cancer in high-risk post-menopausal women with breast cancer is the use of which one of the following?
   A. retinoids
   B. metformin
   C. aromatase inhibitors
   D. Cox-2 inhibitors

5. What type of breast cancer is suggestive of poor prognosis?
   A. ER-positive, PR-positive invasive ductal carcinoma
   B. ER-positive, PR-positive invasive lobular carcinoma
   C. ER-negative, PR-negative, Her-2/Neu-negative breast cancer
   D. T4 tumor between 5 and 10 cm with no lymph nodes positive

6. K.S. is a 54-year-old female with breast cancer and multiple brain metastases is who scheduled to initiate whole-brain radiation therapy (WBRT). The oncology nurse understands the best description of this treatment's intent is which one of the following?
   A. palliative
   B. curative
   C. adjuvant
   D. neoadjuvant

7. D.P. is a 48-year-old woman who was treated 2 years ago for HER2-positive breast cancer with an anthracycline and taxane, as well as trastuzumab for 1 year. She calls the clinic stating she is short of breath. She is scheduled for a follow-up visit immediately. Her oncology team is concerned about which one of the following?
   A. brain and liver metastasis
   B. lung metastasis and cardiac failure
   C. liver and lung metastasis
   D. brain and lung metastasis

8. Diagnostic measures utilized in the diagnosis of breast cancer include which one of the following?
   A. mammography
   B. breast MRI
   C. core needle biopsy
   D. whole-breast ultrasound

9. W. J. is a 56-year-old woman who has just had a mastectomy and was found to have had a positive lymph node. Which one of the following educational points should the nurse perform on the patient's first post-operative visit?
   A. Avoid injury and trauma to the affected arm
   B. Avoid upper extremity exercise
   C. Take temperature and report a temperature of more than 100°F
   D. Reduce sodium intake to less than 1800 mg daily

10. S.L is a 67-year-old women who was recently informed she has stage I ER/PR-positive breast cancer. The patient has a family history of breast, ovarian, and pancreatic cancer. She has an oncotype test which shows a risk score of 24. She asks her nurse what all of this means and the nurse responds with which one of the following statements?
    A. No risk of recurrence
    B. Low risk of recurrence
    C. Intermediate risk of recurrence
    D. High risk of recurrence

11. Which one of the following patients is most likely to develop breast cancer during their lifetime?
    A. T. K., who is a 27-year-old white woman.
    B. J.L, who is a 30-year-old Hispanic woman.
    C. D.C., who is a 25-year-old white male
    D. B.R, who is a 37-year-old African American woman.

12. Breast milk is produced by which one of the following?
    A. terminal duct lobular units
    B. adipose tissue
    C. sebaceous tissue
    D. primary duct units

13. Which one of the following mutations is associated with a hereditary risk for developing lobular breast cancer?
    A. MUTYH
    B. BRCA2
    C. CDH1
    D. PMS2

14. Which one of the following is true about Luminal A tumors?
    A. Luminal A tumors have the highest levels of ER expression: ER positive and/or PR-positive
    B. Luminal A tumors tend to be high grade
    C. Luminal A tumors seldom respond to endocrine therapy
    D. Luminal A tumors have a poor prognosis

15. Histologic characteristics of breast cancer are often determined by the Bloom-Richardson system. Which statement correctly reflects this histologic classification?
    A. Grade 1 - low grade and poorly differentiated
    B. Grade 1 - low grade and well differentiated
    C. Grade 1 - high grade and well differentiated
    D. Grade 1 - high grade and poorly differentiated

# 14 Gastrointestinal Cancers

1. Which one of the following is part of the diagnostic work-up for esophageal cancer?
   A. Colonoscopy
   B. Esophagogastroduodenoscopy
   C. Brain MRI
   D. Abdominal ultrasound

2. Which one of the following is a risk factor for gastric cancer that is considered modifiable?
   A. Alcohol
   B. Family history
   C. Epstein-Barr virus
   D. Lynch syndrome

3. Which one of the following items is a screening technique for colorectal cancer?
   A. Abdominal CT
   B. Abdominal ultrasound
   C. Pelvic CT
   D. Immunochemical fecal occult blood test

4. Molecular classification for metastatic colorectal cancer includes which one of the following?
   A. Programmed death ligand-1
   B. KRAS/NRAS
   C. Estrogen receptor/progesterone receptor
   D. EGFR mutation

5. Which one of the following viruses is most commonly associated with anal cancer?
   A. hepatitis B virus
   B. Epstein-Barr virus
   C. Human papillomavirus (HPV)
   D. Human herpes virus (HHV-8)

6. The virus that is most commonly associated with hepatocellular cancer is which one of the following?
   A. Hepatitis C virus
   B. Influenza
   C. Human papillomavirus infection
   D. Human immunodeficiency virus

7. Which one of the following is a potential curative therapy for hepatocellular carcinoma?
   A. Transarterial chemoembolization
   B. Nivolumab
   C. Sorafenib
   D. Liver transplant

8. What percentage of pancreatic cancers are classified as adenocarcinomas?
   A. 95%
   B. 80%
   C. 25%
   D. 5%

9. Which one of the following is a type of chemotherapy used for cholangiocarcinoma?
   A. Gemcitabine
   B. Methotrexate
   C. Cytoxan
   D. Pembrolizumab

10. Which one of the following is an example of adjuvant chemotherapy therapy for colon cancer?
    A. FOLFOX
    B. Carboplatin/paclitaxel
    C. FOLFIRI
    D. Cetuximab

11. Which one of the following is a significant risk factor for adenocarcinoma of the esophagus?
    A. Smoking
    B. Alcohol
    C. Gastroesophageal reflux disease
    D. Somatic *BRCA1/2* mutation

12. T. J. is a 41-year-old male, in good health, but whose family history of colon cancer has made him concerned about the possibility of developing colorectal cancer. Which one of the following should T.J's nurse recommend to him as a means of cancer prevention?
    A. Treat H. pylori, gastric ulcers
    B. Treat GERD
    C. Limit exposure to cancer-causing chemicals
    D. Limit alcohol intake—fewer than two drinks/day

13. Which one of the following is a modifiable risk for stomach cancer?
    A. Diet high in salted and smoked foods
    B. Gastric polyps
    C. Previous gastric surgery
    D. Family history of the disease

14. Which of the following is a recommended screening for pancreatic cancer?
    A. Ultrasound every 6 months is recommended for high-risk individuals
    B. Routine screening is not recommended for individuals who are not presenting symptoms
    C. EUS or MRI/magnetic resonance cholangiopancreatography (MRCP)
    D. No screening methods are currently identified

# 15 Genitourinary Cancers

1. M. K. is a 59-year old male patient who has been diagnosed with clear-cell carcinoma of the kidney. The nurse caring for him is aware that which one of the following is true about this type of kidney cancer?
   A. The kidney cancer is an unusual type
   B. The kidney cancer is a type of tumor arising in the renal pelvis
   C. Cancer of the kidney has the worst prognosis
   D. Kidney cancer accounts for the majority of cases

2. J.L. is a 63-year-old female patient who has recently been diagnosed with kidney cancer. She is concerned and confused because kidney cancer does not run in her family, and she asks her nurse for an explanation. Her nurse explains that two factors associated with increased risk include which one of the following?
   A. having a history of non-Hodgkin lymphoma and being overweight
   B. being of Asian descent and having a history of kidney stones
   C. consuming processed meats and sedentary occupation
   D. having a tall stature and being underweight

3. T.F. is a 54-year-old female patient who reports episodes of hematuria. The nurse anticipates which one of these diagnostic tests to determine etiology?
   A. Colonoscopy
   B. Kidney biopsy
   C. Intravenous pyelogram
   D. Blood chemistries

4. Diagnostic tests reveal that a patient with limited renal function has developed a primary tumor in the kidney. The nurse should anticipate an order to prepare the patient for which one of the following treatments?
   A. Partial nephrectomy
   B. Cytoreductive nephrectomy
   C. Radiation therapy
   D. Chemotherapy

5. H.R. is a 67-year-old male patient. He arrives at his local infusion center to receive treatment for kidney cancer. Treatment options that have been shown to improve response rates for this type of disease include use of which one of the following?
   A. systemic radiation therapy
   B. antibody-drug conjugates
   C. cytotoxic chemotherapy
   D. immunotherapy agents

6. C. M. is a 47-year-old female patient who has been diagnosed with urothelial carcinoma of the bladder. The nurse educating the patient and her family about this type of bladder cancer explains that urothelial carcinoma of the bladder is:
   A. the least common type of bladder cancer.
   B. responsible for most cases of bladder cancer.
   C. most likely to be invasive at diagnosis.
   D. associated with changes to chromosome 9.

7. T. C. is a 35-year-old son of a patient who has been diagnosed with bladder cancer. During a recent visit, he asks the nurse for advice on which behaviors he should adopt to help him reduce the risk of him becoming diagnosed with cancer, like his father. The nurse explains that factors associated with increased risk include which one of the following?
   A. weight loss
   B. tobacco use
   C. excessive fluid intake
   D. diet low in processed meats

8. J.C. is a 44-year-old man who presents for his annual well-visit examination and asks his nurse about prostate screening. The nurse informs him that guidelines for prostate-specific antigen (PSA) screening in men at average risk of prostate cancer recommend that screening;
   A. begins at age 45 years.
   B. is not useful for men at any age.
   C. should be done between ages 55 to 69 years.
   D. once initiated, should be repeated every year.

9. Grading for prostate cancer is based on the Gleason Score, which is determined by results from which one of the following?
   A. imaging tests using MRI or CT
   B. tissue specimen examination
   C. blood tests for PSA levels
   D. bone marrow aspiration

10. K. L. is a 47-year-old male patient who has been diagnosed with advanced prostate cancer. He arrives at the physician's office to discuss treatment options with his nurse. Options for this patient include which one of the following?
    A. radical prostatectomy
    B. hormonal manipulation
    C. insertion of radioactive seeds into the prostate
    D. cryosurgery to freeze the involved prostatic tissue

11. Potential complications after treatment with radioactive seed placement into the prostate include which one of the following?
    A. decreased libido
    B. constipation
    C. impotence
    D. anemia

12. Which one of the following is a nursing implication when trying to maximize and promote a patient's health and safety after surgery?
    A. Teaching a patient to manage and identify symptoms, including providing recommendations on when to report symptoms.
    B. Monitoring vital signs, hemoglobin, hematocrit, kidney function tests, and urine output.
    C. Teaching patients how to perform coping skills to control anxiety and fear.
    D. Monitoring patients for signs of distress.

13. A patient will be undergoing urologic diagnostic testing. Which one of the following nursing interventions should the nurse perform for a radiographic examination of the kidneys, ureter, and bladder (KUB)?
    A. Assess the patient for history of allergy to iodine dyes or contrast media before performing the test.
    B. Explain to the patient the need to lie flat on examination table.
    C. Observe the patient for a reaction to anesthetic or analgesic.
    D. Monitor the patient for bleeding, and symptoms of a urinary tract infection.

14. Mr. S. is a 60-year old man who has been diagnosed with bladder cancer. His nurse has told him of his options for bladder perseveration therapy, including describing what is considered to be the primary treatment modality being currently offered. After hearing the details, Mr. S. is reluctant to undergo the procedure and eventually declines. Which one of the following bladder preservation therapies did the patient most likely decline?
    A. Radical cystectomy
    B. External beam radiation therapy
    C. Trimodality therapy—transurethral resection (TUR)
    D. Radiation Therapy

# 16 Head and Neck Cancers

1. The classification of head and neck cancers includes which one of the following cancers?
   A. esophagus
   B. thyroid
   C. brain
   D. bone

2. A risk factor for head and neck cancer includes which one of the following?
   A. Human papillomavirus (HPV)
   B. diabetes
   C. menopause
   D. dental implants

3. When preparing to establish a treatment plan for a head and neck cancer patient, the nurse should know that the most essential part of the treatment plan will first require which one of the following?
   A. hereditary genetic test.
   B. detailed family history.
   C. neutrophil count.
   D. biopsy of the tumor.

4. For head and neck cancers, the work-up would most likely include which one of the following?
   A. Chest radiograph and Gallium scan
   B. MRI and CT
   C. Neck ultrasound and intravenous pyelogram
   D. Positron emission tomography and thyroid ultrasound

5. Jill is an oncology nurse focusing on patients with head and neck cancer. Her nursing care of her patients with head and neck cancer should specifically focus on which one of the following?
   A. neutropenia
   B. swallowing
   C. skin care
   D. lymphedema

6. Before a patient's laryngectomy, pre-operative teaching should include which one of the following?
   A. assessment of gait
   B. evaluation of endurance
   C. avoidance of opioid addiction
   D. communication strategies

7. Immediate post-operative care of patients with surgical grafting done during head and neck cancer surgery would include assessment of which one of the following?
   A. perfusion of blood supply to the graft site
   B. range of motion in the shoulders
   C. need for debridement necrotic tissue
   D. blood clots and need for lavage

8. Which one of the following referrals would a patient require after a neck dissection for treatment for head and neck cancer?
   A. occupational therapy
   B. physical therapy
   C. pain management
   D. gastroenterologist

9. A primary nursing concern for a patient who has undergone a supraglottic laryngectomy is the risk for which one of the following?
   A. fall
   B. dehydration
   C. aspiration
   D. somnolence

10. Signs and symptoms of head and neck cancer include which one of the following?
    A. a temperature >100°F accompanied by a sore throat
    B. a lump or sore that does not heal in the mouth or lip
    C. bilateral ear pain with hearing loss
    D. episodic hoarseness that resolves in 1 week

11. Which one of the following descriptions defines the oropharynx?
    A. Extends from the lips to the hard palate above and the circumvallate papillae below, and structures include lips, buccal mucosa, floor of the mouth, and upper and lower alveoli.
    B. Located below the base of the skull and behind the nasal cavity and continuous with the posterior pharyngeal wall.
    C. Extends from the circumvallate papillae below and hard palate above to the level of the hyoid bone.
    D. Extends from the epiglottis to the cricoid cartilage; protected by the thyroid cartilage, which encases it.

12. Which of the following describes the physical alteration and nursing implications for the hemilaryngectomy procedure?
    A. Little to no physical alteration and minimal bleeding.
    B. Vertical excision of one true and one false cord, hoarse voice, and minimal to no swallowing problems.
    C. Partial or total en-bloc resection of the cavity, and may include the ethmoid sinus, and lateral nasal wall, and requires daily care to cavity and placement of obturator.
    D. Surgical approach to inaccessible midfacial and extensive paranasal sinus and nasopharyngeal lesions. May have facial defect and cranial nerve (III, IV, V) deficits.

13. Which one of the following is a definition for the hypopharynx?
    A. Located below the base of the tongue, and extending to but not including the true vocal cord.
    B. Extends from the circumvallate papillae below and hard palate above to the level of the hyoid bone.
    C. Extends from the hyoid bone to the lower border of the cricoid cartilage.
    D. Includes the nasal vestibule; paired maxillary, ethmoid, and frontal sinuses.

14. Which one of the following is the primary treatment for nasopharyngeal cancer?
    A. The primary treatment is radiation
    B. The primary treatment is preoperative radiation or permanently placed iodine-125 seeds
    C. The primary treatment is brachytherapy
    D. The primary treatment is a low dose of radioactive iodine given after surgery

# 17 HIV-Related Cancers

1. The average time from human immunodeficiency virus (HIV) infection to symptomatic disease is best described as which one of the following?
   A. dependent on pre-existing health
   B. approximately 15 years
   C. dependent on age at time of exposure
   D. dependent on number of sexual partner

2. The three stages of HIV are which one of the following? (choose the correct progression of disease):
   A. chronic/progressive disease, acquired immune deficiency syndrome (AIDS), acute infection
   B. acute infection, AIDS, chronic/progressive infection
   C. acute infection, chronic/progressive infection, AIDS
   D. chronic/progressive disease/acute infection

3. Lifestyle factors such as nutrition, health, and smoking may result in infection with other strains of HIV and _____. Choose one of the following that completes the statement.
   A. slow the disease progression
   B. influence the course of infection
   C. may hasten the disease progression
   D. are seen in approximately 37% of cases

4. Which one of the following statements is TRUE regarding the incidence of HIV in the United States?
   A. Incidence among African Americans and white gay males continues to increase.
   B. Diagnoses among young Hispanic/Latino gay and bisexual men has decreased.
   C. Heterosexual contact with HIV-infected individuals accounts for about 34% of new HIV diagnoses.
   D. Those older than 50 years of age are the fastest growing HIV-positive population.

5. A registered nurse at an HIV clinic educates her HIV-positive patients that they are at risk for which one of the following malignancies:
   A. oral and esophageal cancers
   B. prostate and anal cancers
   C. breast and ovarian cancers
   D. B-cell lymphoma and Burkitt lymphoma

6. A nurse is caring for a 29-year-old female patient who was recently diagnosed with AIDS. Her CD4 count is 293, and she is on active antiretroviral therapy. Based on the information provided, the nurse would educate the patient on the fact that she is at increased risk for developing which one of the following types of cancer?
   A. lung cancer
   B. acute myeloid leukemia
   C. cervical cancer
   D. kidney cancer

7. Every attempt should be made to continue chimeric antigen receptor T-cell therapy (cART) through antineoplastic therapy. While a nurse's patient with AIDS-related diffuse large-cell B-cell lymphoma (DLBCL) is receiving R-CHOP, the nurse should do which one of the following?
   A. Monitor for overlapping toxicities that may occur with combination therapy.
   B. Administer steroids to decrease the risk of inflammatory response.
   C. Administer Shingrix to decrease risk of varicella-zoster virus reactivation.
   D. Hold antineoplastic therapy in the setting of low CD4+ counts.

8. A characteristic of HIV-related lymphoma includes which one of the following?
   A. a CD4+ count of 400/mm$^3$
   B. an active EBV infection
   C. the presence of CD20+ marker
   D. an early manifestation of HIV infection

9. HIV-infected patients diagnosed with primary CNS lymphoma have which one of the following?
   A. extensive bone marrow involvement
   B. a normal CD4+ count
   C. a 20% chance of ocular involvement
   D. a concurrent CMV infection

10. J.J. is a 54-year-old HIV-infected male patient who has been admitted for treatment of PCP pneumonia with intravenous Bactrim. On Day 2 of his admission, the patient develops altered mental status, fever, shortness of breath and leukocytosis. His nurse anticipates the patient is experiencing signs and symptoms of which one of the following?
    A. worsening PCP pneumonia.
    B. anaphylactic reaction to Bactrim.
    C. immune reconstitution syndrome.
    D. superimposing infection.

11. Based on a nurse's current knowledge of survival factors in Kaposi sarcoma, the nurse understands that which of the following is true.
    A. there has been a dramatic decrease in survival despite the era of cART.
    B. the median survival is less than six months.
    C. prior or comorbid major opportunistic infections have no impact on survival.
    D. survival is shorter in patients with gastrointestinal lesions or B symptoms.

12. An oncology nurse has volunteered her time at a community health fair and is working a booth on the prevention of various cancers. Included in her materials are teaching materials on how to reduce the possibility of HIV transmission. Which one of the following would most likely be included in any of the educational materials she plans to hand out?
    A. Provide education about the use of latex condom with a water-based lubricant to reduce risk.
    B. Provide education about the use of latex condom with a petroleum-based lubricant to reduce risk.
    C. Provide education about the best way to share household toiletries such as razors and other personal items.
    D. Sharing information on mixing a solution of 1-part household bleach to 10 parts water for use in clean-up of emesis or other body fluid spills, with or without using gloves.

13. As part of any patient education program, an oncology nurse must access the patient's health literacy and ability to comply with complex therapies, and multiple appointments with medical specialists. Which one of the following is an affect that health literacy has on a patient's quality of care?
    A. Low health literacy in patients has little impact on maintaining regular medical care.
    B. Low health literacy is not associated with English not being the first language spoken by a patient since interpreters are readily available at most healthcare institutions.
    C. Only 5% of patients who score low on a health literacy assessment have been found to maintain regular medical care.
    D. Studies of antiretroviral adherence reflect low rates of medication adherence among individuals with low health literacy.

# 18 Leukemia

1. A risk factor for developing acute lymphoblastic leukemia is which one of the following?
   A. exposure to Epstein-Barr virus (EBV)
   B. being of African descent
   C. being of Asian descent
   D. having had a diagnosis of measles as a child

2. A lab value commonly found in a patient diagnosed with acute lymphoblastic leukemia is which one of the following?
   A. the presence of peripheral blasts
   B. a normal blood urea nitrogen (BUN)/creatinine
   C. thrombophilia
   D. a normal prothrombin time (PT)/international normalized ratio (INR)

3. G.R. is a 65-year-old patient who has been newly diagnosed with Philadelphia chromosome-positive acute lymphoblastic leukemia. Induction therapy has been ordered for this patient. Induction therapy would consist of which one of the following?
   A. allogeneic hematopoietic cell transplantation
   B. a pediatric chemotherapy regimen
   C. a monoclonal antibody and corticosteroids
   D. a multi-agent chemotherapy regimen in combination with a tyrosine kinase inhibitor

4. S.T. is a 59-year-old female with newly diagnosed FMS-like tyrosine kinase 3-positive (FLT3+) acute myeloid leukemia. In addition to standard-of-care induction therapy, the nurse caring for her would anticipate for the patient to be on which one of the following oral agents?
   A. venetoclax
   B. enasidenib
   C. ivosidenib
   D. midostaurin

5. D.R. is a 44-year-old male who has a new diagnosis of high-risk acute promyelocytic leukemia. D.R. has no known comorbidities. His nurse knows he will begin treatment with a regimen of; all-trans-retinoic acid (ATRA) plus which one of the following?
   A. arsenic trioxide
   B. arsenic trioxide plus anthracycline
   C. arsenic trioxide plus gemtuzumab ozogamycin
   D. arsenic trioxide plus intrathecal chemotherapy

6. Chronic lymphocytic leukemia accounts for 25% of all diagnosed leukemias. Which one of the following statements is also true regarding chronic lymphocytic leukemia?
   A. Chronic lymphocytic leukemia is the second most frequent form of leukemia.
   B. Chronic lymphocytic leukemia is more frequently seen in those of Hispanic and Asian than those of Caucasian descent.
   C. Chronic lymphocytic leukemia is most commonly diagnosed at 60 years of age, with less than 15% diagnosed under age 50 years.
   D. Chronic lymphocytic leukemia is a leukemia that originates from immature B lymphocytes.

7. S.W. is a 60-year-old female patient with a diagnosis of chronic lymphocytic leukemia. Upon review of the patient's medication list, her nurse notes that this patient is taking ibrutinib for her diagnosis. The nurse would expect for her patient to have which one of the following markers?
   A. 17p deletion
   B. TP53 mutation
   C. CD20 antigen
   D. CD52 antigen

8. Mr. W is a 67-year-old male patient who has been newly diagnosed with chronic myelocytic leukemia. Upon review of his chart, his nurse finds that he has been diagnosed with Rai stage III, high-risk disease based on his clinical findings. His nurse anticipates that he presented with lymphocytosis and which one of the following?
   A. adenopathy
   B. thrombocytopenia <100,000 μl
   C. splenomegaly
   D. anemia hemoglobin <11 g/dl

9. J.T. is a 68-year-old man who has recently been diagnosed with acute myeloid leukemia (AML). Which one of the following risk factors most likely contributed to his developing the disease?
   A. Radiation Therapy
   B. Long-term exposure to benzene
   C. Heavy usage of alcohol
   D. A diet rich in red meats

**35**

10. Which statement is accurate regarding the epidemiology of leukemia?
   A. The most common type of leukemia in children is acute lymphocytic leukemia.
   B. The most common type of leukemia in children is chronic myelogenous leukemia.
   C. The most common type of leukemia in children is chronic lymphocytic leukemia.
   D. The most common type of leukemia in adults is acute lymphocytic leukemia.

11. Mr. M., a 69-year-old male, has a lymphocyte count greater than 6000 B lymphocytes/μL. His other laboratory results reveal thrombocytopenia with a platelet count of 86,000. The patient also reports he has noticed some swollen lymph nodes in the groin and the left axilla area. He also reports he has early satiety. Using the Rai staging system for CLL, the nurse determines that his extent of disease is which one of the following?
   A. low
   B. medium
   C. intermediate
   D. high

12. Chronic myelogenous leukemia (CML) is a clonal disorder that originates from which one of the following?
   A. Philadelphia chromosome
   B. ataxia telangiectasia mutated (ATM) gene
   C. germline tp53 mutated gene
   D. trisomy 21

# 19 Lung Cancer

1. An oncology nurse is caring for a patient with lung cancer who is exhibiting intrathoracic effects of his disease. The nurse is aware that the signs and symptoms of this disease include which one of the following?
   A. shoulder pain
   B. neuropathy in bilateral lower extremities
   C. hypomagnesia
   D. darkening of the skin

2. F.R. is a 52-year-old male who arrives on the oncology unit with a diagnosis of extensive small-cell carcinoma of the lung. The nurse assigned to the patient is aware that this type of lung cancer is which one of the following statements?
   A. is slow growing and less likely to metastasize
   B. has a more aggressive course
   C. has a better prognosis than the other forms of lung cancer
   D. has multiple surgical options

3. T.C. is a 44-year-old female, who is a newly diagnosed patient with lung cancer. Her nurse, working in an outpatient oncology clinic, reviews her chart prior to the patient visit. She is trying to determine the patient's highest risk for developing lung cancer. Which of one of the following actions would give her the best information regarding the patient's risk?
   A. questions the patient about the age when they first started smoking
   B. assesses the frequency of cigarettes smoked during a day
   C. assesses the number of packs of cigarettes smoked daily and years of smoking
   D. reviews the family history of smoking and passive smoke exposure

4. Attending a local health fair, an oncology nurse is staffing a booth promoting cancer prevention. A man comes to her booth and questions whether or not he should have screening for lung cancer. She instructs him that the guidelines for screening include which one of the following?
   A. ≥30 pack-years
   B. age 70 years or greater
   C. use of inhaled marijuana
   D. vaporized cigarette use

5. C.R. is a 50-year-old male who has been a smoker all of his adult life, and now has developed lung cancer. Admitting he must make a lifestyle change, C.R. asks his oncology nurse who is caring for him about smoking cessation. The type of smoking cessation education she may provide to him includes which one of the following?
   A. gestalt therapy techniques
   B. ice chips to minimize cravings
   C. taking vitamin E daily
   D. nicotine replacement products

6. An oncology nurse is reviewing a patient with lung cancer's pathology report and notes that the patient has the presence of the KRAS mutation. She knows that having this mutation:
   A. has a very good response to tyrosine kinase inhibitors.
   B. determines a poorer survival rate than those without it.
   C. is associated with response to monoclonal antibodies.
   D. allows the patient to only take oral medications as part of their treatment.

7. G.L. is a 60-year-old male patient with Stage I lung cancer. He is seen in the outpatient clinic to evaluate treatment options, including surgery. The nurse caring for him knows that the type of treatment with the least risk for morbidity includes which one of the following?
   A. pneumonectomy with wedge resection
   B. sleeve resection
   C. resuscitative thoracotomy
   D. video-assisted thoracic surgery with wedge resection

8. H.M. is a 47-year-old female who has been newly diagnosed with stage IIa lung cancer. After consultation with her oncology health care team, she has decided against having surgery. The oncology nurse caring for the patient knows that the next best treatment for this patient would be which one of the following?
   A. stereotactic ablative radiotherapy (SABR)
   B. oral chemotherapy
   C. low-energy radiation
   D. immunotherapy

9. A nurse on an oncology unit is administering Pembrolizumab to a patient with lung cancer. The nurse understands that this medication:
   A. blocks enzymes to prevent cancer cells from growing and dividing.
   B. is a second-line therapy for patients with advanced non–small-cell lung cancer.
   C. is an immune-checkpoint inhibitor.
   D. harbors molecules which break down cancer cells.

10. An oncology nurse caring for a patient with small-cell lung cancer is aware that, with this type of lung cancer, which one of the following is correct?
    A. brain radiation therapy is given to prevent metastasis
    B. there is greater than 5-year survival with response to treatment
    C. KRAS mutations are present, which guides treatment choice
    D. a lobectomy is often performed

11. D.J. is a 52-year-old male with a diagnosis of non-small cell lung cancer (NSCLC). He will begin treatment with molecular targeted therapy. The nurse treating him understands that molecular targeted therapy has which one of the following considerations?
    A. Is not known to be effective in treating individuals with genetic mutations.
    B. Erlotinib is now considered first-line therapy for individuals with advanced, recurrent, or metastatic non–squamous NSCLC.
    C. Bevacizumab is recommended in select patients with advanced NSCLC.
    D. Does not seem likely to impact therapies for pathways of mutation.

12. E.W. is a 59-year-old man who has worked in construction doing home remodeling, renovation, and demolition for the past 25 years. He was a smoker for a brief time as a teenager but quit after only a few years and has not touched a tobacco product in the intervening years. And, yet, despite being successful in his efforts for long-term smoking cessation, he has developed lung cancer. He is overweight and has been trying unsuccessfully to control his weight for the past few years. He is confused. He only thought he could develop lung cancer from smoking. The nurse reviews his chart and decides which one of the following could have contributed to his developing of the disease?
    A. His gender and age.
    B. His weight, which is above the average for his age.
    C. His exposure to paint and paint thinners on the job.
    D. His exposure to asbestos in his career in home construction.

# 20 Lymphoma

1. An oncology nurse is caring for L.J, a 25-year-old male with favorable Hodgkin's Lymphoma diagnosis. After speaking with his healthcare provider, L.J. asks the nurse about his standard course of treatment. The nurse explains that he will receive which one of the following?
   A. five cycles of chemotherapy plus radiation therapy
   B. two to three cycles chemotherapy, plus radiation therapy
   C. high-dose chemotherapy and autologous bone marrow transplant
   D. Palliative chemotherapy and radiation therapy

2. R.K.is a male, 46-year-old patient with Stage II diffuse large B-cell lymphoma, who has been admitted for treatment. The oncology nurse caring for him knows that the standard treatment for a patient with this diagnosis is which one of the following?
   A. autologous peripheral blood stem cell transplant
   B. rituximab, cyclophosphamide, doxorubicin, vincristine, prednisone
   C. salvage radiation therapy with 6000 cGy
   D. ifosfamide, carboplatin, etoposide, prednisone

3. A 37-year-old female patient presents to the clinic with signs of Hodgkin's Lymphoma. The patient undergoes testing and her oncology nurse should anticipate seeing results confirming this diagnosis would include one of which of the following?
   A. reed-Steenberg cells
   B. bone marrow involvement
   C. extranodal involvement in distal sites
   D. metastases to the long bones

4. An oncology nurse is caring for a 36-year-old female who is newly diagnosed patient with Hodgkin lymphoma. The staging system most commonly used for this type of lymphoma is which one of the following?
   A. the Tumor Nodes Metastasis staging system
   B. the Rai staging system of leukemia and lymphoma
   C. the Reed-Steenberg pathologic staging system
   D. the Ann Arbor Staging system

5. S.D. is a 49-year-old man who has come to the clinic for treatment. An oncology nurse is assessing this patient's past medical history and discovers that the patient has a history of *Helicobacter pylori* bacterial infection. The nurse reports this finding, as this is a significant risk factor for the development of which one of the following?
   A. breast cancer
   B. cancer of the distal colon
   C. mucosa-associated lymphoid tissue (MALT) lymphoma
   D. Burkitt lymphoma

6. A nurse is caring for G.F., a 37-year-old male patient, who has a high-grade non-Hodgkin lymphoma with localized disease. In a meeting with the physician, the patient asks about his prognosis. The nurse caring for G.F. would most likely expect the provider to respond that the disease:
   A. "We could achieve a cure with combination therapy and you have an overall survival of 5 years."
   B. "You will most likely relapse within two years, and, unfortunately, your overall cure rate is only 10%."
   C. "We have encouraging news. You have a greater than 80% cure rate and a survival time of more than 20 years."
   D. "This disease is completely curable, after you have undergone an autologous stem cell transplant."

7. T.J. is a 22-year-old male who makes an appointment with the clinic after complaining of systemic symptoms that have gotten his clinician concerned about the possibility that he could be diagnosed with a lymphoma. Reading over his chart, the attending nurse would be likely suspicious of which one of the following systemic symptoms?
   A. Fever, weight loss, fatigue, and night sweats
   B. Pain in the chest area
   C. Swelling of the limbs
   D. Extreme thirst and frequent urination

8. J.B. is a 46-year-old male patient, whose chest radiography done in the emergency department reveals mediastinal widening. A chest CT is done, and a large mediastinal mass is detected. Upon axillary lymph node biopsy, a large cell follicular lymphoma is diagnosed. Which one of the following diagnostic tests is not necessary to determine treatment options?

A. Obtain a 24-hour urine.
B. Determine whether he lymph node biopsy is CD 20+.
C. Obtain a CT scan of the abdomen and pelvis.
D. Perform a bilateral bone marrow biopsy and aspirate.

# 21 Multiple Myeloma

1. Which one of the following risk factors have been found to be associated with the incidence of newly diagnosed multiple myeloma (MM)?
   A. employment status
   B. history of monoclonal gammopathy of undetermined significance (MGUS)
   C. female gender
   D. exposure to Epstein-Barr virus

2. The three pathognomonic features of MM are which one of the following set of examples?
   A. renal disease, anemia, hypocalcemia.
   B. monoclonal plasmacytosis, excess production of M protein, osteolytic bone lesions.
   C. anemia, hypocalcemia, immunodeficiency.
   D. low production of M protein, osteolytic bone lesions, anemia.

3. The diagnosis of multiple myeloma is confirmed by:
   A. bone scan
   B. complete blood count
   C. bone marrow biopsy
   D. renal ultrasound

4. According to the 2013 Mayo Clinic Stratification of Myeloma and Risk-Adapted Therapy (mSMART), a patient with symptomatic MM and genetic abnormalities such as of chromosome 17p, translocation of chromosomes 14 and 16, and 14 and 20 will be classified as which one of the following?
   A. low-risk MM
   B. standard-risk MM
   C. intermediate-risk MM
   D. high-risk MM

5. Pain in a person with MM is most commonly due to which one of the following conditions?
   A. anemia
   B. neural infiltration of plasma cells
   C. intestinal obstruction due to an abdominal mass
   D. lytic bone lesions

6. J.M. is a 67-year-old male patient, with a newly diagnosed, symptomatic multiple myeloma. The patient has started on a triple regimen with bortezomib, lenalidomide, and low dose dexamethasone. Which one of the following is a key nursing consideration for educating the patient on chemotherapy?
   A. Intravenous aprepitant on day 1 of each cycle
   B. Allopurinol prophylaxis
   C. Acyclovir prophylaxis
   D. Intravenous fluid hydration three times a week

7. S.T. is a 70-year-old male, who has been recently diagnosed with multiple myeloma and is having a difficult time coming to terms with his diagnosis. He is a veteran of the Vietnam War, and has lived a mostly healthy lifestyle. He is not someone who is interested in sharing his feelings yet the nurse caring for him understands he needs nursing intervention related to physical, emotional, psychological, social, and spiritual distress as he is about to embark on a long journey filled with extensive diagnostic testing and treatment regimens. Which one of the following interventions should his nurse utilize in managing his psychosocial issues?
   A. Encourage the patient to verbalize his feelings about the disease and the treatment
   B. Encourage the patient to talk with his family since his loved ones know him best
   C. Refer the patient to pastoral care
   D. Tell the patient there is "noting to worry about" so there is no sense in getting worked up

8. According to the SLiM CRAB criteria myeloma-related organ dysfunction requires which one of the following diagnostic criteria for active or symptomatic multiple myeloma requiring therapy?
   A. Seventy percent clonal bone marrow plasma cells
   B. Serum-free Light chain ration Kappa: lambda < 100
   C. Magnetic resonance imaging (MRI) studies with < 1 focal lesion (>8 mm in size)
   D. Calcium elevation in blood, with a calcium level greater than 10.5 ng/L or the upper limit of normal

9. D.L. is a 50-year-old patient who presents to the oncology clinic with a new diagnosis of multiple myeloma. Which one of the following results is a poor prognostic indicator in this patient?
   A. hypocalcemia
   B. elevated creatinine
   C. normal bone scan
   D. plasma cells in bone marrow

10. A patient presents to the clinic to discuss treatment for his new diagnosis of multiple myeloma and is ruled out as candidate for transplant. The patient asks the nurse if he has been diagnosed with a terminal disease. The nurse responds with the understanding that medication treatment in multiple myeloma:
    A. has a high likelihood of cure
    B. is curable in some trisomy translocations
    C. is used prior to surgery
    D. is aimed at controlling disease

# 22 Neurologic System Cancers

1. An oncology nurse working with a pediatric patient population recognizes that which one of the following statements on pediatric brain and spinal cord tumors is true? Brain and spinal cord tumors are:
   A. the second most commonly diagnosed pediatric cancer.
   B. a rare diagnostic occurrence.
   C. the most frequently diagnosed pediatric cancer.
   D. most often diagnosed as benign tumors.

2. A patient with cancer who has undergone a craniotomy and tumor resection and the nurse caring for the patient understands that the best practice for a new baseline MRI or CT to be completed post-operatively within which one of the following time frames?
   A. 12 hours
   B. 24 hours
   C. 48 hours
   D. 72 hours

3. The oncology nurse recognizes that the most important first-line treatment for a malignant primary brain tumor is which one of the following?
   A. maximal surgical tumor resection
   B. chemotherapy
   C. antiepileptic medications
   D. corticosteroids

4. The mother of a child diagnosed with a primary central nervous system tumor asks the nurse about her child's chances of survival. The nurse responds to the mother with an understanding that the 5-year survival rate for children and teens diagnosed with a primary central nervous system tumor is which one of the following?
   A. 25%
   B. 50%
   C. 75%
   D. 90%

5. A 27-year-old male patient has been newly diagnosed with grade III oligodendroglioma and is scheduled to receive chemotherapy teaching from his oncology nurse. The most important time sensitive educational intervention that she can provide him would include which one of the following?
   A. sperm banking
   B. lifting of driving restrictions
   C. obtaining a second opinion
   D. hospice services

6. A patient with a progressive malignant brain tumor reports to the oncology nursing caring for him that he is having symptoms of hyperglycemia, myopathy, lymphopenia, and osteoporosis. The nurse understands these symptoms are most likely related to which one of the following?
   A. bone resorption inhibitors
   B. anticonvulsants
   C. corticosteroids
   D. immunosuppressants

7. The tumor type with the highest predilection to metastasize the central nervous system is which one of the following?
   A. colorectal
   B. melanoma
   C. breast
   D. renal cell

8. The tumor type most frequently associated with leptomeningeal carcinomatosis originates from which one of the following?
   A. breast
   B. lung
   C. hematologic malignancies
   D. prostate

9. Which one of the following is the most common and severe symptom reported by a patient with a primary brain tumor?
   A. fatigue
   B. headache
   C. seizures
   D. constipation

10. When caring for a patient with brain cancer, treatment with anti-epileptic medication is indicated:
    A. for driving
    B. with radiation
    C. peri-operatively
    D. at diagnosis

11. Primary central nervous system tumors are staged according to which one of the following?
    A. World Health Organization (WHO) classifications
    B. Tumor Node Metastasis (TNM) criteria
    C. National Comprehensive Cancer Network (NCCN) criteria
    D. American Joint Committee on Cancer (AJCC) classifications

12. Which one of the following sections of the brain would the oncology nurse most likely identify as being responsible for a person's personality? The section of the brain responsible for personality is the:
    A. temporal lobe
    B. occipital lobe
    C. parietal lobe
    D. frontal lobe

13. Among the following types of spinal tumors, which one, is the least common?
    A. Sarcomas
    B. Astrocytomas
    C. Chordomas
    D. Schwannomas

14. Which one of the following sections of the brain is responsible for a person's coordination and balance?
    A. temporal lobe.
    B. pituitary gland.
    C. brain stem.
    D. cerebellum.

15. Risk factors for central nervous system tumors can be known intrinsic, known situational, known extrinsic, and genetic/inherited risk. Of the following risk factors, which one is a known extrinsic risk factor?
    A. Immunocompromised, including HIV/AIDS, immunosuppressive medical therapies, and congenital immunodeficiency.
    B. Exposure to pesticides, vinyl chloride and petrochemicals.
    C. Ionizing radiation (IR), with a causal relationship between therapeutic irradiation of doses >2500 cGy and development of brain tumors.
    D. Race/ethnicity, with Caucasian northern European most common and meningioma more common in African American populations.

# 23 Reproductive Cancers

1. Prevention of cervical cancer deaths is addressed through all of the following except:
   A. Papanicolaou test and human immunodeficiency virus (HIV) screening in female patients over age 21 years as per American Cancer Society (ACS), US Preventive Services Task Force (USPTF), or American College of Obstetricians and Gynecologists (ACOG) guidelines.
   B. vaccination against oncogenic (high-risk) hepatitis C virus subtypes.
   C. Attempting to conceive after the patient's hCG levels have normalized for 6-8 weeks and menses have become regular.
   D. addressing risk factors including encouraging regular screening exams, discussing risks of multiple partners, and discouraging tobacco use.

2. Major risk factors for endometrial cancer include increasing age, obesity, and which one of the following?
   A. early menopause
   B. hereditary nonpolyposis colorectal cancer/Lynch syndrome
   C. aromatase inhibitor use
   D. late menarche

3. G.T. is a 35-year-old patient, who is a one-half pack-per-day smoker with a history of PID. She was recently diagnosed with advanced ovarian cancer. She states that "cancer always happens to us," in reference to her elder sister whom is a breast cancer survivor. She is concerned that her 10-year-old daughter could be at risk for ovarian cancer in the future, and asks her oncology nurse for advice. The nurse knows which one of the following is true?
   A. Patients should have routine ovarian cancer screening for early detection.
   B. Tobacco use and history of PID are risk factors for ovarian cancer, but does not outweigh the need for a genetics referral for this patient.
   C. A new diagnosis of ovarian cancer is more common in premenopausal than in postmenopausal women.
   D. Her daughter should start hormone-replacement therapy after menopause to decrease her ovarian cancer risk.

4. When is it safe for a patient with a history of gestational trophoblastic neoplasia to attempt to conceive? Choose from one of the following statements.
   A. It is safe to attempt to conceive as soon as the patient's human chorionic gonadotropin (hCG) levels have started to respond to chemotherapy.
   B. It is safe to attempt to conceive after the patient has completed one year of surveillance.
   C. It is safe to attempt to conceive after the patient's hCG levels have normalized for 6-8 weeks and menses have become regular.
   D. It is safe to attempt to conceive as soon as the patient's menses are regular, however, the patient will most likely experience difficulty conceiving at all due to the chemotherapy treatment's deleterious effects on fertility.

5. Oncogenic human papillomavirus (HPV) infection and smoking have been associated with an increased risk of developing cervical cancer, vaginal cancer, and vulvar cancer. Which one of the following additional risk factors would be correctly considered for the patients below?
   A. An additional risk factor would be diethylstilbestrol use by the mother of a patient diagnosed with vaginal cancer.
   B. An additional risk factor would be breast cancer in a first degree relative of a patient diagnosed with cervical cancer.
   C. An additional risk factor would be asbestos exposure in the mother of a patient diagnosed with vulvar cancer.
   D. An additional risk factor would be personal use of hormone replacement therapy by a patient diagnosed with vulvar cancer.

6. Which one of the following is statistically more likely to be diagnosed with testicular cancer?
   A. 65-year-old while male with a weak urinary stream and a history of well-controlled HIV infection.
   B. A 32-year-old Hispanic male with a history of painless unilateral testicular swelling.
   C. A 25-year-old male of Pacific Islander descent with a history of recurrent herpes simplex virus-2 infection.
   D. A 50-year-old African American male with two first-degree relatives with a history of colorectal cancer.

**45**

7. Modifiable risk factors for penile cancer include which one of the following?
   A. hepatitis B vaccination
   B. tobacco cessation
   C. circumcision is recommended after puberty
   D. avoid retracting the foreskin while cleaning the glans

8. Typical signs and symptoms of recurrent ovarian cancer include which one of the following?
   A. rising CA125 tumor marker
   B. weight gain
   C. increased appetite
   D. vaginal discharge or bleeding

9. The standard treatment for most patients with newly diagnosed endometrial cancer is which one of the following?
   A. fertility sparing whenever possible
   B. oral hormonal therapy for 10 years for estrogen suppression
   C. upfront hysterectomy and bilateral salpingo-oophorectomy
   D. D&C followed by close observation for endometrial thickening

10. Which one of the following is a treatment for early-stage (IA1–IB1) cervical cancer?
    A. Radical hysterectomy, lymph node evaluation
    B. Definitive chemoradiation (with or without ovarian transposition if premenopausal), possibly neoadjuvant chemotherapy followed by resection
    C. Fertility sparing, including conization with cold knife or LEEP procedure, lymph node evaluation if lymphovascular space invasion (LVSI) is present, radical trachelectomy
    D. Primary treatment followed by observation, external beam radiation therapy (EBRT), and/or adjuvant chemotherapy

11. L.J. is a 47-year-old female patient with metastatic cervical cancer. Which one of the following would her nurse know to be a treatment for metastatic cervical cancer?
    A. Simple or modified radical hysterectomy with or without lymph node evaluation
    B. External beam radiation therapy (EBRT) and neoadjuvant chemotherapy
    C. Radiation therapy with or without chemotherapy, palliative systemic agents, and supportive care
    D. Radiation therapy, systemic therapy, local ablation, and surgical resection

12. Which one of the following stages of testicular cancer has the best five-year survival rate in the United States?
    A. Distant
    B. Un-staged
    C. Regional
    D. Localized

13. Mr. H. and his wife are distressed with his recent diagnosis of testicular cancer. During the course of the assessment, it becomes clear to his oncology nurse that some of this distress is related to fertility concerns. His nurse discusses sperm banking with the couple. The nurse explains that sperm banking should be completed:
    A. before surgery.
    B. before chemotherapy.
    C. after surgery.
    D. after chemotherapy.

14. F.D. is a 45-year-old woman having a TAH BSO for ovarian cancer. She has been experiencing irregular menses prior to surgery. Possible complications she might experience include which one of the following?
    A. alternating constipation and diarrhea
    B. vaginal drying and pelvic tissue atrophy
    C. decreased risk of cardiovascular disease
    D. changes in urinary function

# 24 Skin Cancer

1. A nurse is caring for N.M., who is a 72-year-old female patient, and has had several basal cell carcinomas (BCC) diagnosed on her face and arms over the years. The nurse knows that the predominant risk factor for developing BCC is which one of the following?
   A. sunlight overexposure
   B. tobacco smoking
   C. family history
   D. young age

2. A nurse is assessing a patient in the clinic who has a history of non-melanoma skin cancer. Which one of the following findings would be considered a precursor for squamous cell carcinoma?
   A. Atypical nevi
   B. Multiple moles
   C. Actinic keratoses
   D. Skin viral infection

3. A Mohs procedure is recommended to treat a patient with a non-melanoma skin cancer. In teaching the patient about what to expect, the nurse explains to the patient which one of the following?
   A. subzero temperature swabs will be applied to the area
   B. the area will be injected with a chemotherapy drug
   C. a curette will be used to scrape away tumor cells, then the area will be cauterized
   D. thin layers will be removed from the area and examined under a microscope

4. J. R. is a 40-year-old female kidney transplant patient who is being treated for Merkel cell carcinoma. During an office visit, she begins showing signs of distress and asks the oncology nurse "Why me"? The nurse explains that which one of the following factors is associated with increased risk?
   A. Female gender
   B. Organ transplant
   C. African American descent
   D. Age between 35 and 50 years

5. The oncology nurse is teaching K.T, a 40-year-old female patient, how to recognize skin signs that could indicate a need for melanoma assessment by a specialist. The nurse should instruct the patient to report the sighting of a mole showing signs of which one of the following?
   A. regular border
   B. symmetrical shape
   C. tendency to bleed
   D. uniform brown color

6. F.R. is a 60-year-old male patient, who has been diagnosed with metastatic melanoma. During an office visit, F.R. asks the nurse, "What will happen to me next?" In answering his question, his nurse anticipates what his standard treatment will include. In her explanation, she includes which one of the following treatments?
   A. isolated limb perfusion
   B. immunotherapy
   C. cranial radiation therapy
   D. photodynamic therapy

7. Which one of the following is a characteristic of Merkel cell carcinoma?
   A. Develops primarily on sun-exposed skin; rarely found on palmoplantar surfaces and never appears on the mucosa
   B. Presents as papules, plaques, and cyst-like structures or pruritic tumors on the lower extremities
   C. Often presents as a new or enlarging lesion that may bleed, weep, be tender, or be painful
   D. Can develop at sites of chemical exposure or chronic trauma

8. Which one of the following statements about basel cell carcinoma is true?
   A. Major risk factor is exposure to UVR, especially intermittent exposure early in life
   B. Most commonly presents as an erythematous or violaceous, tender, dome-shaped nodule on sun-exposed areas on the head or neck of an elderly white male
   C. Typically, these are slow growing, however, those arising in in non–sun-exposed sites (i.e., lips, genitalia, perianal areas) are more aggressive with a higher risk of metastases
   D. Most lesions are <2 cm in diameter at the time of diagnosis; rapid growth is common

# 25 Surgery

1. D. J. is a 45-year-old male patient, who is on a surgical oncology unit. He is scheduled for surgery the following day for removal of a malignant tumor. The nurse caring for the patient understands that prior to surgery, it is most important to define whether which one of the following is happening?
   A. Is the organ being removed necessary for bodily function?
   B. Will there will be placement of a jugular venous catheter during surgery?
   C. Will the physician involved be engaged in proper positioning of the patient?
   D. Will the wound be prepared and irrigated during the procedure?

2. T.G. is a 40-year-old male, who has a wide excision of the left axilla. After the procedure, the patient askes the nurse taking care of him asks her, "What has happened to me? What is a wide excision?" As part of her answer, the nurse offers him which one of the following explanations?
   A. "Your cancer has been removed and a large margin of the surrounding tissue was also removed."
   B. "Your cancer was removed, along with some adjacent tissue, and your regional lymph nodes."
   C. "There was removal of a very small amount of cancerous tissue but they also took out many lymph nodes."
   D. "The procedure that you underwent involved removal of the entire lesion along with your upper pectoris muscle."

3. H. R. is a 50-year-old male patient with cancer. He presents for presurgical evaluation and, during the assessment, he reports to the nurse that he has been diagnosed with uncontrolled diabetes. The nurse is aware that the patient is at risk for developing which one of the following conditions?
   A. kidney disease
   B. hypertension post-operatively
   C. electrolyte disturbances
   D. hypoglycemia post-operatively

4. C. K. is a 45-year-old patient with breast cancer. She has an appointment in the breast clinic to discuss with her nurse the management of her breast cancer. The physician has recommended conservative therapy and post-surgical radiation with the patient. The oncology nurse working with C.K. understands that the purpose of this type of management of this patient's disease is to do which one of the following?
   A. The purpose of the disease management is to block the action of proteins to prevent the growth of cancer cells.
   B. The purpose of the disease management is to treat potentially microscopic diseases after conservative therapy.
   C. The purpose of the disease management is to fight cancer cells using the patient's own immune system.
   D. The purpose of the disease management is to conserve the patient's breast tissue for later reconstruction.

5. A nurse is preparing one of her patients for surgery in the perioperative suite. The nurse maintains standards of care through the World Health Organization, which ensure which one of the following?
   A. there is a "pause" completed, and that staff are in position for surgery.
   B. safety standards are met to decrease the length and cost of surgery.
   C. consent for treatment is completed, and there is team collaboration.
   D. hazardous drugs are properly used and disposed of.

6. Which one of the following is a definition of a laparoscopic surgical approach?
   A. A procedure in which surgical tools are passed through an existing orifice (mouth, nares, anus, urethra) without external incision/scar
   B. A procedure requiring extended, full-thickness incision to allow thorough exploration and manipulation of tissues
   C. A procedure in which multiple small incisions ("ports"') are made for surgical camera insertion and application of operative tools allowing less tissue manipulation
   D. A procedure in which remotely controlled instruments allowing less invasion, improved optics, finer control, and ergonomics to lessen tissue manipulation

7. Which one of the following defines the characteristics of palliative cancer surgery?
   A. This type of surgery removes primary tumor, lymph nodes, adjacent affected organs with negative margins attained via the least invasive means available
   B. This type of surgery improves function or appearance of a surgical defect improving the quality of life
   C. This type of surgery improves comfort when curative resection is not possible; includes surgical debulking or decompression or diversion via stent or ostomy (e.g., gastrojejunostomy, colostomy)
   D. This type of surgery is performed for issues such hemorrhage, organ ischemia or perforation, drainage/washout for abscess or infection, and cord compression

# 26 Blood and Marrow Transplantation

1. Which one of the following statements is true regarding allogeneic hematopoietic stem cell transplantation?
   A. The recipient receives his or her own procured stem cells after high-dose chemotherapy.
   B. Immunosuppression is not required to prevent graft-versus-host disease (GVHD).
   C. Human leukocyte antigen (HLA) matching is not required as part of pre-transplantation workup.
   D. The recipient receives hematopoietic stem cells from a healthy related or unrelated donor.

2. The use of post-transplant immunosuppression in allogeneic hematopoietic stem cell transplantation (HSCT) is to prevent which one of the following:
   A. Donor T lymphocytes mounting an immune response against the stem cell recipient.
   B. Relapse due to a low undetectable level of tumor cells persisting in the infusing cells.
   C. Damage to the small sinusoid of the liver from pre-transplant conditioning regimen.
   D. Post-transplant infectious complications with viral, bacterial, or fungal organisms.

3. Which one of the following factors significantly impacts determination in the type of transplant a patient is to undergo?
   A. Underlying malignancy or non-malignant hematologic disease
   B. Availability of an ABO-matched donor
   C. Donor's disease status
   D. Donor's physical and psychosocial status

4. G. L. is a 47-year-old female patient with acute myeloid leukemia (AML), who underwent a HSCT a month ago. The patient now is presenting with new onset of erythematous skin on her face, palms of hands, and soles of feet. The nurse caring for this patient is concerned about the development of which one of the following post-transplant complications?
   A. hepatic sinusoidal obstruction syndrome
   B. hand-foot-mouth disease
   C. GVHD
   D. graft-versus-leukemia effect

5. The nurse should assess which one of the following for hepatic sinusoidal obstruction syndrome?
   A. tacrolimus levels
   B. abdominal girth daily
   C. characteristics of stool
   D. skin conditions

6. Which one of the following medications is often used to treat cytomegalovirus (CMV) infection?
   A. Voriconazole
   B. Posaconazole
   C. Foscarnet
   D. Acyclovir

7. Reduced-intensity or non-myeloablative regimens are used in the setting of HSCT when the patient presents which one of the following traits?
   A. The patient is less than 60 years old
   B. The patient has no pre-existing comorbidities
   C. The patient has excellent organ function status
   D. The patient has a disease that will benefit from a graft-versus-tumor (GVT) immunologic effect

8. Which one of the following statements is true regarding autologous HSCT?
   A. Autografting is most frequently used for the treatment of AML and aplastic anemia.
   B. Autologous HSCT can be effective in treating some autoimmune diseases.
   C. Immunosuppressant agents are routinely used in autologous stem cell transplantation.
   D. A conditioning regimen is not required prior to stem cell transplantation.

9. Preventative measures for idiopathic pulmonary interstitial pneumonitis include the use of which one of the following?
   A. a filtered air system and high-dose steroid
   B. a filtered air system and CMV sero-negative blood products
   C. mycophenolate and depletion of T cells from marrow
   D. Trimethoprim/sulfamethoxazole and tacrolimus

10. Which one of the following medications is used to prevent sinusoidal obstruction syndrome (SOS)?
    A. Ursodiol
    B. Lovenox
    C. Pantoprazole
    D. Bactrim DS

11. J.R. is a 56-year-old male patient with hx of AML s/p Allo transplant day +48 presented with total bilirubin of 4 with more than 1000ml of stool per day. The nurse grades his GVHD as:
    A. acute GVHD, overall clinical Grade II.
    B. acute GVHD, overall clinical Grade III.
    C. chronic GVHD, overall clinical Grade II.
    D. chronic GVHD, overall clinical Grade III.

12. One of the risk factors for the development of SOS is which one of the following?
    A. Karnofsky score >90% before transplantation
    B. First transplantation
    C. Pre-transplantation hepatotoxic drug therapy
    D. 10/10 HLA-matched unrelated allogeneic transplantation

13. Which one of the following medications has a narrow drug therapeutic window?
    A. acyclovir
    B. ursodil
    C. alemtuzumab
    D. tacrolimus

14. Which one of the following statements is true regarding survivorship?
    A. Long-term follow up is not required.
    B. Delayed organ dysfunction is uncommon.
    C. Post-transplantation vaccinations are required.
    D. Evaluation of chronic GVHD is not required.

15. Which one of the following statements is true regarding goals of a pre-transplant conditioning regimen?
    A. To boost the patient's immune system to allow for marrow engraftment.
    B. To eradicate remaining malignancy and to open spaces within marrow.
    C. To prevent GVHD and promote a graft-versus-tumor effect.
    D. To prevent post-transplant complications such as infections and SOS.

16. Which one of the following is a nursing implication for the management of graft-versus-host disease (GVHD), both acute and chronic?
    A. Implement routine of coughing, and deep breathing.
    B. Monitor reports on patient's vision acuity.
    C. Monitor patients' weight gain.
    D. Evaluate the patient's cyclosporine or tacrolimus levels and notify practitioner of significant abnormalities.

17. Which one of the following is true regarding an infection in a patient with idiopathic pulmonary interstitial pneumonitis (infectious)?
    A. Occurs most frequently in patients > 30 years old with a history of chest irradiation or previous bleomycin therapy
    B. Results from engraftment of immunocompetent donor T lymphocytes
    C. Occurs in 30% to 60% of all autologous bone marrow transplant recipients
    D. Occurs most commonly in women < 30 years of age with a history of anthracycline therapy

18. Which one of the following is a fungal infection complication that occurs in HSCT recipients one to four months after transplantation?
    A. Gram-positive organisms
    B. Parainfluenza
    C. *Aspergillus* species
    D. *Pneumocystis jiroveci* (*carinii*)

19. Which one of the following is a bacterial infection complication that occurs in HSCT recipients four to twelve months after transplantation?
    A. Varicella-zoster
    B. *P. jiroveci* (*carinii*)
    C. *Streptococcus pneumoniae*
    D. Coccidioidomycosis

20. Which one of the following is a social evaluation during assessment for a potential recipient of a HSCT?
    A. Number, type, effectiveness of coping mechanisms used in past stressful situations (before transplantation therapy) by patient and family members
    B. Perceptions of patient and family about isolation, prolonged hospitalization, living will, use of life-support technology, and potential death or survival
    C. Understanding of treatment aggressiveness, goals of therapy, chances of survival
    D. Type, number, and history of use of support systems in the family and community

# 27 The Practice and Principles of Radiation Oncology

1. The oncology nurse caring for the patient receiving external beam radiation is aware of safety measures that need to be taken, such as which one of the following?
   A. wearing silicone ring badges to monitor radiation exposure
   B. full understanding of radiation effects, risk of exposure, and safety practices
   C. adhering to principles of time, exposure, and distance
   D. ensuring that radiation beams turn on when entering rooms

2. C.K. is 60-year-old female patient with cervical cancer. She will be receiving external beam radiation as well as brachytherapy as part of her treatment. The patient asks the oncology nurse caring for her why she would be required to have both types of radiation therapy. The nurse tells C.K. which one of the following?
   A. "You are receiving combined therapy because this type of therapy treats bulky local disease and improves local control."
   B. "You are receiving brachytherapy because this type of therapy uses a lower dose, whereas the external uses higher doses in a small area."
   C. "Combining the two therapies will result in virtually no side effects for you."
   D. "Receiving both external and internal radiation will decrease the need for you to undergo surgery."

3. J.S. is a 48-year-old female with cancer. J.S. is undergoing external beam radiation therapy to the chest wall and who has moist desquamation in her skin folds. A nurse caring for this patient knows interventions to manage side effects for this type of treatment includes which one of the following?
   A. cleansing the area with hydrogen peroxide and applying an adhesive dressing over the site
   B. instructing the patient to massage the area when pruritis becomes a problem
   C. applying an ice pack on the area to decrease pain and swelling
   D. using hydrocolloid or hydrogel dressings to maintain a moist healing environment

4. An oncology nurse is caring for a patient who has been diagnosed with lung cancer. This patient will be treated with stereotactic body radiation therapy (SBRT). The nurse knows that with this type of therapy which one of the following statements is true?
   A. Normal tissues and organs are not spared treatment-related toxicity.
   B. The patient will receive anywhere between 1 and 10 treatments.
   C. Immobilization is not required for this type of treatment.
   D. Doses are higher than conventional radiation treatments.

5. G.D. is a 62-year-old male patient with prostate cancer who is currently on a surgical oncology unit awaiting a procedure. He is scheduled to have image guided radiation (IGRT). The nurse is aware that the type of IGRT the patient will be having includes which one of the following?
   A. cone beam CT
   B. fiducial markers
   C. stereotactic radiosurgery
   D. brachytherapy

6. D.K. is a 56-year-old female patient who has had radiation therapy to the head and neck. In caring for this patient, the oncology nurse instructs the patient about the long-term side effects of radiation that includes which one of the following?
   A. xerostomia
   B. secondary cancers such as acute myeloid leukemia
   C. esophageal narrowing
   D. neurologic effects

7. After a multidisciplinary team meeting regarding radiation therapy treatment for a 60-year-old male patient with pancreatic cancer, the oncology nurse is aware that the next step in the process of treatment includes which one of the following?
   A. administering the actual radiation therapy
   B. using three-dimensional conformal radiotherapy (3D-CRT) treatment planning
   C. Calculating the dose to target and tolerated dose to surrounding structures
   D. Protecting the organs with the use of slings and contours to minimize movement

8. An oncology nurse is caring for a patient with central nervous system disease. The patient is receiving proton therapy. The nurse educates the patient that the advantage of proton beam therapy is which one of the following?
   A. the tumor is targeted and well controlled
   B. its ability to cut and destroy tumors into small particles
   C. it shapes the beam to fit the targeted area
   D. the protons combine with neurons to maximize cell kill

9. An experienced nurse is educating a new nurse on an oncology unit regarding the guidelines for radiation safety while caring for a patient who has had Iodine 131. The experienced nurse instructs the novice nurse that barriers to exposure include which one of the following?
   A. the use of insulating materials to protect against the effects of radiation
   B. wearing gloves to protect against radioisotopes excreted through body fluids
   C. the use of fluid-resistant materials to prevent sweat from evaporating and igniting radioactive ions
   D. the use of respiratory equipment to protect from fumes emitted from radioactive isotopes

10. L.M. is a 63-year-old female patient on an oncology unit is receiving image guided radiation (IGRT) for lung cancer. The nurse caring for the patient is aware that management of side effects includes which one of the following?
    A. teaching the patient about oxygen conservation
    B. administering Cepacol mouth rinses
    C. placing the patient on seizure precautions
    D. NSAIDs for chest pain

11. Radiation therapy dosing is based on medical physics and depends upon which one of the following?
    A. Density of the bone type to be penetrated
    B. Distance from the radiation source to the skin
    C. Energy and circumference of the beam
    D. Density and type of skin surface

12. Which of the following statements is true regarding the use or characteristics of stereotactic radiotherapy (SRT)?
    A. Frames or thermoplastic masks may be used for CNS tumors, body frames are used for extracranial sites when using SRT
    B. SRT is less precise than stereotactic radiosurgery (SRS)
    C. SRT allows for a large target/treatment volume and can treat any size of lesion
    D. SRT treats a wide target area of the body

13. Which of the following is a characteristic for moist desquamation?
    A. The rate of repair of basal cells is inadequate for replacement of epidermis
    B. Skin can feel taut reports of "awareness of skin"
    C. Red or tan appearance
    D. Drying of the skin surface with associated itching

14. Which one of the following statements correctly reflects the principles of the 5 R's of radiation therapy?
    A. "Reassortment" refers to the tumor cell proliferation that occurs during radiation.
    B. "Radiosensitizing" refers to the concept that ionizing radiation therapy is most effective on cells that are undifferentiated and undergoing active mitosis.
    C. "Repair" refers to radioresistant cells that synchronize into a more radiosensitive phase of the cell cycle after a fraction of radiation.
    D. "Reassortment" refers to the importance of oxygen in mediating the cytotoxic effects of radiation due to free radical production.

15. Which one of the following does not influence the biologic response to radiation?
    A. Level of DNA damage
    B. Oxygen effect
    C. Sensitivity of cells to radiation
    D. Ability of the body to clear toxins

16. Which of the following statements is true about the reasoning behind why the delivery of radiation is divided into small fractions?
    A. Delivering the same total dose of radiation at one time can only be done by use of brachytherapy technique.
    B. Fractionation allows for recovery of the surrounding nonmalignant tissues and in some tissues promotes recruitment of the malignant cells into the cell cycle for an improved cell kill.
    C. Daily treatments over several weeks allow for the development of a therapeutic relationship between the health care providers and the individual undergoing treatment.
    D. Fractionation helps to deoxygenate the malignant cells in the radiation field, making them more sensitive to the radiation.

**53**

# 28 Chemotherapy and Hormonal Therapy

1. Both normal and malignant cells pass through the five-stages of the cell cycle in order to reproduce and proliferate. In the synthesis phase of the cell cycle which one of the following is correct?
   A. cellular DNA is replicated
   B. cells are ready for division or mitosis
   C. cells are resting and are not dividing
   D. cellular ribonucleic acid (RNA) is being produced

2. Cells from different organs reproduce at different rates depending on the type of cell. The amount of time required for a cell to move from one mitosis to the next mitosis is termed as which one of the following?
   A. cell cycle time
   B. tumor burden
   C. growth fraction
   D. cell cycle phase

3. In combination chemotherapy, different agents are used simultaneously. The advantage of combination chemotherapy is which one of the following?
   A. Combination chemotherapy increases the number of cells exposed to cytotoxic effects
   B. Combination chemotherapy increases the opportunity for drug resistance
   C. Combination chemotherapy is limited to the recurrent setting
   D. Combination chemotherapy is limited to the recurrent setting

4. All of the following are chemotherapy agents used as radiosensitizers, except for which one of the following?
   A. cisplatin
   B. 5-fluorouracil
   C. mitomycin C
   D. protein-bound paclitaxel

5. Chemotherapy can be administered to a patient in a variety of ways. The method of delivering doses of chemotherapy to the specific site of the tumor is called which one of the following?
   A. systemic chemotherapy
   B. regional chemotherapy
   C. high-dose chemotherapy
   D. dose-dense chemotherapy

6. An example of a cell cycle-specific chemotherapy drug is:
   A. gemcitabine
   B. cyclophosphamide
   C. busulfan
   D. cisplatin

7. Chemotherapy drugs that exert their cytotoxic effects on cells that are in any phase of the cell cycle, even those in the resting, non-dividing phase, are called cell cycle-nonspecific agents. An example of this type of chemotherapy drug is which one of the following?
   A. faslodex
   B. carboplatin
   C. goserelin
   D. paclitaxel

8. Chemotherapy drugs are classified into five different groups based on their mechanism of action. Fluorouracil which is used to treat many types of solid tumors is an example of which one of the following classes of chemotherapy?
   A. Nitrogen mustards
   B. Nitrosoureas
   C. Antimetabolite
   D. Platinum compounds

9. Aromatase inhibitors are a type of:
   A. differentiating agent.
   B. hormonal therapy.
   C. alkylating agent.
   D. immunotherapy.

10. Side effects of hormonal therapy include all of the following except which one of the following?
    A. vaginal discharge
    B. increased libido
    C. weight gain
    D. acne

11. Nurses need to be alert to the potential for hypersensitivity reactions in patients receiving infusions of certain chemotherapy agents. For patients receiving paclitaxel and docetaxel, nurses need to assess for anaphylaxis-type reactions that are known to occur most frequently during which one of the following?
    A. first infusion
    B. third infusion
    C. fifth infusion
    D. seventh infusion

12. Chemotherapy precautions for handling body fluids and soiled linens should remain in effect for what period of time after chemotherapy administration is complete?
    A. 24 hours
    B. 48 hours
    C. 2 weeks
    D. 4 weeks

13. Mesna is an agent that is administered in conjunction with some chemotherapy drugs to protect against which one of the following toxicities?
    A. cardiotoxicity in patients who require more than 300 mg/m$^2$ of doxorubicin
    B. renal toxicity from cisplatin therapy
    C. bladder toxicity from ifosfamide
    D. ototoxicity from carboplatin dosage greater than 60-75 mg/m$^2$

14. Extravasation can cause serious injury to tissues in the arm in which it occurs. Recommendations to avoid the risk of extravasation include which one of the following?
    A. use the biggest vein in the antecubital area
    B. select distal sites before proximal sites
    C. use veins on the dorsal side of the hand
    D. select IV sites that have been in place at least 24 hours

15. Nurses may not administer chemotherapy via the following route:
    A. intravenous
    B. intraperitoneal
    C. subcutaneous
    D. intrapleural

16. Every precaution should be taken to avoid a drug extravasation during chemotherapy administration. If an extravasation of a vinca alkaloid occurs or is suspected, the infusion should be stopped immediately and the area be treated with which one of the following?
    A. cold compress
    B. hyaluronidase
    C. sodium thiosulfate
    D. dexrazoxane

17. Side effects of cisplatin include all of the following except:
    A. rash
    B. peripheral neuropathy
    C. ototoxicity
    D. renal toxicity

18. Which one of the following chemotherapy agents has the ability to cause "wasabi nose"?
    A. Etoposide
    B. Cyclophosphamide
    C. Carboplatin
    D. Doxorubicin

19. The nurse is caring for a patient with colon cancer who is receiving oxaliplatin. Patient education about potential side effects of this drug should focus on providing teaching about which one of the following complications?
    A. Heat sensitivity
    B. Cardiotoxicity
    C. Hypersensitivity reaction with the first dose
    D. Peripheral neuropathy

20. A patient has been diagnosed with HER2-positive breast cancer. Assessment of her cardiac function is essential prior to initiating therapy with which one of the following drugs?
    A. Cisplatin
    B. Trastuzumab
    C. Vincristine
    D. Irinotecan

21. Over time, as a tumor increases in size and volume, changes occur in the cells within the tumor mass. This property is taken into account when planning for the most effective type of anti-tumor therapy. The cellular changes in the cancer cells of an enlarging tumor include which one of the following?
    A. decrease in the number of actively dividing cells
    B. increase in the number of cells undergoing mitosis
    C. decreased cellular heterogeneity
    D. increased cellular growth rate

22. Chemotherapy treatments can be given for different purposes at different points of time over the course of a malignant disease. Ms. M, a 68-year-old woman, has been diagnosed with a 4.5 cm tumor in the left upper quadrant of her left breast. Her surgeon consults with the medical oncologist about the feasibility of reducing the size of the malignant mass so that subsequent breast surgery can be limited to a lumpectomy. The type of chemotherapy treatment that is given prior to surgery to shrink the size of a tumor is called which one of the following?
    A. adjuvant
    B. neoadjuvant
    C. consolidation
    D. concurrent

23. Ms. M. is also scheduled to receive doxorubicin as part of her combination chemotherapy regimen. The nurse is aware that Ms. M. should be assessed for signs of which one of these adverse side effects most likely related to doxorubicin?
    A. cardiotoxicity
    B. hemorrhagic cystitis
    C. ototoxicity
    D. neurotoxicity

24. Hormonal therapy may be used in patients with breast cancers to inhibit the actions of hormones that stimulate malignant cell growth. A class of hormonal agents that is used to prevent estrogen production in the breast and other body tissues, is which one of the following?
    A. adrenocorticoids
    B. aromatase inhibitors (AIs)
    C. selective estrogen receptor modulators (SERMS)
    D. gonadotropin-releasing hormone (GnRH) agonists

25. Hormonal therapy used in the treatment of patients with breast cancer or prostate cancer can lead to side effects that are most likely to include which one of the following?
    A. increased libido
    B. hypoglycemia
    C. weight loss
    D. hot flashes

26. Which one of the following is an advantage of oral administration of antineoplastic agents?
    A. Requires adequate muscle mass and tissue for absorption
    B. Ease of administration and gives patients a sense of control and independence
    C. Provides increased dose to the tumor with decreased systemic side effects
    D. Ease of administration and rapid absorption

27. Which one of the following is a disadvantage of intrapleural administration of antineoplastic agents?
    A. Requires placement of Tenckhoff catheter or intraperitoneal port
    B. Requires lumbar puncture or surgical placement of reservoir or implanted pump
    C. Requires insertion of a thoracotomy tube, and the Nurse Practice Act may not allow the nurse to administer the drug via this method
    D. Requires insertion of indwelling catheter

28. Which one of the following is a nursing implication of subcutaneous or intramuscular administration of antineoplastic agents?
    A. Evaluate the patient's platelet count before administration as needed and use smallest gauge needle as possible
    B. Monitor for signs and symptoms of bleeding or occlusion
    C. Use smallest catheter available and avoid areas of flection, lower extremities, and arms where lymph nodes have been removed
    D. Administer at room temperature, and place patient in semi-Fowler's position

# 29 Biotherapy, Immunotherapy, and Targeted Therapies

1. Before placing a patient on treatment for colon cancer, the oncologist asks about the results of *KRAS* and epidermal growth factor receptor (EGFR) testing. The nurse responds with the understanding that which one of the following is true about testing?
   A. KRAS and EGFR testing is necessary prior to beginning therapy for those most likely to benefit from treatment in some cancer types
   B. KRAS and EGFR testing is an United States Food and Drug Administration (FDA)-approved test used prior to starting targeted treatment for all types of cancers
   C. KRAS and EGFR testing is designed to be paired with a specific drug, but does not have to be FDA approved
   D. KRAS and EGFR testing can only test one biomarker at a time and generally does not improve outcomes

2. H.L. is a 60-year-old patient with cancer. She expresses to her oncology nurse that she is concerned about beginning treatment with Crizotinib, worrying that the drug will not be effective. The oncology nurse explains which one of the following is true about Crizotinib?
   A. "Crizotinib is an oral chemotherapy medication that will directly kill your cancer cells."
   B. "Crizotinib acts to block defective genes that caused your cancer."
   C. "Crizotinib works by replacing the defective genes identified in your cancer with genes that are healthy."
   D. "Crizotinib works quickly and has fewer side effects than chemotherapy."

3. It is important to assess and monitor blood pressure levels in a patient being placed on bevacizumab because which one of the following statements is true about hypertension?
   A. Hypertension will result in seizures
   B. Hypertension can be the first sign of cardiomyopathy
   C. Hypertension is a common problem with this drug that can be managed
   D. Hypertension is most likely to occur in patients without risk factors

4. Targeted therapies work in several ways to stop cancer growth. Which one of the following is a way that targeted therapies work?
   A. deregulating cell signaling pathways
   B. oncogene activation
   C. inhibiting excessive growth factors
   D. blocking apoptosis

5. J.R. is a 60-year-old male patient with cancer who is receiving a treatment of gemtuzumab ozogamicin. Which one of the following statements is true regarding this agent?
   A. Gemtuzumab ozogamicin is a conjugated monoclonal antibody that is chemically linked to a chemotherapy agent
   B. Gemtuzumab ozogamicin is an unconjugated monoclonal antibody that is linked to a radioisotope
   C. Gemtuzumab ozogamicin is a chimeric conjugated monoclonal antibody linked to a chemotherapy agent
   D. Gemtuzumab ozogamicin is a conjugated monoclonal antibody that has several antigens as targets

6. An oncology nurse's patient is being placed on a monoclonal antibody in addition to chemotherapy. The patient is wondering why she needs both types of treatment. The oncology nurse caring for her replies that the monoclonal antibody:
   A. results in immediate cell death while chemotherapy blocks intracellular signaling.
   B. flags cancer cells for destruction by the immune system and chemotherapy initiates the complement cascade.
   C. targets primarily the nucleus of the cancer cell to stop proliferation.
   D. targets a specific protein that is driving the growth of the cancer.

**57**

7. S. J. is a 44-year-old female patient with cancer with a known BRCA mutation. She is being treated with olaparib. The oncology nurse caring for her is teaching her about her disease. As part of her teaching, the nurse most likely explains which one of the following?
   A. Genetically mutated ovarian cancer cells are sensitive to poly-ADP ribose polymerase (PARP) inhibition.
   B. PARP inhibitors repair damaged DNA single-strand breaks.
   C. Cyclin-dependent kinase inhibitors are used in the treatment of estrogen receptor–negative breast cancers.
   D. Proteasome inhibitors are effective in the treatment of BRCA-mutated breast cancer.

8. H. K. is a 57-year-old patient with cancer, who is about to start adjuvant treatment with chemotherapy, pertuzumab, and trastuzumab. His baseline blood pressure is 140/88. Which one of the following test results would be of concern and should be investigated prior to him starting treatment?
   A. Liver enzymes indicate an aspartate transaminase of 35 µ/L and alanine aminotransferase of 40 µ/L.
   B. A left ventricular ejection fraction (LVEF) of 45%.
   C. Hemoglobin A1c (HbA1c) is 5.0%.
   D. Creatinine clearance is 100 mL/min.

9. An oncology nurse is caring for a patient with cancer who is about to start treatment with rituximab. Which one of the following medical diagnoses would be a concern?
   A. Hypertension
   B. Type 2 diabetes
   C. Hepatitis B
   D. Basal cell carcinomas

10. G.K. is a 50-year-old female patient who will be started on an EGFR Inhibitor for treatment of her cancer. Which one of the following statements indicates that the patient understands the oncology nurse's education regarding rash?
    A. "If I do develop an acne-like condition, I know that it is OK to use an over-the-counter product containing benzoyl peroxide."
    B. "I should apply a moisturizer once a day after taking a hot shower."
    C. "If I develop a rash, that means that the drug is working effectively."
    D. "I need to avoid sun exposure as much as possible and use sunscreens that contain zinc oxide."

11. J. L. is a 61-year-old male patient with cancer who is on treatment with bevacizumab. It is most important for the nurse to do which one of the following?
    A. monitor for signs and symptoms of hypertension
    B. schedule treatment 1 week after surgery
    C. ensure that the patient takes one tablet daily with water
    D. take medication on an empty stomach

12. L.T. is a 48-year-old male patient being treated with an EGFR inhibitor who comes into the clinic complaining of diarrhea. He reports having six unformed, watery stools per day. Infection has been ruled out through testing. Which one of the following is an appropriate intervention for management of the patient's diarrhea?
    A. Administer loperamide and instruct the patient on a high-fat, high-fiber diet.
    B. Administer loperamide to the patient and monitor the patient for signs and symptoms of dehydration.
    C. Instruct the patient to take probiotics and modify his diet by increasing fiber and fats.
    D. Instruct the patient to increase hypotonic fluids to at least 1 liter per day and report any fever.

13. A patient is receiving everolimus. An appropriate pharmacologic intervention would include which one of the following?
    A. a steroid-based mouthwash to reduce the incidence and severity of stomatitis
    B. an oral hypoglycemic agent to prevent hyperglycemia
    C. prophylactic loperamide to prevent diarrhea
    D. prophylaxis with trimethoprim-sulfamethoxazole to prevent pneumocystis pneumonia

14. Immunotherapy offers the ability for potential effectiveness after treatment has ended. This may best be explained by which one of the following statements?
    A. the use of antibodies to direct activity against tumors
    B. the ability of the immune system to distinguish between healthy tissue and tumor
    C. the immune system's unique memory abilities
    D. immune-mediated cytotoxicity against cancer cells

15. D.W. is a 48-year-old male patient with cancer who will be starting treatment with a checkpoint inhibitor. His oncology nurse explains that this type of treatment works by:
    A. blocking links between proteins and receptors that cancer cells use to turn off the immune system.
    B. tagging a protein produced by the tumor to allow the immune system to recognize the protein and destroy it, leading to tumor cell death.
    C. using viruses to directly infect tumor cells.
    D. binding with antibodies to directly attack tumors.

16. Adverse events (AEs) with immunotherapy differ from those associated with cytotoxic therapy in that AEs associated with immunotherapy are which one of the following?
    A. AEs associated with immunotherapy are predictable and limited in duration.
    B. AEs associated with immunotherapy are unpredictable and prolonged.
    C. AEs associated with immunotherapy are treated with supportive care measures that target the AE.
    D. AEs associated with immunotherapy are prolonged in duration and "off-target."

17. S. K. is a 52-year-old female patient who has received chimeric antigen receptor T-cell (CAR-T) cell therapy 5 days ago. She now presents with a fever of 104°F, and complains of fatigue and headache. Her heart rate is 90 beats/min and blood pressure is 100/60 mmHg. The oncology nurse caring for her suspects that she has which one of the following?
    A. capillary leak syndrome
    B. pseudoprogression
    C. central nervous system metastases
    D. cytokine release syndrome

18. An oncology nurse is caring for a patient who is experiencing Grade 2 pneumonitis from treatment with a checkpoint inhibitor. The oncology nurse anticipates that the healthcare provider will order which one of the following?
    A. hold the checkpoint inhibitor therapy and initiate corticosteroids
    B. keep the patient on the checkpoint inhibitor and initiate corticosteroids
    C. permanently discontinue the checkpoint inhibitor
    D. initiate empiric antibiotics keep the patient on the checkpoint inhibitor

19. A patient with cancer who is receiving a programmed death-1 (PD-1) therapy tells her oncology nurse that she is experiencing some fatigue and flu-like symptoms. The oncology nurse recommends that the patient do which one of the following?
    A. Go to Urgent Care if her symptoms become worse.
    B. Report this symptom to her primary care physician at her upcoming appointment.
    C. Document her symptoms and only seek medical attention if a fever develops.
    D. Report this symptom to the healthcare team who prescribed the PD-1 treatment.

20. Patients who have received immunotherapy should alert all of their healthcare providers because of which one of the following?
    A. each provider should be aware of the potential for immune-related adverse events
    B. most providers know how to manage long-term effects of immunotherapy
    C. adverse events generally occur while patients are receiving immunotherapy
    D. most adverse events are short-term and require management by a multidisciplinary team

21. S.E. is a 47-year-old female patient with metastatic ovarian cancer. She has had genetic testing done due to an extensive family history of breast and ovarian cancer and is found to have a mutation in the BRCA1 gene. The genetic testing results may also influence treatment decisions. Her treatment might include which one of the following?
    A. Olaparib or Rucaprib
    B. Niraparib or Ceritinib
    C. Erlotinib or Olaparib
    D. Alectinib or Ceritinib

22. Which one of the following statements is true about monoclonal antibodies?
    A. Monoclonal antibodies are intracellular enzymes that control DNA repair and cellular apoptosis
    B. Monoclonal antibodies bind to only one specific target substance with exceptional specificity
    C. Monoclonal antibodies are circulating growth factors in serum that stimulate growth
    D. Monoclonal antibodies block the binding site the intracellular portion of a receptor

23. Companion tests are ordered to do which one of the following?
    A. evaluate for germline genetic mutations
    B. evaluate for somatic genetic mutations
    C. determine the appropriate dose of a targeted therapy
    D. determine the stage of the tumor

24. An oncology patient is receiving a targeted therapy that ends with the suffix –**ximab**. This suffix refers to which one of the following?
    A. a monoclonal antibody that is fully human
    B. a monoclonal antibody that is mouse (murine)
    C. a monoclonal antibody that is chimeric human
    D. a monoclonal antibody that is humanized mouse

25. Infusion reactions most commonly occur with which one of the following?
    A. EGFR targeted therapies
    B. anti-VEGFR therapies
    C. mTOR therapies
    D. monoclonal antibody therapies

59

# 30 Support Therapies and Access Devices

1. A patient with acute leukemia had a previous febrile reaction to platelets and is scheduled for another platelet transfusion. Which one of the following platelet products should be used?
   A. Human leukocyte antigen (HLA) -matched platelets
   B. single-donor platelets
   C. pooled platelets
   D. leukocyte-reduced platelets

2. W. K. is a 46-year-old female patient with colon cancer who is undergoing surgical resection of her mass and may need red blood cells (RBCs) during her surgery. Which one of the following is the method of RBC collection to ensure that the correct component will be available?
   A. Whole blood
   B. Homologous blood
   C. Autologous blood
   D. Directly donated blood

3. After a transfusion of platelets, the patient should expect correction of which one of the following conditions?
   A. anemia
   B. thrombocytopenia
   C. hypogammaglobulinemia
   D. clotting factors

4. A nurse began an RBC transfusion and, during the follow-up assessment, the nurse notes that the patient has a temperature of 102°F degrees, taken orally, along with chills and is complaining of nausea. Which type of reaction is this patient exhibiting?
   A. Febrile nonhemolytic reaction
   B. Hemolytic reaction
   C. Transfusion-related acute lung injury (TRALI)
   D. Iron overload

5. S. L. is a 65-year-old male patient with lung cancer who is undergoing chemotherapy. He presents to the clinic for lab work, 10 days after treatment. A Complete Blood Count reveals his absolute neutrophil count to be 1000/mm$^3$, hemoglobin 6.8g/dl, and platelets 30,000/mm$^3$. Which one of the following blood products will be ordered for this patient?
   A. Platelets
   B. Neutrophils
   C. RBCs
   D. Immunoglobulin

6. G. R. is a 49-year-old female patient who presents to the clinic with a report that, during her last platelet transfusion, the patient exhibited a mild case of hives with itching. Which one of the following premedication choices will be ordered prior to future platelet transfusions?
   A. Diphenhydramine
   B. Meperidine
   C. Hydrocortisone
   D. Diuretic

7. To decrease the incidence and severity of a transfusion reaction, which one of the following is the best nursing intervention to follow?
   A. Use of normal saline as a diluent during the transfusion
   B. Use the maximum number of units according to the lab value
   C. Attach an appropriate filter to the blood product
   D. Monitor patients for 4 hours after transfusion

8. A husband is asking which blood product is the safest should his wife require a blood product for an upcoming elective surgery. The nurse caring for his wife explains that blood received from an autologous donor is the safest and also is which one of the following?
   A. HLA matched
   B. Collected during a blood drive
   C. Collected from the intended recipient
   D. Directly donated blood

9. V. K. is a 59-year-old female patient who presents to the clinic seven days after receiving a chemotherapy treatment, and states that her gums have been bleeding. Complete blood count reveals a platelet count of 38,000/mm$^3$ and hemoglobin of 8.5 g/dL. Which one of the following blood component therapies would the nurse anticipate being ordered for this patient?
   A. Red blood cells
   B. Plasma
   C. No blood product
   D. Platelets

10. Which one of the following techniques can be used to minimize blood loss in a patient who refuses blood component therapy while undergoing cancer treatment?
    A. Routinely check complete blood counts
    B. Administer iron and vitamin supplementation
    C. Use of histamine-2 antagonist
    D. Use of regular blood collection tubes

11. A patient receiving red blood cells begins to demonstrate uncontrolled shaking chills, shortness of breath, and wheezing. Which one of the following would be the appropriate initial intervention?
    A. Notify the provider and blood bank of potential reaction
    B. Administer diphenhydramine intravenously
    C. Administer meperidine intravenously
    D. Stop the infusion immediately and start intravenous normal saline

12. A nurse is teaching her patient and the patient's family about a peripherally inserted central catheter (PICC). The nurse knows the patient needs more teaching when the patient describes the PICC as:
    A. inserted into a central vein.
    B. available in single, double, or triple lumens.
    C. inserted at the antecubital fossa.
    D. inserted for 6 months and removed.

13. J. D. is a 62-year-old male patient who returns from surgery after a tunneled venous catheter has been inserted. The nurse caring for him can begin chemotherapy treatments when which one of the following is performed?
    A. computed tomography CT scan
    B. clood return on aspiration
    C. chest x-ray
    D. fluids infuse without difficulty

14. Bundled care is incorporated upon insertion of venous catheters to decrease risk of which one of the following?
    A. bleeding
    B. infection
    C. catheter dislodgement
    D. catheter migration

15. A patient presents to clinic for chemotherapy infusion and the nurse caring for the patient accesses the implantable port and attempts to flush. The port flushes easily, however, a blood return is unobtainable. Which one of the following is the most common cause for no blood return?
    A. Precipitation
    B. Deep vein thrombosis
    C. Fibrin sheath
    D. Intraluminal blood clot

16. T. S. is a 57-year-old male patient who will be discharged from the hospital to receive intravenous antibiotics at home for the next 10 days. Which of the following pumps is not equipped with audible alarms?
    A. Peristaltic
    B. Syringe
    C. Smart pump
    D. Elastomeric

17. A patient has been diagnosed with leptomeningeal disease requiring frequent administration of chemotherapy into the cerebral spinal fluid. Which one of the following devices would be implanted?
    A. Intraventricular catheter
    B. Peritoneal catheter
    C. Epidural long-term catheter
    D. Intrapleural catheter

18. Which one of the following is an example of an intervention of the prevention of a mechanical complication of an access device?
    A. Maintain flushing routine, flush with pulsatile (push-pause) method to cause swirling action in device
    B. Change intrathoracic pressures: have the patient inhale fully and hold breath or exhale fully and hold breath
    C. Surgical removal, as indicated, to avoid fracture
    D. Remove needle, and re-access port using a non-coring needle

19. Which one of the following is an example of a restoration of a problem for a mechanical complication of an access device?
    A. Monitor the length of the catheter (tunnel, midline, PICC) to ensure placement is intact
    B. Refer to the physician for repositioning the catheter using a fluoroscopy
    C. Avoid placing the port at the sites of actual or potential tissue damage (in radiation field)
    D. High-pressure infusions or flushing with 1- or 3-mL

20. Which one of the following is a characteristic of a short-term or intermediate-term peripheral catheter?
    A. Insertion is done centrally into the jugular vein, subclavian vein, superior vena cava (SVC), or inferior vena cava
    B. Available with a pressure-activated safety valve (PASV) located in the catheter hub and designed to permit fluid infusion and decrease risk of blood reflux
    C. Catheter tip must be confirmed before initial use by ultrasound (during placement if used), fluoroscopy, or chest x-ray
    D. Infuses fluids, medications, blood products, and peripheral total parenteral nutrition (TPN) and to obtain blood specimens

21. In addition to febrile complications of BCT, an oncology nurse monitors the recipient's response for which one of the following?
    A. Allergic reactions, hypothermia, and hemolytic reactions
    B. Fluid volume overload and deep vein thrombosis (DVT) caused by the platelet increase
    C. DVT and other coagulation problems
    D. Bone marrow reaction to the unrelated presence of unrelated stem cells

**61**

22. The nurse is preparing a BCT infusion. She knows that which one of the following guidelines maximizes patient safety?
   A. Using a gravity-flow infusion line
   B. Adding medications slowly through the Y-port
   C. Using the smallest gauge intravenous (IV) catheter available
   D. Together with a second registered nurse, checking BCT product with the patient's ID

23. An oncology nurse is evaluating the potential for a patient with cancer to receive an implanted venous access device. Which one of the following best supports the decision for the patient to have this type of device?
   A. The patient demonstrates the ability to care for the device
   B. The patient needs chemotherapy infusions and blood samples
   C. The patient expresses concerns about implantation of the device
   D. The patient and the patient's family are reluctant to care for an external device

24. K. R. is a 60-year-old male who is being discharged from the ambulatory infusion center with an infusion system for continuous chemotherapy infusion. Which one of the following would indicate that the patient and his family are adequately prepared for use of the infusion system?
   A. If they acknowledge understanding of how to flush the line with sterile water every 12 hours
   B. If they acknowledge understanding of how to monitor the infusion system for proper functioning
   C. If they acknowledge understanding of how to attach a second line to the infusion system for pain control
   D. If they acknowledge understanding of how to change the dose of the drug whenever the patient is sleeping

# 31 Medication Management

1. A patient who received chemotherapy 7 days ago presents to the emergency department (ED) with a fever of 102°F and chills. His absolute neutrophil count is 500 cells/μL. His spouse asks the nurse why he is being admitted to the hospital since he "doesn't look that sick". The nurse explains that which one of the following is true?
   A. The patient's fever might be an early sign of infection.
   B. The patient is dehydrated and requires IV hydration.
   C. The patient needs a platelet transfusion.
   D. Fever might be a sign of an allergic drug reaction.

2. Which one of the following antimicrobial agents is appropriate for the treatment of cytomegalovirus (CMV)?
   A. Ganciclovir
   B. Levofloxacin
   C. Acyclovir
   D. Fluconazole

3. Patients who are considered high risk for febrile neutropenia should avoid which one of the following medications?
   A. Antipyretics
   B. Antibiotics
   C. Antivirals
   D. Antifungals

4. Which one of the following statements regarding vancomycin as an empiric therapy is true?
   A. Dose adjustments per pharmacy are not required prior to initiation.
   B. Vancomycin provides appropriate empiric coverage of gram-negative bacteria.
   C. Empiric vancomycin is recommended for low-risk patients.
   D. Routine use of empiric vancomycin should be avoided.

5. Adverse reactions associated with amphotericin B (deoxycholate) include which one of the following?
   A. nephrotoxicity and electrolyte wasting.
   B. myelosuppression and central nervous system (CNS) toxicity.
   C. ocular toxicity and prolonged QTc.
   D. serotonin syndrome and ototoxicity.

6. A patient with cancer complains of burning on urination. Microbiology results show the urinalysis with leuko-esterase, white blood cell (WBC) and nitrate positivity, and it is positive for *Escherichia coli*. Which one of the following nursing actions would be indicated?
   A. Encourage patient to drink fluids in order to prevent antibiotic use.
   B. Ensure the patient has an order for prophylactic antibiotics upon discharge to prevent future urinary tract infections (UTIs).
   C. Report culture results to provider and anticipate orders for antibiotics.
   D. No further action is needed.

7. G. T. is a 58-year-old male who is in the clinic receiving chemotherapy for lung cancer and is inquiring about whether he can receive the flu vaccine before he leaves clinic today. The nurse caring for him responds to him with which one of the following?
   A. influenza vaccines contain live virus and should be avoided.
   B. the influenza vaccine can be administered between chemotherapy cycles.
   C. receiving the influenza vaccine may increase the risk for infection.
   D. the vaccination schedule is dependent on his CD34 counts.

8. Anti-inflammatory agents are effective in treating pain and inflammation because they do which one of the following?
   A. block major nerve pathways and conduction.
   B. inhibit cyclooxygenase and prostaglandin production.
   C. decrease platelet function and bleeding risk.
   D. lower temperature threshold and signs of infection.

9. A patient has returned to clinic for a follow up appointment and reports that she has been taking an over-the-counter NSAID for the mild bone pain she has been experiencing. Which other reported medication should prompt the nurse to notify the medical team?
   A. Metoprolol
   B. Clopidogrel
   C. Multivitamin
   D. Ciprofloxacin

10. A patient is prescribed corticosteroids for the treatment of multiple myeloma. The nurse caring for the patient knows to monitor for which one of the following?
    A. Signs of bleeding
    B. Renal and hepatic failure
    C. Nausea and vomiting
    D. Muscle weakness

11. Ondansetron and granisetron disrupt signaling pathways by targeting which neurotransmitter?
    A. Serotonin
    B. Dopamine
    C. Histamine
    D. Neurokinin

12. During a follow-up visit, a patient reports that she is experiencing breakthrough chemotherapy-induced nausea and vomiting despite receiving palonosetron 0.25 mg PO prior to her chemotherapy infusion. The nurse should anticipate administering which one of the following antiemetics?
    A. Ondansteron 8 mg IV
    B. Dexamethasone 12 mg IV
    C. Granisetron 2 mg PO
    D. Repeat dose of palonosetron

13. Metoclopramide has a black box warning for which adverse reaction?
    A. Drug-drug interactions
    B. Prolongation of QT interval
    C. Extrapyramidal symptoms
    D. Orthostatic hypotension

14. The nurse understands which one of the following is an essential principle of analgesic medication management?
    A. For chronic pain, patients should have long-acting and breakthrough options available.
    B. Patients with acute pain should avoid opioids to prevent physical dependence.
    C. Opioid tolerance means the patient has developed a psychological addiction to the drug.
    D. Stool softeners should only be administered once the patient reports changes in bowel movements.

15. S. L. is a 48-year-old male patient who arrives to the clinic with complaints of nausea, sweating, and insomnia. During the medication reconciliation, he states that he recently stopped taking his prescribed morphine sulfate. The nurse suspects he is experiencing which one of the following?
    A. poor pain control
    B. constipation
    C. addiction
    D. withdrawal

16. Which one of the following medications would be appropriate for a patient experiencing somnolence from opioid use?
    A. Methyphenidate
    B. Metoclopramide
    C. Micafungin
    D. Mithramycin

17. A patient with cancer has just been prescribed oral oxycodone. The nurse caring for the patient knows that teaching for the patient will include which one of the following?
    A. avoid grapefruit juice.
    B. take medication with food.
    C. take medication on an empty stomach.
    D. medication should be taken in combination with acetaminophen.

18. Anxiolytics can be used as supportive treatment for patients with cancer to do which one of the following?
    A. prevent or manage anticipatory nausea.
    B. replace the need for narcotic pain control.
    C. prevent opportunistic infection.
    D. treat clinical depression.

19. A patient has just been prescribed Lexapro 10 mg to manage depression. Which one of the following statements would most likely indicate that the patient needs additional teaching?
   A. "I should take this medication with food."
   B. "If I experience any side effects, I will discontinue and follow up at my next appointment."
   C. "I will carry a bottle of water with me to help relieve dry mouth."
   D. "My mood should be better by the end of the week."

20. Which one of the following medications is an appropriate option for managing sleeping disorders?
   A. Linezolid
   B. Posaconazole
   C. Zolpidem
   D. Temozolomide

21. A cancer patient who has been diagnosed with a major depressive disorder has recently been prescribed an antidepressant. Which one of the following is the most important question to ask during the patient's follow up appointment?
   A. "Is your pain being well controlled?"
   B. "Are you having any thoughts of harming yourself?"
   C. "How would you describe your sleep pattern over the last few nights?"
   D. "Did you drive yourself to clinic today?"

22. Which one of the following antidepressants is associated with a higher risk of anticholinergic effects (blurred vision, dry mouth, and constipation)?
   A. Fluoxetine
   B. Sertraline
   C. Citalopram
   D. Amitriptyline

23. Which one of the following chemotherapy drugs has the potential to lower the seizure threshold?
   A. Cytarabine
   B. Melphalan
   C. Carmustine
   D. Mitoxantrone

24. Levetiracetam is associated with which one of the following side effects?
   A. Somnolence
   B. Hepatotoxicity
   C. Nausea
   D. Hallucinations

25. Anticonvulsants have the potential to change drug metabolism and drug-drug interactions through which mechanism of action? because they are categorized as which one of the following types of enzymes?
   A. Inducers
   B. Substrates
   C. Inhibitors
   D. Receptors

26. T.W.is a 60-year-old male patient who has received an autologous stem cell transplant 5 days ago and has an order for filgrastim. The nurse caring for him understands this medication is used to do which one of the following?
   A. Filgrastim is used to prevent veno-occlusive disease.
   B. Filgrastim is used to support neutrophil engraftment.
   C. Filgrastim is used to reduce the need for red blood cell transfusions.
   D. Filgrastim is used to prevent delayed nausea and vomiting.

27. Myeloid growth factors are used to stimulate production of which one of the following?
   A. neutrophils and macrophages
   B. natural killer cells
   C. B lymphocytes
   D. plasma cells

28. Erythropoietin can increase the risk of which adverse event?
   A. Bone pain
   B. Deep vein thrombosis
   C. Splenic rupture
   D. Peripheral neuropathy

29. In the neutropenic patient with cancer, which one of the following surgeries may impact the treatment of active infections?
   A. Lobectomy
   B. Appendectomy
   C. Splenectomy
   D. Cholecystectomy

30. S. R. is a 62-year-old male patient with cancer is experiencing anxiety. The nurse caring for him relays the patient assessment to the physician who orders a serotonin selective reuptake inhibitors (SSRI) to begin while the patient remains hospitalized. The nurse would understand that SSRI do which one of the following?
    A. relieves anxiety symptoms early in therapy
    B. have an optimal effect when starting at the maximum dose and then taper down and then decreased to optimal dose for each unique patient
    C. effect will be seen in first seven days
    D. abrupt discontinuation may precipitate withdrawal syndrome

31. A patient with cancer is diagnosed with major depressive disorder which is characterized by which one of the following?
    A. sad, empty and irritable mood occurring late in the day.
    B. higher use of healthcare services.
    C. occurs in about 75% of patients with cancer.
    D. depressive symptoms occur daily for at least 5 days.

32. Which one of the following types of antidepressants would the patient with cancer be counseled to make dietary modifications to avoid tyramine?
    A. Serotonin selective reuptake inhibitors (SSRIs)
    B. Serotonin and norepinephrine reuptake inhibitors (SNRIs)
    C. Tricyclic antidepressants (TCA)
    D. Monoamine oxidase inhibitors (MAOIs)

33. S. R. is the 62-year-old male patient with cancer who was diagnosed with depression. He was recently started on an antidepressant. If improvement in symptoms occur, which one of the following is true about the therapy?
    A. The therapy should be continued for six months.
    B. The therapy should be continued for six weeks.
    C. The therapy should be discontinued.
    D. The patient should begin gradual tapering until off medication.

34. When applying the principles of medical management with myeloid growth factors (MGFs), the risk of neutropenia is increased in which one of the following patient populations?
    A. patients with endocrine dysfunction
    B. patients with recent surgery or open wounds
    C. pediatric patients
    D. patients with pulmonary hypertension

35. When evaluating the patient with cancer's iron stores prior to use of erythropoiesis-stimulating agents (ESA) or erythropoetin (EPO), such as epoetin alfa, epoetin alfa-epbx, and darbpoetin, the oncology nurse should consider which one of the following statements?
    A. patients who are iron-deficient will respond best to EPO.
    B. this medication is warranted in patients with hemoglobin greater than 16 g/dL.
    C. the increased risk of venous thromboembolism.
    D. the increased number of RBC transfusions to treat anemia.

36. When performing the medication reconciliation for the neutropenic patient, the oncology nurse would expect the cell nadir to occur during which one of the following?
    A. The cell nadir would occur the day after the last chemotherapy dose.
    B. The cell nadir would occur at the beginning of the third chemotherapy cycle.
    C. The cell nadir would occur when the absolute neutrophil count is greater than 500/mm$^3$.
    D. The cell nadir would occur in 7-14 days after chemotherapy treatment.

37. The potential for "Disturbed Body Image" would be important for the oncology nurse to assess and document with which one of the following drug classification?
    A. Corticosteroids
    B. NSAIDS: Cox-2 selective agent
    C. Salicylates
    D. Aminoglycosides

38. When requesting a prescription from the provider for Morphine to control pain, the oncology nurse should consider which one of the following?
    A. Morphine 30 mg IV has equivalent potency as Morphine 10 mg oral
    B. Onset of effect for oral Morphine is 30 minutes
    C. Peak effect is 60 minutes with Morphine IV
    D. Morphine IV and oral have a duration of effect of 4-8 hours

39. Temperature threshold for neutropenic patients is defined as which one of the following?
    A. Multiple axillary temperatures over 37.5°C (99.5°F)
    B. Two consecutive rectal temps over 36.8°C (98.2°F)
    C. Single oral temperature of 38.3°C (101°F)
    D. Sustained temperature of 38°C (100.4°F) over three hours.

40. A patient with lymphoma, who is currently receiving chemotherapy, presents to the urgent clinic complaining of fever and aching for past 36 hours. The patient has a central line with no redness, tenderness or edema at the insertion site. Skin is warm and intact. The patient is tolerating oral fluids without nausea or vomiting. The physician orders blood cultures. When obtaining the blood cultures, the gold standard for diagnosis is to draw which one of the following?
    A. two peripheral cultures
    B. two central line cultures
    C. no cultures until 48 hours for duration of symptoms
    D. one peripheral and one from the central line

41. In a low-risk patient with febrile neutropenia, the provider may prescribe viral prophylaxis in patients with which one of the following prior conditions?
    A. herpes simplex virus (HSV)
    B. human immunodeficiency virus (HIV)
    C. pseudomonas
    D. respiratory syncytial virus (RSV)

42. During which one of the following time frames would the nurse anticipate discontinuation of antimicrobial therapy for the resolution of a fever in a low risk patient that is clinically stable with negative cultures but with an ANC remaining less than 500?
    A. after a total of 14 days
    B. after a total of 5 to 7 days
    C. after a total of 17 to 21 days
    D. after the ANC is above 500 for 7 consecutive days

43. Stevens-Johnson syndrome is an adverse effect of antimicrobial therapy impacting which one of the following areas?
    A. hepatic
    B. cardiovascular
    C. gastrointestinal
    D. dermatologic

44. A patient who is on a chemotherapy regimen is requesting the measles, mumps, and rubella (MMR) vaccine since her grandchildren have been exposed to measles in school. If the provider warrants this as necessary, the vaccine should be administered:
    A. more than 2 weeks prior to chemotherapy.
    B. one month after the chemotherapy regimen completed.
    C. greater that 4 weeks prior to chemotherapy.
    D. at the next chemotherapy appointment since it is not a live virus.

45. Which one of the following may be used as a means of timing vaccine administration in a patient that is post-transplant?
    A. human leukocyte antigen-DR
    B. CD34
    C. vascular endothelial growth factor receptor (VEGFR)
    D. complete blood count (CBC)

46. F. L. is a 75-year-old patient who presents in the cancer center with a history of renal insufficiency and cardiovascular disease and is complaining of musculoskeletal pain. The medication list also reveals the patient is prescribed coumadin. When prescribing a medication for the patient's pain, which one of the following would put the patient be at high risk for toxicity?
    A. NSAIDs
    B. anti-convulsants
    C. acetaminophen
    D. corticosteroids

47. Which one of the following describes the use of Cannabis for chemotherapy-induced nausea and vomiting?
    A. Cannabis is used as an agent for highly emetogenic intravenous chemotherapy.
    B. Cannabis is legal in every state for medical use only with chemotherapy.
    C. Cannabis is not prescribed due to prolonged, irreversible side effects.
    D. Cannabis is used as an agent for breakthrough nausea and vomiting.

48. Fat-to lean body ratio is important to assess when prescribing pain medication by which one of the following routes?
    A. buccal
    B. transdermal
    C. subcutaneous
    D. rectal

49. G. H. is a 50-year-old male patient with cancer who has just been diagnosed as having a *Candida* infection. Which one of the following medications does his oncology nurse expect the primary practitioner to order?
    A. Amphotericin B or fluconazole (Diflucan)
    B. Caspofungin (Cancidas) or ciprofloxacin (Cipro)
    C. Voriconazole (Vfend) or fluconazole (Diflucan)

50. Administration for the management of acyclovir include which one of the following?
   A. Dosing should be based on the patient's actual body weight to ensure adequate blood levels.
   B. It is an effective preemptive therapy for cytomegalo-virus (CMV) in high-risk patients with cancer.
   C. Probenecid is given to patients to prevent renal reabsorption and related toxicities.
   D. Fluid hydration is necessary if therapeutic IV doses are used.

51. Antiemetics that belong to the same class as Zofran affect nausea and vomiting by acting as which one of the following?
   A. 5 HT3 agonists
   B. D2 antagonists
   C. NK-1 antagonists
   D. 5 HT3 antagonists

52. Which one of the following statements places antiemetics with the appropriate neurotransmitter agent?
   A. Serotonin – aprepitant
   B. Cannabinoid agonist – dronabinol
   C. Histamine H1 antagonist – prochlorperazine
   D. Dopamine D2 antagonist – promethazine

53. Which one of the following is true related to the onset of action for fentanyl?
   A. IV 2 to 3 minutes
   B. IV 5 to 6 minutes
   C. Patch 8 to 10 hours
   D. Buccal 15 to 30 minutes

54. Which one of the following is a common side effect of concern for patients receiving serotonin reuptake inhibitors?
   A. Hot flashes
   B. Neuropathy
   C. Sexual dysfunction
   D. Increased appetite

55. A common side effect of filgrastim (G-CSF) is which one of the following?
   A. sedation
   B. liver dysfunction
   C. constipation
   D. bone pain

# 32 Complimentary and Alternative Modalities

1. Which one of the following classes describes the entire domain of therapies that are independent of conventional medicine?
   A. Integrative
   B. Complementary and alternative
   C. Allopathic
   D. Mind body

2. The two broad subgroups of complementary health approaches defined by National Center for Complementary and Integrative Health (NCCIH) are which one of the following?
   A. massage and acupuncture.
   B. Tai chi and healing touch.
   C. chiropractic and osteopathic manipulation.
   D. natural products and mind and body practices.

3. When an oncology nurse is discussing safety and risks with a patient, which of the following factors is true regarding herbal and botanical medicine?
   A. United States Food and Drug Administration (FDA) approved
   B. Tightly regulated in the United States
   C. Efficacy ensured
   D. Interacts with prescribed medication

4. Art and music therapy are modalities labeled as which one of the following?
   A. mind body
   B. whole medicine
   C. biologically based
   D. manipulative

5. Which one of the following is an appropriate response by the oncology nurse when assessing the patient's use of complementary and alternative medicine at the patient's initial appointment?
   A. "We only need to know the medicines prescribed by your primary physician for your medical record."
   B. "Complementary therapy will be assessed at the end of your treatment visit."
   C. "If there are cultural or religious practices that you incorporate for your health, it should be noted for your oncology team."
   D. "Biologically based therapies are not part of your cancer care so they do not need be addressed at this time."

6. Which one of the following chemotherapy agents is commonly impacted by natural products and would warrant a review of the patient's medication and complementary and alternative medicine (CAM) list in their electronic medical record (EMR) to ensure safety?
   A. Adriamycin
   B. Docetaxel
   C. Lupron
   D. Bleomycin

7. Massage therapy is therapeutic to decrease emotional and physical tension, and is appropriate if which one of the following conditions is met?
   A. platelets <50,000.
   B. applied directly at the bone metastatic site.
   C. peripheral neuropathy grade 3 or less.
   D. white blood cell (WBC) count is <1500.

8. Which one of the following descriptions defines the mind-body modality of neurolinguistic programming (NLP)?
   A. This modality has a meditative component that brings harmony to body, mind, and spirit.
   B. With this modality, the patient focuses on positive aspects of his or her life to promote a positive outlook over time.
   C. Practices within this modality share characteristics and often involve focused breathing and a relaxed yet alert state that promotes control over thoughts and feelings.
   D. This is a modality with a structured process that uses live or recorded readings describing different scenarios or detailed images to guide the patient through a certain process.

9. Which one of the following descriptions defines the mind-body modality of guided imagery?
   A. A technique within this modality trains patients to develop awareness of experiences moment by moment and in the context of all senses.
   B. Enhances coordination and balance and promotes physical, emotional, and spiritual well-being.
   C. May lead the patient through progressive muscle relaxation or visualization of a treatment process (e.g., visualization of chemotherapy entering the body and seeking out cancer cells to remove them from the body).
   D. A psychotherapy technique based on the concept that distressing events are associated with specific rapid eye movements.

**69**

10. Which one of the following descriptions defines the manipulative and body-based practice of acupressure?
    A. the use of vigorous massage to stimulate flow of lymphatic fluid.
    B. the use of manual pressure and strokes on muscle tissue.
    C. an ancient Oriental technique associated with traditional Chinese medicine (TCM), used to restore or promote health and well-being using fine-gauge needles inserted into specific points on the body to stimulate or disperse the flow of energy.
    D. the use of finger or hand pressure over specific points on the body to relieve symptoms or to influence specific organ function.

11. Which one of the following is a safety issue when using aromatherapy?
    A. Standardization is lacking in the preparation and clinical use of essential oils.
    B. Use of aromatherapy can trigger depression, and these agents can target psychological well-being.
    C. Agents have a narrow range of safe applicability.
    D. Patients frequently develop an allergy to the transporter.

12. The term Feldenkrais refers to which one of the following?
    A. Gentle manipulation of the skull to reestablish natural configuration and movement.
    B. The use of vigorous massage to stimulate the flow of lymphatic fluid out of an area of the body.
    C. A somatic education system that teaches movement and gentle manipulation to increase body awareness and function.
    D. A technique that uses movement and touch to restore balance to the body.

13. Which one of the following terms defines reiki?
    A. A technique for balancing the flow of energy in the body through the transfer of human energy.
    B. An energy healing technique that uses nursing process and specific protocols.
    C. The use of magnetic fields to positively impact the body to stimulate healing.
    D. An energy healing modality in which the practitioner directs the flow of energy to various parts of the body to facilitate healing and relaxation.

14. Acupuncture is often successful in alleviating pain because of which one of the following?
    A. Acupuncture is often successful in alleviating pain because of the placebo effect in which patients expect pain relief and, therefore, feel less pain.
    B. Acupuncture is often successful in alleviating pain because the introduction of pain at the insertion site allows the patient to refocus his or her perception of the original site of pain.
    C. Acupuncture is often successful in alleviating pain because the stimulation of the nerve fibers entering the dorsal horn of the spinal cord, which mediates the impulses of the other parts of the body, and allows the patient to experience less at pain at the original site.
    D. Acupuncture is often successful in alleviating pain because the pressure applied by exerting a finger and thumb on the specific point on the surface of the skin acts as an entrance and an exit for an internal healing force, thereby eliminating the overall sensation of pain.

# 33 Cardiovascular Symptoms

1. Which one of the following is a treatment related risk factor for lymphedema?
   A. Lowered body mass index (BMI)
   B. Tumor invasion
   C. Prolonged immobilization
   D. Lymph node dissection

2. Which one of the following interventions would be an urgent priority for medical management of lymphedema?
   A. Treatment of suspected infection
   B. Weight management
   C. Exercise program
   D. Axillary reverse mapping (ARM)

3. When caring for the patient with lymphedema, the nurse would expect to see which one of the following interventions in the plan of care?
   A. Restrict exercise
   B. Dangle extremities
   C. Apply extreme heat
   D. Complete decongestive therapy

4. H. K. is a 50-year-old female with breast cancer, who has been suffering from lymphedema. When the oncology nurse in her care is educating the patient about lymphedema management at home, which one of the following is an appropriate point for her to convey?
   A. Wear tight fitting clothes
   B. Consume diet high in sodium and low in fiber
   C. Maintain healthy weight
   D. Follow-up with health care team for 1 month

5. Movement of fluid from the vascular space into the interstitial space causing edema would occur by which one of the following?
   A. decreased capillary pressure.
   B. increased capillary permeability.
   C. increased plasma oncotic pressure.
   D. lowered hydrostatic pressure.

6. B. L is a 62-year-old patient who experiences edema after receiving plasma expanders. This condition would be documented as being caused by which one of the following?
   A. medication related
   B. allergic
   C. systemic
   D. iatrogenic

7. Which one of the following is a risk factors for edema?
   A. Increase in mobility
   B. Absent history of edema
   C. Long distance travel
   D. Hypotension

8. The primary medical management of edema is to do which one of the following;
   A. treat the underlying cause.
   B. restrict beta blockers.
   C. increase sodium in diet.
   D. force fluids.

9. A primary diagnosis that commonly results in malignant pericardial effusion is which one of the following?
   A. basal cell skin cancer
   B. mesothelioma
   C. brain tumor
   D. amyloidosis

10. A risk factor for malignant pericardial effusion is which one of the following?
    A. a fractionated radiation dose of 30 cGy/day to the iliac crest.
    B. simultaneous cancer treatment with hormones.
    C. coexisting renal infection.
    D. radiation targeted to more than 33% of the heart.

11. The most common characteristic or symptom of malignancy-related pericardial disease is which one of the following?
    A. gradual onset
    B. dyspnea
    C. productive cough
    D. abdominal distention

12. Normal pericardial fluid volume is which one of the following measurements?
    A. 15-50 ml
    B. 50-80 ml
    C. 900-1000 ml
    D. 1-5 ml

13. A patient's blood pressure (BP) is 120/80, pulse 60 and respirations 12. Thirty minutes later, the BP is 106/76, pulse 64, respirations 14. This difference in BP demonstrates which one of the following?
    A. imminent stroke
    B. narrowing pulse pressure
    C. widening pulse pressure
    D. pulsus paradoxus

**71**

14. Which one of the following drug classifications is associated with the cardiovascular toxicity that can cause coronary artery spasm?
    A. Alkylating agents
    B. Anthracyclines
    C. Antimetabolites
    D. Angiogenesis inhibitors

15. Which of the following is a characteristic of an acute cardiovascular toxicity from chemotherapy?
    A. frequently occur.
    B. occurs within 7 days of drug administration.
    C. is usually reversible.
    D. requires discontinuation of the drug.

16. Prevention of cardiotoxicity would include which one of the following nursing interventions for a patient receiving doxorubicin?
    A. Ensure patient treated for hyperlipidemia.
    B. Prescribe a beta blocker.
    C. Prescribe a calcium channel blocker.
    D. Document total cumulative dose of chemotherapy.

17. A 70-year-old patient with advanced stomach cancer presents to the clinic with an infection. The nurse's assessment reveals poor performance status, presence of a venous access device, and lymphadenopathy. The nurse would recognize that the patient is at high risk for which one of the following conditions?
    A. a thrombotic event
    B. lymphedema
    C. malignant pericardial effusion
    D. cardiovascular toxicity

18. A 61-year-old patient with cancer presents to the clinic. A physical examination reveals severe pain in the patient's right leg. The right leg is also cool with a decreased pulse. This exam describes which one of the following conditions?
    A. venous occlusion
    B. arterial embolus
    C. pulmonary embolus
    D. valvular abnormality

19. Mild, spontaneously reversible, and slight heaviness of the extremity with smooth skin texture with pitting edema. Pain and erythema may be present. These characteristics of lymphedema describe which one of the following stages?
    A. 0
    B. 1
    C. 2
    D. 3

20. When the limb starts to look disfigured with over 30% difference in size at the greatest point of the limb and interferes with activities of daily living, which of the following grades of lymphedema would this be?
    A. 1
    B. 2
    C. 3
    D. 4

21. Which of the following descriptions of cardiovascular toxicities is associated with the drug class of anthracyclines?
    A. Associated with toxicity from injury of free radicals that result in myocardial cell loss, fibrosis, and loss of contractility resulting in left ventricular dysfunction (LVD), HF, myopericarditis
    B. Associated with acute myopericarditis, pericardial effusions, arrhythmias, HTN, thromboembolism, and heart failure
    C. Associated with bradycardia, thromboembolism, and HTN may be seen
    D. Associated with coronary artery spasm resulting in angina, arrhythmia, myocardial infarction, cardiac arrest, and sudden death; coronary artery thrombosis and apoptosis of myocardial cells

22. Which one of the following techniques should oncology nurses use for the prevention of thrombotic events in high risk patients?
    A. Elevate the patient's foot with their knee extended.
    B. Elevate the patient's knee with their foot extended.
    C. Employ constant pneumatic compression device.
    D. Ambulate frequently, and implement leg exercises if the patient is bedridden.

23. Nursing management for treatment and prevention of issues related to lymphedema includes which one of the following?
    A. Implementing sterile technique before the administration of antineoplastic agents in the limb.
    B. Using an electronic or automated, rather than a manual, blood pressure cuff.
    C. Using massage therapy on and vigorous weight-lifting with the affected limb.
    D. Recording regular measurement of extremities and elevating the affected limb.

24. If a patient with breast cancer has not developed lymphedema in the first three years after surgery, which one of the following statements is true?
    A. She will probably not develop lymphedema in the arm.
    B. She must be instructed that the potential for lymphedema exists and she should report any issues.
    C. She probably had sentinel node mapping at the time of her initial surgery.
    D. She most likely benefited from breast conservation and radiation therapy.

25. Findings related to edema of cancer include which one of the following?
    A. The presence of S2 heart sound.
    B. Decreased levels of serum albumin and protein.
    C. Increased peripheral pulses.
    D. Decreased blood pressure and heart rate.

# 34 Cognitive Symptoms

1. S.L. is a 45-year-old breast cancer survivor who has undergone treatment with multimodal therapies. She is reporting having difficulty juggling multiple tasks at work. She is likely experiencing which one of the following?
   A. cognitive impairment
   B. decreased self-confidence
   C. delirium
   D. post-traumatic stress

2. Which one of the following treatment modalities has the potential to stimulate cytokine dysregulation, resulting in cognitive impairment?
   A. Surgery
   B. Radiation therapy
   C. Chemotherapy
   D. Hormonal therapy

3. B. H. is a 50-year-old male patient with metastatic prostate cancer. He reports bilateral decreased strength in his lower extremities. The nurse caring for him would anticipate receiving an order for which one of the following procedures?
   A. bone scan
   B. electrolytes, including calcium
   C. liver function tests
   D. magnetic resonance imaging

4. J. L. is a 43-year-old colon cancer survivor who has completed treatment but is concerned about "chemo brain" affecting his work performance. Which one of the following interventions could be recommended for management of chemotherapy-induced impairment?
   A. Cognitive training
   B. Mindfulness stress reduction
   C. Donzepezil
   D. Methylphenidate

5. One of the hallmark symptoms in a patient with delirium when compared with other cognitive impairment is the presence of:
   A. decreased motor function
   B. hypervigilance
   C. impaired concentration
   D. memory changes

6. Which one of the following is a risk factor for delirium in the cancer patient?
   A. Multimodality therapy
   B. Sensory impairments
   C. Metabolic abnormalities
   D. Genetic polymorphism

7. The most appropriate initial step in assessing a patient with delirium would be to do which one of the following?
   A. review current medications.
   B. obtain an MRI of the brain.
   C. consider CBC with differential.
   D. perform a lumbar puncture.

8. Mr. R. is an 80-year-old male patient with delirium. He becomes severely agitated. The nurse caring for him would anticipate an initial order for administration of which one of the following options?
   A. Lorazepam 0.5 mg PO
   B. Haloperidol 0.5 mg PO
   C. Risperidone 0.5 mg PO
   D. Olanzapine 5 mg PO

9. In the patient with delirium, low dose anti-psychotics may be useful to which one of the following?
   A. treat metabolic imbalances.
   B. minimize sensory deficits.
   C. promote uninterrupted sleep.
   D. manage severe agitation.

10. Which one of the following is a nursing management technique for cancer- and cancer treatment-related cognitive impairment?
    A. Avoid excessive sensory stimulation and/or restraints
    B. Incorporate environmental strategies such as having a visible clock or calendar available and keep a room well-lit and surrounded by familiar objects
    C. Provide frequent reorientation and reassurance
    D. Reinforce cognitive and exercise training plans

11. Ms. B. is an 87-year-old patient with breast cancer who has been diagnosed with delirium. In planning her care, the oncology nurse would do which one of the following?

A. Remove calendars from the patient's environment because they increase confusion.

B. Allow family photos only if the patient can identify the people depicted in the photos.

C. Encourage the patient to consistently use assistive devices such as eyeglasses and hearing aids.

D. Maximize the patient's exposure to environmental sounds, such as alarms, to remind her that she is in a hospital room and not in her own home.

# 35 Endocrine Symptoms

1. The adrenal gland produces which one of the following hormones?
   A. Antidiuretic hormone
   B. Luteinizing hormone
   C. Thyroxine
   D. Cortisol

2. F. H. is a 70-year-old female patient with cancer who arrives at the infusion center with reports of weakness, depression, and feeling cold most of the time. The nurse caring for her is aware that these symptoms most likely represent the presence of which one of the following?
   A. hypothyroidism
   B. hyperthyroidism
   C. hypoparathyroidism
   D. adrenal insufficiency

3. A patient with a history of coronary artery disease has a new diagnosis of treatment related hyperthyroidism secondary to an immune checkpoint inhibitor. He is admitted to the oncology unit. The oncology nurse caring for him should anticipate receiving an order for which one of the following?
   A. methylprednisolone
   B. dexamethasone
   C. levothyroxine
   D. cinacalcet

4. The oncology nurse is caring for a patient who is to begin levothyroxine therapy after being treated with radioactive iodine for a malignant thyroid nodule. The nurse should expect that levels of thyroid stimulating hormone (TSH) and thyroxine (T4) will be monitored on which one of the following schedules?
   A. Every week for a month
   B. Every 4-6 weeks until stable
   C. On an annual basis
   D. Daily for 6 months

5. An oncology nurse provides teaching to a patient diagnosed with asymptomatic primary hyperparathyroidism. Education should include instructions on which one of the following?
   A. initiating thiazide diuretics
   B. how to take phosphate binders
   C. a low calcium, high phosphate diet
   D. a diet rich in calcium-containing foods

6. An oncology nurse is caring for a 54-year-old male patient following surgical removal of the parathyroid glands. The nurse anticipates that medication management of resulting hypoparathyroidism will be based on the level of which serum electrolyte?
   A. Potassium
   B. Chloride
   C. Sodium
   D. Calcium

7. S. L. is a 60-year-old male patient who is undergoing radiation for brain metastases. He presents to the clinic with reports of feeling thirsty much of the time and having to urinate frequently during the day and night. The nurse suspects that the patient is demonstrating signs of which one of the following?
   A. hypothyroidism
   B. diabetes insipidus
   C. adrenal insufficiency
   D. hyperparathyroidism

8. An oncology nurse is caring for a 62-year-old patient who is being treated for adrenal insufficiency. Patient education should include which one of the following?
   A. wear an alert bracelet indicating steroid stress doses
   B. decrease steroid doses prior to surgical procedures
   C. increase steroid doses five-fold for a head cold
   D. adjust the steroid doses on a weekly basis

9. Which one of the following scenarios most likely describes a patient who would be diagnosed with hyperthyroidism/thyrotoxicosis?
   A. The patient presents with symptoms of anxiety, agitation, weakness, and heat intolerance. A physical examination shows the patient has lost weight and is hyperactive.
   B. The patient complains of bone pain, and is fatigued, weak, and is presenting with signs of anorexia. A physical examination reveals hypertension and bradycardia.
   C. The patient presents with fatigue, anxiety, depression, and irritability. The patient's physical examination reveals chronic skeletal abnormalities.
   D. The patient presents with visual changes, headache, and myalgias. A physical examination shows the patient has experienced weight loss and is showing signs of hypotension.

# 36 Fatigue

1. Which one of the following factors is an underlying physiologic mechanism of fatigue?
   A. Low levels of pro-inflammatory cytokines, interleukins, tumor necrosis factor
   B. 5-Hydroxytryptophan autoregulation
   C. Hypothalamic-pituitary-adrenal axis dysfunction
   D. Circadian rhythms that reflect a desire to stay up late in the evening

2. J. L. is a 65-year-old woman with a Grade IV glioblastoma who is undergoing radiation therapy. She presents in a wheelchair due to increased weakness and a complaint of severe fatigue. Which one of the following factors can significantly increase the risk of this patient's fatigue?
   A. Older age
   B. Female sex
   C. Low performance status
   D. High doses of ondansetron

3. Which one of the following is the best measurement strategy for a patient experiencing fatigue?
   A. Provider assessment
   B. Patient-reported questionnaire
   C. An Eastern Cooperative Oncology Group (ECOG) score
   D. Nurse-reported distress screening tool

4. Which one of the following laboratory analyses should be considered initially to evaluate potential underlying causes of fatigue?
   A. Thyroid function
   B. Serum protein electrophoresis (SPEP)
   C. Tumor markers
   D. Platelet count

5. A 59-year-old patient with Stage II breast cancer reports significant fatigue and has been struggling with pancytopenia during treatment. Medical management of her fatigue should include which one of the following?
   A. blood transfusions for severe anemia
   B. routine use of erythropoiesis-stimulating agents
   C. high-dose dexamethasone for severe fatigue
   D. benzodiazepines for fatigue

6. Which one of the following interventions has the strongest evidence for the management of cancer-related fatigue?
   A. Blood transfusions
   B. Dexamethasone
   C. Patient education on priority setting
   D. Exercise

7. An oncology nurse is meeting with T. K., a young adult patient who has just completed treatment for acute myelogenous leukemia. He is feeling better, but his primary complaint is fatigue. Which one of the following educational information statements should the nurse include for management of this patient's fatigue?
   A. Because of the patient's age, high-intensity exercise is recommended.
   B. Depression can mimic fatigue and referral to psychosocial resources can be important.
   C. Increasing environmental stimuli can help alleviate fatigue.
   D. Fatigue is likely to resolve within 2 months.

8. Fatigue can be caused by a variety of disease-related factors, from fatigue caused by disease-related anemia to fatigue caused by comorbidities and underlying diseases. Which one of the following percentage of patients with cancer experience cancer-related fatigue?
   A. 20% to 30%
   B. 50% to 60%
   C. 40% to 50%
   D. 70% to 80%

9. Fatigue is often seen with other symptoms related to cancer. Which one of the following have been found to cluster with fatigue?
   A. anxiety
   B. dietary changes
   C. cognitive changes
   D. sleep disturbances

# 37 Gastrointestinal Symptoms

1. J. R. is 50-year-old male patient with head and neck cancer who is undergoing radiation therapy after surgery. The oncology nurse is aware that during the initiation phase of the pathogenesis of mucositis which one of the following statements is true?
   A. Cytokines and modulators produced are associated with mucositis production
   B. Signs and symptoms are already present within the oral mucosa
   C. Angiogenesis is absent, leading to the development of small nodules
   D. Interferons and tumor necrosis factor (TNF) cells proliferate, leading to the development of mucositis

2. M. K. is a 46-year-old male patient with cancer who arrives in the clinic for evaluation prior to the start of chemotherapy. Upon reviewing the patient's medical record, the oncology nurse finds that the patient is at risk for developing mucositis due to which one of the following?
   A. a body mass index (BMI) of 19.0
   B. past history of alcohol use
   C. a serum creatinine level of 2.7
   D. use of alcohol-based mouth wash

3. A nurse is caring for a 45-year-old female patient with acute myelocytic leukemia on a hematopoietic stem cell transplant unit. She will soon be undergoing chemotherapy, along with TBI for an autologous HSCT. The physician has ordered Palifermin. The nurse instructs the patient that this drug has been ordered to do one of the following?
   A. decrease nausea and vomiting during treatment
   B. elevate blood counts after transplant
   C. alleviate painful cramping during treatment
   D. reduce the incidence and severity of mucositis

4. A patient is admitted to the hospital for his course of chemotherapy. The treatment includes cisplatin. The oncology nurse caring for him is aware that when acute chemotherapy-induced nausea and vomiting (CINV) occurs which one of the following is true?
   A. the vagus nerve is stimulated by 5-HT3 agonists and CINV occurs within 24 hours
   B. receptors in the brain send an intense emetic message and CINV occurs within 48 hours
   C. the small intestine is stimulated and CINV persists from a few to many days
   D. abdominal muscle contraction leads to CINV within hours to days

5. An oncology nurse is caring for a 56-year-old female patient on an oncology unit who is due to receive her first dose of chemotherapy. What finding in the patient's history puts the patient at risk for chemotherapy-induced nausea and vomiting (CINV)?
   A. Use of NSAIDs
   B. History of smoking
   C. History of gastroesophageal reflux disease (GERD)
   D. No previous alcohol use

6. T. J. is a 42-year-old male patient who arrives in the clinic for his first infusion of chemotherapy. The patient inquires what treatment he will receive for nausea and vomiting. The oncology nurse is aware that the standard of care antiemetic the patient would receive includes which one of the following?
   A. 5-HT3 antagonist
   B. dopamine
   C. benzodiazapine
   D. antisecretory drugs

7. An oncology nurse is caring for a patient with ovarian cancer on a gynecology unit who has malignant ascites. The nurse understands that this is due to which one of the following?
   A. increased drainage from malignant tumor, leading to accumulation of fluid
   B. lymphatic cells draining fluid into the peritoneum
   C. seeding by malignant cells within the peritoneal cavity
   D. fluid moving from the intravascular space into the interstitial space

8. K. M. is a 58-year-old female patient on an oncology unit who has malignant ascites. The patient has been scheduled for a paracentesis. Her oncology nurse instructs the patient which one of the following?
   A. "With your procedure, there is the potential for cardiac effects."
   B. "Your procedure comes with a high risk for bowel obstruction."
   C. "The procedure requires deep sedation."
   D. "With this procedure, you will feel a decreased abdominal distension discomfort."

**78**

9. G. L., a 62-year-old male patient, arrives in the oncology clinic with complaints of constipation. The patient, who is a diabetic, states that he has not been drinking much and a urine sample shows indication of uremia. The etiology of this patient's constipation is most likely due to which one of the following?
   A. metabolic causes
   B. dietary causes
   C. kidney stones
   D. a urinary fistula

10. A nurse is caring for a 70-year-old male patient on an oncology unit who is suffering from fecal impaction. An enema has been ordered for the patient. The patient asks why he can't have an oral agent. His nurse explains to the patient which one of the following?
   A. the liquid in the enema has a fiber-forming agent which softens the stool
   B. an enema is the preferred method and more predictable for the discharge of stool
   C. oral stool softeners will cause further constipation without removing the stool
   D. water taken along with the oral medications will cause cramping and bloating

11. A patient arrives in the clinic with complaints of diarrhea after receiving a course of chemotherapy. After reviewing the patient's medical record, the nurse believes the diarrhea may be caused by which one of the following?
   A. a bacterial infection such as *Escherichia coli*
   B. malabsorption due to chemicals in etoposide
   C. recent treatment with methotrexate
   D. recent constipation

12. The nurse caring for a patient on an oncology unit is discharging a patient home who has been admitted for diarrhea. The patient inquires as to what he should eat and drink. The nurse responds by explaining to the patient which one of the following?
   A. drink plenty of apple juice for rehydration
   B. eat high-fiber foods cereals to bulk up stool
   C. eat fruits such as peaches and nectarines
   D. eat a low-fat, high-potassium diet, with small frequent meals

13. A patient with asthma is receiving radiation therapy with concurrent chemotherapy for head and neck cancer. The radiation field includes the salivary glands. The physical assessment reveals the patient's complaint of dry mouth; difficult chewing, eating with and wearing their dentures; difficulty swallowing and altered taste. Medical management of this patient could include an agent to increase saliva secretion. With this patient's history and physical assessment, which of the following drugs would be avoided in the plan of care for xerostomia?
   A. Cevimeline (Evoxac)
   B. Pilocarpine (Salagen)
   C. Aquoral
   D. Xero-Lube

14. A patient with cancer arrives at the urgent care clinic with complaints of nausea, frequent vomiting, and inadequate fluid and food intake. A feeding tube had been placed 2 days prior. The physician determines the patient should be admitted to the hospital and begin total parenteral nutrition (TPN). Using the National Cancer Institute, Common Terminology Criteria for Adverse Events (NCI-CTCAE) for gastrointestinal symptoms, the patient's vomiting would be rated as which one of the following?
   A. Grade 1
   B. Grade 2
   C. Grade 3
   D. Grade 4

15. A patient with cancer presents to the nurse with symptoms of dysphagia. Symptoms reported include cough, a sense of choking with swallowing, voice change, frequent throat clearing, and earache. Which type of dysphagia is the patient most likely experiencing?
   A. Oropharyngeal dysphagia (OD)
   B. Mechanical dysphagia
   C. Esophageal dysphagia (ED)
   D. Radiation dysphagia

16. Which one of the following would be considered a lifestyle factor that could cause xerostomia?
   A. Use of an antihistamine
   B. Caffeinated beverage consumption
   C. Secondary Sjogren syndrome
   D. Use of anticholinergic agents

17. The patient with head and neck cancer is scheduled for a sialometry and the RN is to instruct the patient before the procedure. Which of the following would be an accurate statement about this test?
   A. The evaluation is done at normal bedtime.
   B. The test is performed after an 8-hour fast.
   C. This test is a measure of regurgitation.
   D. The patient is sitting upright for the procedure.

18. Which one of the following is a preventative nursing management measure for oral mucositis?
    A. Have the patient apply a topical protective or coating agent to the affected area
    B. Remind the patient to avoid spicy food, or hot drinks
    C. Have the patient use a solution of normal saline, salt, and baking soda
    D. Request the patient to make a pretreatment dental examination and provide them with instructions for an oral hygiene regimen

19. S. L. is a 50-year-old male patient who complains of dry mouth after treatment. Within several weeks, he develops thick, ropy saliva. He also has trouble chewing his food. His oncology nurse suspects he has developed which one of the following?
    A. dysphagia
    B. xerostomia
    C. mucositis
    D. trismus

20. Which one of the following interventions are appropriate for patients with xerostomia?
    A. Decrease patient intake of liquids
    B. Encourage the patient to eat popsicles
    C. Encourage the patient to eat dry and spicy foods
    D. Encourage the patient to rinse with commercial mouthwashes frequently to increase moisture

21. Ascites is most likely linked to which one of the following cancer types?
    A. Cervical cancer
    B. Ovarian cancer
    C. Malignant melanoma
    D. Head and neck cancer

22. T. H. is a 53-year-old patient with cancer who is complaining of abdominal bloating and cramping with no bowel movement for the past 5 days. She has reported that she normally has a bowel movement daily. Bowel sounds are present. She has completed her last dose of chemotherapy (doxorubicin and cyclophosphamide) approximately 10 days ago. Which one of the following actions should be recommended to alleviate her constipation?
    A. A glycerin suppository
    B. A Fleet enema to stimulate peristalsis
    C. A stimulate laxative until the bowel movement occurs, then evaluation, as needed, for daily stool softeners or lubricant laxatives
    D. Begin bulk-forming laxatives for constipation, and a mild narcotic for her pain

23. A patient is receiving radiation therapy to her abdomen and asks for dietary instructions to decrease her diarrhea. Which one of the following would the nurse not include in the patient's dietary teaching?
    A. Eat a high-fiber diet that is high in protein.
    B. Begin a low-residue diet that is high in protein.
    C. Avoid spicy, fried, or fatty foods.
    D. If the patient has a known or temporary lactose intolerance, recommend that they keep to a low-lactose diet.

# 38 Genitourinary Symptoms

1. The nurse on the oncology unit notes that a patient in her care has a history of urinary stress incontinence. The nurse is aware that this type of incontinence is caused by which one of the following?
   A. intensified psychological concerns
   B. intrinsic urinary sphincter dysfunction
   C. impaired reflexes controlling bladder emptying
   D. physical activities that increase abdominal pressure

2. P. R. is a male patient who is receiving radiation therapy to the bladder. He reports frequent involuntary loss of urine. The oncology nurse caring for him is aware that this condition is most likely due to which one of the following?
   A. treatment-induced bladder inflammation
   B. reduced size of the bladder tumor
   C. advanced age of the patient
   D. presence of kidney stones

3. F. R. is a 60-year-old female patient with cancer. The patient has been experiencing recent onset urinary incontinence. The nurse caring for her explains that the best diagnostic testing for this condition would include which one of the following?
   A. determination of amount of residual urine after voiding
   B. review of the patient's bladder diary of the past 2 weeks
   C. colonoscopy if not performed in the previous 5 years
   D. gathering information about usual voiding habits

4. J. T. is a 55-year-old female patient with cancer who is dealing with urinary incontinence. She asks the nurse in the outpatient oncology clinic about management of uncontrolled loss of urine. Appropriate nursing education might include which one of the following?
   A. minimizing trips outside the house as much as possible
   B. scheduled voiding at the same time daily
   C. increase in fluid intake during the day
   D. learning bladder self-catheterization

5. An oncology nurse is caring for a 57-year-old male patient who is scheduled for surgery to remove his bladder and create a continent urinary diversion with a stoma in the skin. In teaching the patient about what to expect after the procedure, the nurse should explain which one of the following?
   A. An external urine collection device will be required.
   B. It is possible that some urine will dribble continuously.
   C. Catheterization of urine will need to be done every 4-6 hours.
   D. The pouch will need to emptied before each chemotherapy treatment.

6. The nurse is caring for a patient who has a newly created ileal conduit after removal of a malignant bladder. Patient teaching should include instructions to do which one of the following?
   A. Avoid eating cruciferous vegetables.
   B. Use alcohol to clean the peristomal skin.
   C. Catheterize the stoma several times per day.
   D. Empty the collection pouch when it is half full.

7. K. L. is a 58-year-old male patient with a history of melanoma who presents for a follow-up visit. The patient reports nocturia, lethargy, difficulty concentrating at work, and refractory nausea. The nurse caring for him suspects the patient is experiencing signs of which one of the following?
   A. renal dysfunction
   B. prostatic hypertrophy
   C. metastasis to the brain
   D. delayed hypersensitivity reaction

8. Laboratory test results reveal that a patient on the oncology unit has developed Stage 2 renal dysfunction. The nurse caring for the patient should anticipate an order for which one of the following?
   A. reduce fluid intake
   B. record daily weights
   C. initiate oxygen via nasal cannula
   D. administer diphenhydramine by mouth

9. S. H. is a 44-year-old patient with breast cancer who has widespread bone metastasis. She is now undergoing radiation therapy. Since radiation therapy has started, she reports a recent change in output of large amounts of urine. The nurse caring for her suspects that this change may be caused by which one of the following?
   A. decreased renal blood flow
   B. pelvic lymph nodes obstructed by tumor
   C. hypercalcemia of malignancy
   D. nephrotoxicity associated with radiation therapy

10. L. R. is a 58-year-old female patient with cancer. The patient comes into a visit to the infusion center and reports that she is been experiencing the involuntary loss of urine, with an abrupt and strong desire to void her bladder. The nurse is aware that this type of incontinence is most likely which one of the following?
    A. stress incontinence
    B. reflex incontinence
    C. functional incontinence
    D. urge incontinence

11. Which one of the following is an example of a pharmacologic intervention for a patient with cancer diagnosed with renal dysfunction?
    A. Anticholinergics
    B. Amifostine and sodium thiosulfate for cisplatin nephrotoxicity
    C. Tricyclic antidepressants
    D. Potassium channel openers

12. Which one of the following is an example of medical management of urinary incontinence?
    A. Saline hydration with appropriate diuretic
    B. Oral or intravenous (IV) sodium bicarbonate to maintain alkaline urine
    C. Replacement of electrolytes
    D. Electrostimulation

13. Which one of the following types of patients would be suitable candidates for neobladder surgery?
    A. A patient with a history of benign prostatic hypertrophy (BPH)
    B. A patient with inflammatory bowel disease
    C. A patient who has received radiation therapy
    D. A patient with urethral cancer

14. Which one of the following chemotherapy agents requires aggressive hydration before, during, and after therapy to prevent renal toxicity?
    A. Daunorubicin (Cerubidine)
    B. 5-FU
    C. Cisplatin (Platinol)
    D. Flutamide (Eulexin)

# 39 Hematologic and Immune Symptoms

1. Granulocyte cell counts include which one of the following types of cells?
   A. Red blood cells
   B. Platelets
   C. Monocytes
   D. Lymphocytes

2. When reviewing a patient's lab work, the nurse knows that the patient's risk of infection is increased when which one of the following is true?
   A. absolute neutrophil count rises above 2500/mm$^3$
   B. absolute neutrophil count falls below 1500/mm$^3$
   C. white blood cell count decreases to $4.3 \times 10^9$/L
   D. absolute basophil count increases above normal limits

3. A patient who received chemotherapy last week calls the infusion unit to report a temperature of 100.9°F. The nurse is concerned that the patient is a risk for which one of the following?
   A. febrile neutropenia
   B. thrombocytopenia
   C. hypercalcemia
   D. hemolytic anemia

4. A patient at high risk for chemotherapy-induced neutropenia has an order for prophylactic injections of a granulocyte colony-stimulating factor (G-CSF) agent. The nurse anticipates monitoring the patient for G-CSF-related adverse events, which include which one of the following?
   A. eye inflammation
   B. acne-like rash
   C. lung fibrosis
   D. bone pain

5. A patient with metastatic prostate cancer who is undergoing radiation to the pelvis, ischium, and left femur at increased risk for which one of the following?
   A. bone marrow suppression
   B. peripheral neuropathy
   C. wet desquamation
   D. urinary retention

6. The oncology nurse is caring for an immunosuppressed patient who is being treated with concomitant chemotherapy and radiation therapy. Nursing interventions to minimize infection risk in this patient might include which one of the following?
   A. avoid frequent bathing as it is drying to the skin
   B. change water in pitchers every 4 hours
   C. prohibit visits from family members
   D. restrict delivery of fresh flowers

7. Patient education to minimize infection risk should include instructions to call the healthcare provider to report which one of the following?
   A. dry mouth
   B. sore throat
   C. temperature of 99.8°F
   D. urinary hesitancy

8. Results of a complete blood count in a patient being treated for esophageal cancer reveal anemia. Further work-up might include tests to determine which one of the following?
   A. iron overload
   B. platelet function
   C. gastrointestinal blood loss
   D. estrogen level

9. A patient arrives at the chemotherapy infusion unit complaining of fatigue and dyspnea. A rapid heart rate is noted. The nurse is aware that the patient is most likely exhibiting signs of which one of the following?
   A. anemia
   B. neutropenia
   C. lymphocytopenia
   D. thrombocytopenia

10. When receiving a transfusion of packed red blood cells, the optimal goal for a patient with symptomatic anemia would be to maintain a:
   A. hemoglobin level that is greater than 10 g/dL
   B. red blood cell count that is greater than 6.2 mcL
   C. heart rate lower than 90 beats/min
   D. glomerular filtration rate of 90 mL/min/1.73 m$^2$

11. A patient being treated for prostate cancer develops disseminated intravascular coagulation. The oncology nurse anticipates an order to monitor which one of the following?
    A. the patient's red blood cell count
    B. the patient's hemoglobin level
    C. the patient's platelet count
    D. the patient's ferritin level

12. The oncology nurse provides teaching about bleeding precautions to a patient who is newly diagnosed with myelodysplastic syndrome. Education should include which one of the following?
    A. prevention of falls
    B. use of enemas for constipation
    C. shave with a straight-edge razor
    D. apply warm packs to cuts in the skin

13. A patient who is being treated with cytotoxic chemotherapy develops a urinary tract infection. Which one of the following findings, if recorded by the oncology nurse, indicate high risk for clinical deterioration?
    A. Blood pressure of 86/50 mmHg and respiratory rate of 26
    B. Blood pressure of 155/90 mmHg and respiratory rate of 20
    C. Temperature of 100.1°F and depression
    D. Heart rate of 80 beats/min and sleepiness

14. The oncology nurse is caring for a patient who underwent biopsy for suspected kidney cancer. During rounds, the oncology nurse notices that the patient has become pale, has a weak, irregular pulse, and has moist skin. The patient is exhibiting signs of which one of the following?
    A. anemia
    B. neutropenia
    C. hemorrhage
    D. thrombocytopenia

15. A patient on the oncology unit has developed fever and chills following completion of chemotherapy administration. Appropriate nursing interventions to promote comfort for this patient include which one of the following?
    A. provide heating blankets
    B. give tepid sponge baths
    C. limit warm fluids by mouth
    D. immerse in ice bath

16. Which one of the following factors is a disease and treatment-related risk factor associated with chemotherapy-induced myeloid toxicity?
    A. Decreased immune function
    B. Recently completed surgery
    C. Drug-drug interactions
    D. Dose intensity

17. Colony-stimulating growth factor administration is initiated when which one of the following occurs?
    A. A chemotherapy dose has been reduced.
    B. A patient has experienced a previous anemia with chemotherapy administration.
    C. A patient is undergoing radiation therapy for cancer treatment.
    D. A patient is at risk of grade 3/4 chemotherapy-induced neutropenia or is febrile. Febrile neutropenia with dose intense treatment planned.

18. Which one of the following places the patient with cancer at risk for opportunistic infection?
    A. Basophilia
    B. Lymphopenia
    C. Thrombocytopenia
    D. Anemia

19. How is an ANC calculated? Chose one of the following that best represents the correct calculation.
    A. % neutrophils (segmented neutrophils + bands) divided by total WBC
    B. Total WBC divided by % neutrophils (segmented neutrophils + bands)
    C. % neutrophils (segmented neutrophils + bands) multiplied by WBC
    D. Actual number of neutrophils (segmented neutrophils + bands) multiplied by WBC

20. From which one of the following do platelets arise?
    A. Lymphoid stem cells
    B. Megakaryocyte stem cells
    C. Myeloid stem cells
    D. Epithelial stem cells

21. Granulocytes collectively include which one of the following?
    A. basophils, eosinophils, and neutrophils
    B. basophils, lymphocytes, and neutrophils
    C. eosinophils, lymphocytes, and monocytes
    D. basophils, lymphocytes, and monocytes

22. Patients with cancer are at a severe risk for bleeding when which one of the following occurs?
    A. Neutrophils are at 50%
    B. Lymphocytes are at 30%
    C. Platelets are less than 20,000 mm$^3$
    D. Erythrocytes are at 20%

23. Which one of the following statements is true about nadir?
    A. Nadir is the highest point the WBC's reach after cancer treatment and occurs 7 to 14 days after treatment.
    B. Nadir is WBC lysis related to chemotherapy administration.
    C. Nadir is the lowest point blood cells reach after a cancer treatment and occurs 7 to 14 days after treatment.
    D. Nadir regularly occurs after biotherapy administration.

24. Thrombocytopenia describes a decrease in the circulating
    A. Platelets below 100,000/mm$^3$
    B. WBCs below 1500/mm$^3$
    C. Neutrophils below 1000/mm$^3$
    D. RBCs below 1000/mm$^3$

1. Which one of the following layers of skin serves as an insulator to temperature changes?
   A. The dermis
   B. The subcutaneous tissue
   C. The epidermis
   D. The inner connective tissue

2. R. K. is a 50-year-old patient who presents to clinic with disease-related pruritus on the upper extremities. The oncology nurse caring for the patient knows that the patient's condition will require pharmacologic management. Which one of the following drugs utilized to treat the patient's pruritus are most likely to cause drowsiness?
   A. Corticosteroids
   B. H1 and H2 antagonists
   C. Capsaicin
   D. Calamine lotion

3. F. M. is a 60-year-old man who has been diagnosed with colon cancer. He is receiving irinotecan and reports to the oncology nurse in his care that he is experiencing frequent diarrhea on Day 2 after receiving treatment. When providing education for the patient, which one of the following measures related to perineal hygiene should be avoided?
   A. Use alcohol wipes to cleanse the affected area.
   B. Frequent hand washing.
   C. Mild soap, rinsing thoroughly, pat dry.
   D. Apply a skin barrier after each stool.

4. Graft-versus-host disease is most often related to which one of the following?
   A. a skin graft
   B. a bone marrow transplant
   C. melanoma
   D. malnutrition

5. H. W. is a 57-year-old male patient who has just completed radiation therapy. He was diagnosed with acute radiation dermatitis, and the oncology nurse caring for him recognizes that symptoms for his condition include which one of the following?
   A. circular red scaly rash
   B. rash involving extremities, including palms and soles
   C. thinning of skin, scarring and contractures, and telanglectasias
   D. erythema, pain, dermal swelling, itching, and necrosis

6. A skin reaction commonly seen in a patient is receiving an epidermal growth factor receptor (EGFR) inhibitor is which one of the following?
   A. oncholysis
   B. acneiform rash without comedones
   C. erythema of hands and feet
   D. permanent hyperpigmentation of gums

7. The nurse is teaching her 52-year-old patient who is receiving chemotherapy about the importance of reducing ultraviolet light exposure during chemotherapy because many agents are photosensitizing. The photosensitizing of chemotherapy agents often manifests as which one of the following?
   A. several days after sunburn, causing the sunburn to reappear
   B. transverse lines in nails with bands corresponding to when drug was given
   C. a moderate-to-severe sunburn in sun-exposed areas
   D. paronychia

8. Which one of the following is a description of symptoms related to chronic radiation dermatitis?
   A. Thinning of skin, scarring and contractures, telangiectasias, and long-term skin sensitivity to irritants and environmental agents
   B. Occurs in previously irradiated skin within 1-2 weeks after chemotherapy; erythema, edema, superficial ulcerations, and superficial skin sloughing
   C. Immediate dermatitis occurring in radiated areas with erythema, pain, dermal swelling, itching, and necrosis
   D. Allergic response where drug touches skin (erythema, local swelling, desquamation, blistering, and necrosis is possible)

9. Which one of the following is a description of symptoms related to erythema multiforme (antigen–antibody complexes) skin reaction?
   A. Itching, redness, and swelling within one hour after infusion has begun
   B. Outbreak of rash with typical target lesions involving extremities, including palms of the hands and soles of the feet, can progress to a generalized rash
   C. Occurs in previously irradiated skin within 1-2 weeks after chemotherapy and symptoms include erythema, edema, andansuperficial ulcerations

D. Involves generalized vascular inflammation with end organ damage

10. Which one of the following skin reactions is known to be caused by treatment through platinum derivatives (cisplatin, carboplatin)?
    A. Contact allergy
    B. Acute radiation dermatitis
    C. Immunoglobulin E (IgE) mediated
    D. Vasculitis

11. After receiving radiation therapy treatment, J. T., a 47-year-old male patient with cancer, experiences a skin reaction involving blistering, local swelling, and erythema outside of the radiation field. The nurse caring for him suspects that a contact allergy could be to blame for his symptoms. Which one of the following could have been responsible?
    A. Reaction to his premedication
    B. Reaction to something he had eaten earlier in the day
    C. Reaction to the radiation therapy
    D. Latex found in gloves or rubberized protective clothing

12. Which one of the following is a description of symptoms related to recall radiation dermatitis?
    A. Reaction occurs in previously irradiated skin within 1-2 weeks after chemotherapy, and is associated with erythema, edema, superficial ulcerations, and superficial skin sloughing
    B. Rash with typical target lesions involving extremities, including palms and soles; can progress to generalized
    C. Thinning of skin, scarring and contractures, telangiectasias, and long-term skin sensitivity to irritants and environmental agents
    D. Flulike symptoms, which may progress to life threatening

# 41 Musculoskeletal Symptoms

1. When assessing a patient with sarcopenia, the oncology nurse would expect to see which one of the following?
   A. loss of skeletal muscle mass
   B. bone marrow suppression
   C. joint contractures
   D. muscle spasticity

2. W. R. is a 61-year-old female patient with a history of lymphoma. She arrives at the oncology clinic and reports difficulty standing after using the toilet. Which one of the following factors is most likely to increase risk for musculoskeletal alterations?
   A. Medical marijuana use
   B. Enteral tube feedings
   C. Vegetarian diet
   D. Increased bed rest

3. The nurse is caring for a 58-year-old male patient on the oncology unit who has a Karnofsky performance status (KPS) of 50. The nurse caring for him anticipates which of the following to be true?
   A. The patient will be able to participate in self-care independently.
   B. The patient will need considerable assistance with daily activities.
   C. The patient will show minor signs and symptoms of disease.
   D. The patient will be disabled and require complete care.

4. During a clinic visit the nurse assesses a patient's musculoskeletal status by observing which of the following traits of the patient?
   A. Cleanliness
   B. Gait
   C. Body language
   D. Habitus

5. G. K. is a 47-year-old female patient who has completed a course of cisplatin two weeks ago. She arrives at the oncology clinic complaining of muscle weakness in her legs. The nurse anticipates that blood tests will be ordered to assess for which one of the following?
   A. neutrophilia
   B. hypermagnesemia
   C. hypokalemia
   D. thrombocytopenia

6. The nurse is caring for a patient on the oncology unit who has impaired mobility. Appropriate nursing measures for this patient include which one of the following?
   A. changing the patient's position every shift
   B. instituting soft lighting during the day
   C. placing a soft restraint vest while in bed to prevent falls
   D. encouraging an active range of motion exercises every 4 hours

7. J. B. is a 49-year-old male patient with cancer on the oncology unit who has an Eastern Cooperative Oncology Group (ECOG) Performance Status score of 3. The nurse caring for him anticipates which of the following to be true?
   A. The patient is disabled and unable to carry out any activities related to self-care.
   B. The patient is fully active and able to carry on all normal activities as he would have before his diagnosis.
   C. The patient is restricted in strenuous activity such as heavy lifting or vigorous aerobic workouts.
   D. The patient is capable of limited self-care and is restricted to a bed or chair during half of his waking hours.

8. F. R. is a 67-year-old female patient with cancer. She is reporting to the clinic with complaints of pain and numbness in her extremities and muscle contractions in her legs. The oncology nurse caring for her knows she will be getting orders for a laboratory workup. Which one of the following electrolyte abnormalities might the nurse expect to find in the results?
   A. An abnormality in her potassium level
   B. An abnormality in her calcium level
   C. An abnormality in her chloride level
   D. An abnormality in her sodium level

9. H. R. is a 69-year-old female patient with cancer on the oncology unit who has an Eastern Cooperative Oncology Group (ECOG) Performance Status score of 1. The nurse caring for her anticipates which of the following to be true?
   A. The patient is capable of performing light activities such as housework.
   B. The patient is restricted to a bed or chair during half of his waking hours and capable of limited self-care.
   C. The patient is fully disabled with no capability for self-care.
   D. The patient has died.

10. An oncology nurse is caring for a 62-year-old male patient with cancer who reports to the clinic with complaints of a fast or irregular heartbeat and some pain in his legs. The oncology nurse caring for him knows she will be getting orders for a laboratory workup. Which one of the following electrolyte abnormalities might the nurse expect to find in the results?
    A. An abnormality in his chloride level
    B. An abnormality in his calcium level
    C. An abnormality in his potassium level
    D. An abnormality in his phosphate level

# 42 Neurological Symptoms

1. Factors that may put patients at increased risk for neuropathies include which one of the following?
   A. A diagnosis of cancer under the age of 60 years.
   B. A diagnosis of anxiety and depression.
   C. A history of vitamin B complex deficiency.
   D. A history of a lumpectomy for breast cancer.

2. Seizures, encephalopathy, and cerebellar dysfunction in a patient with cancer are symptoms most likely to be attributed to which one of the following?
   A. neuropathies of the central nervous system (CNS)
   B. anxiety and depression
   C. a past medical history of childhood epilepsy
   D. damage to the peripheral nervous system (PNS)

3. Medical management for cancer-related neuropathies include which one of the following?
   A. fentanyl patch
   B. solumedrol
   C. pregabalin
   D. alprazolam

4. Nursing management for cancer-related neuropathies includes instructing the patient on which one of the following?
   A. the use of massage and lotions on hands and feet
   B. refrain from exercise
   C. avoid using assistive devices so muscle strength can be restored
   D. stimulate the skin of affected area often

5. F. N. is a 51-year-old female patient with cancer, who has been receiving chemotherapy, and is complaining of decreased sensation in her hands. An appropriate intervention would include which one of the following?
   A. engage in a hand-strengthening program
   B. wear gloves to protect from cold
   C. apply hand sanitizer at least hourly
   D. use a three point cane for ambulation

6. S. W. is a 52-year-old female patient with cancer who is receiving a chemotherapy agent known to increase the risk of neuropathy. To assess proprioception, the nurse would do which one of the following?
   A. check vibration using a tuning fork
   B. assess for discrimination between sharp and dull sensations
   C. check for clonus
   D. evaluate balance using a Romberg test

7. When assessing for neuropathy, the patient will be evaluated for cerebellar and proprioception, sensory function, and deep tendon reflexes. Which one of the following would be the procedure for assessing sensory function related to neuropathy?
   A. Observe for accurate movement of extremities.
   B. Assess for discrimination between sharp and dull sensations.
   C. Have patient stand with feet together, arms at side with eyes closed. A slight sway is normal.
   D. Evaluate rapid alternating movement of hands.

8. G. R. is a 64-year-old male patient with cancer who has been experiencing a decline in mobility and struggling with caring for himself. The nurse caring for him knows that to increase mobility impairment and allow the patient to improve self-care which one of the following interventions would be appropriate?
   A. Develop an exercise and muscle-strengthening program.
   B. Offer the patient access to acupressure and acupuncture services.
   C. Encourage the patient to implement relaxation techniques.
   D. Refer the patient for biofeedback.

9. R. H. is a 61-year-old female with cancer. She presents to the clinic with increased pain and signs of depression and anxiety. R. H. is not interested in any medications to alleviate pain or other symptoms and is seeking alternative solutions. The nurse caring for understands that which one of the following would be an appropriate nonpharmacologic intervention for this patient?
   A. Teach the patient about the side effects of treatments.
   B. Provide assistive services for the patient in performing daily activities, as needed.
   C. Empower the patient to communicate with her physician and caregivers regarding the severity of her symptoms.
   D. Encourage the patient to enroll in a yoga class.

# 43 Nutritional Issues

1. Mr. Johns, a 75-year-old male patient, is currently undergoing treatment for tonsillar cancer and has a gastrostomy tube for tube feedings. Which one of the following symptoms might be assessed in the patient's enteral therapy?
   A. Confusion
   B. Constipation
   C. Bradycardia
   D. Bradypnea

2. E. N. is a 51-year-old female patient with Stage IV cancer. She is currently undergoing chemotherapy and reports no appetite, significant muscle weakness, and fatigue. The oncology nurse caring for her determines that she has lost 5% of her baseline weight over the past 6 months. Based on this assessment, E. N.'s signs and symptoms are most consistent with which one of the following?
   A. malnutrition
   B. anorexia
   C. cachexia
   D. depression

3. To minimize risk of the occurrence and severity of taste alterations during chemotherapy treatment, the oncology nurse should do which one of the following?
   A. Encourage the use of salt and pepper to enhance taste.
   B. Encourage the patient to drink one glass of alcoholic beverage prior to dinner.
   C. Instruct the patient to perform oral hygiene in the morning and at bedtime.
   D. Instruct the patient to suck on smooth, flat, tart candies or lozenges.

4. A risk factor for weight gain in patients with cancer is which one of the following?
   A. a multi-agent chemotherapy regimen
   B. immunotherapy
   C. adjuvant chemotherapy for lung cancer
   D. bisphosphonate therapy

5. In patients with weight loss, an intervention to promote comfort while eating is which one of the following?
   A. Administer pain medications if needed, 3 hours before eating.
   B. Encourage patients to perform oral hygiene only after meals.
   C. Encourage patients to consume cold foods.
   D. Administer nystatin suspension 5 minutes prior to eating.

6. Dysgeusia is defined as which one of the following?
   A. the loss of taste
   B. an unpleasant taste sensation
   C. a decrease in acuity in taste sensation
   D. an increase in acuity in taste sensation

7. D. R. is a 51-year-old female patient with cancer who comes to the clinic with a 5-pound weight loss since her last treatment 4 weeks ago. The patient states that she has lost her sense of taste. A recommendation that may help this symptom may include that the patient should do which one of the following?
   A. Have a glass of wine before dinner.
   B. Participate in cooking of meals.
   C. Encourage food intake without gravy; and sauces.
   D. Avoid chewing gum.

8. Anorexia can be caused by which one of the following?
   A. hypercalcemia
   B. hyperkalemia
   C. hypermagnesemia
   D. hypernatremia

9. Enteral nutrition therapy is given by which one of these approaches?
   A. Nephrostomy tube
   B. Tracheostomy tube
   C. Urostomy tube
   D. Naso-gastric tube

10. A risk factor for weight loss in a patient with cancer would include which one of the following?
    A. chemotherapy regimens containing steroids
    B. use of biologic medications
    C. diagnosis of non-Hodgkin lymphoma
    D. pleural effusions

11. Taste alterations may be due to which one of the following?
    A. thin saliva following radiation therapy
    B. excess zinc levels
    C. tamoxifen therapy
    D. candidiasis

12. Potential complications can arise from central line insertion for parenteral nutrition. Which one of the following is a nursing intervention for management of a pneumothorax?
    A. Perform chest radiography after insertion of subclavian catheter to verify placement.
    B. Regulate infusion on a volumetric pump for accuracy.
    C. Monitor the catheter for migration from the superior vena cava to another vein, while making a notation of patient complaint of pain in the neck and shoulder, as well as swelling in the surrounding area.
    D. Check each bottle or bag before and during infusion for color and clarity of solution.

13. A patient developed an air embolus as a complication from central line insertion for the use of parenteral therapy. Which one of the following is a nursing intervention for management of an air emboli?
    A. Observe for bright red blood pulsating from catheter.
    B. Clamp IV tubing immediately and place patient on left side in the Trendelenburg position.
    C. Infuse 10% dextrose in water solution peripherally or through other lumen of catheter at the same rate as with total parenteral nutrition (TPN) to prevent hypoglycemia.
    D. If sudden cessation of TPN occurs, infuse 10% dextrose in water solution peripherally at same rate as TPN.

14. Which one of the following nursing interventions would be most effective in the prevention of infection when administering parenteral nutrition?
    A. Check each bottle or bag before and during infusion for color and clarity of solution.
    B. Change all IV tubing per institutional or agency procedure, using aseptic technique, and avoid interrupting TPN for other infusions or blood collection.
    C. Change dressing, using clean technique, and following institutional procedure, while observing the site for redness, tenderness, swelling, and exudates.
    D. Check urine for sugar, ketones, and acetone every 6 hours.

15. Potential complications can arise from enteral tube placement and feedings. Which one of the following is a nursing intervention for prevention of abdominal distention, and for symptoms such as vomiting and diarrhea?
    A. Give continuous rather than bolus feeding.
    B. Flush nasogastric tube with hot water or pulsating motions.
    C. Give formula at room temperature.
    D. Verify proper placement via chest radiography and check placement each time using tube.

16. Controversies exist abound on how nutritional support therapy should be managed long-term for patients with cancer. Which one of the following is an example of a controversial stance on long-term nutritional support for patients with cancer?
    A. The benefits of nutritional support can be sustained over a long time period.
    B. Nourishing a patient with cancer may enhance tumor growth, rather than slow it, by improving the supply of nutrients to the body.
    C. The psychological impact of the patient's family is severe.
    D. Legality comes into question when providing long-term nutrition.

17. Which one of the following is an example of physical assessment a patient with cancer might undergo as part of an overall nutritional assessment?
    A. Measure of daily caloric intake
    B. Blood pressure and heart rate
    C. Measures of serum prealbumin, total protein, and serum transferrin to assess protein stores
    D. Weight in comparison with ideal body weight

18. Which one of the following is an example of laboratory data that could be collected for a patient with cancer as part of an overall nutritional assessment?
    A. Measure of allergic reactions to proteins in certain foods
    B. Skin turgor
    C. Muscle mass
    D. Nitrogen balance

19. A patient visits the clinic and expresses concerns about metabolic changes caused by cancer. To best answer the question, the nurse explains to the patient the impact of malignancy on the metabolism of which one of the following?
    A. vitamins and minerals
    B. pharmacologic agents including chemotherapy
    C. protein and calories
    D. mono- and polyunsaturated fats

20. Which one of the following medications may stimulate a person's appetite?
    A. Dexamethasone and opioids
    B. Megestrol acetate and dexamethasone
    C. Muscle relaxants and methylphenidate
    D. Opioids and metoclopramide

# 44 | Pain

1. A patient with metastatic cancer is currently receiving MS Contin twice a day and morphine immediate release every 4 hours as needed for bone pain with good control of symptoms. The patient's pain is best categorized as which one of the following?
   A. neuropathic pain with insidious breakthrough pain episodes
   B. chronic cancer-related pain
   C. acute cancer pain
   D. a combination of visceral, somatic, and neuropathic cancer-related pain

2. Which one of the following types of pain is poorly localized and results from nociceptor activation related to distention, compression, or infiltration of the thoracic or abdominal tissue?
   A. Somatic pain
   B. Sympathetically maintained pain
   C. Visceral pain
   D. Peripherally mediated neuropathic pain

3. Which part of the pain pathway involves the brain's attempt to modify the pain experience through the release of endogenous opioids, norepinephrine, and serotonin?
   A. Transduction
   B. Transmission
   C. Perception
   D. Modulation

4. An oncology nurse is seeing a patient who has been diagnosed with Stage III esophageal cancer. The patient has recently completed combined neoadjuvant therapy with chemotherapy and radiation. The oncology nurse would anticipate that the patient may experience the most pain symptoms from which one of the following?
   A. post-surgical incision
   B. lymphedema
   C. mucositis
   D. sinusitis

5. An oncology nurse is seeing a patient who has been diagnosed with Stage III esophageal cancer. The patient has recently completed combined neoadjuvant therapy with chemotherapy and radiation complicated by a shingles outbreak. The oncology nurse would anticipate that the patient may experience the most pain symptoms from which one of the following?
   A. post-herpetic neuralgia
   B. chemotherapy-induced peripheral neuropathy (CIPN)
   C. chemotherapy-induced lymphedema
   D. complex regional pain syndrome (CRPS)

6. J. M. is a 16-year-old male patient with acute leukemia who has just undergone intrathecal chemotherapy administration and is now complaining of a headache. When assessing the patient's pain, which one of the following scales would be most appropriate for pain assessment?
   A. Pain faces
   B. "0-10" scale
   C. Verbal descriptor – mild, moderate, severe
   D. Checklist of nonverbal pain indicators

7. D. V. is a 62-year-old male patient with lung cancer and multiple liver metastasis. He reports intermittent pain rated 6 out of 10 in the area of the tumor. He has a history of renal failure and diabetes. Using the World Health Organization's analgesic ladder, which one of the following may be considered the best initial treatment for this patient's pain?
   A. Acetaminophen 1000 mg four times per day
   B. Morphine 15 mg every 3 hours as needed
   C. Fentanyl patch 25 mcg/hour
   D. Oxycodone 5 mg/acetaminophen 325 mg combination (1-2 tablets) every 4 hours as needed

8. L. M. is a 59-year-old male patient with end stage pancreatic cancer. He is admitted to the hospital with intractable pain and is being treated with opioids. His wife has concerns of addiction and worries about withdrawal. The nurse's best response to L. M.'s wife is which one of the following?
   A. "While addiction is a risk, the drugs are useful, and we consider them to be the primary method for pain control."
   B. "There is no need for you to worry about addiction because of your husband's advanced cancer."
   C. "The patient is experiencing tolerance, which means he has increased needs of medication due to his disease."
   D. "The patient will not go through withdrawal because he is not addicted to the medicine."

9. Which one of the following best reflects an existential concern when conducting a comprehensive pain assessment?
   A. Fear of addiction with the use of opioids due to recent media attention.
   B. Depression related to the fatigue caused by the pain.
   C. Lack of mobility caused by the pain.
   D. Perception that pain is a punishment.

10. Which of the following categories of antidepressants do not have pain relieving properties?
   A. Mood stabilizers
   B. Serotonin-specific reuptake inhibitors
   C. Serotonin and norepinephrine reuptake inhibitors
   D. Tricyclic agents

11. Which one of the following best reflects a psychological concern when conducting a comprehensive pain assessment?
   A. Financial hardship as a result of paying for pain medication
   B. Influence of religion and prayer on coping with pain
   C. Use of traditional medicine in healing
   D. The patient's history of illnesses such as anxiety and depression

12. Which one of the following best reflects a social concern when conducting a comprehensive pain assessment?
   A. The patient's experience with coping with pain in the past.
   B. The patient's willingness to try non-traditional medicines.
   C. How a family caregiver responds to a patient's pain.
   D. The role of a spiritual community in a patient's ability to cope with pain.

13. Which one of the following best reflects a psychological concern when conducting a comprehensive pain assessment?
   A. The role of pain in the everyday life of the patient
   B. Definition of how patient differentiates pain and suffering
   C. The amount of support a patient receives, either at home or through their community
   D. Level of cognition, including any signs of confusion or delirium

14. In the pain assessment known as PQRST, which one of the following represents the "P" in the acronym?
   A. Pain
   B. Position
   C. Proximity
   D. Provocation/Palliation

15. In the pain assessment known as OLDCART, which one of the following represents the "R" in the acronym?
   A. Region
   B. Radiation
   C. Relation
   D. Relieving

# 45 Respiratory Symptoms

1. A nurse is administering a monoclonal antibody to a patient who develops a hypersensitivity reaction to include bronchospasm. The nurse understands that the mechanism of action in bronchospasm is due to:
   A. abnormal fluid accumulation in the lung
   B. compression of tracheobronchial tree
   C. aveolar hemorrhage
   D. bronchitis

2. K. L. is a 64-year-old female patient with a diagnosis of breast cancer 8 years ago. The nurse caring for her on an oncology unit reviews her medical history, and is aware that the patient is at risk for developing respiratory problems due to which one of the following?
   A. The patient's history of radiation therapy to the right breast.
   B. The patient's recent upper respiratory disease.
   C. The patient's history of axillary lymph node dissection.
   D. The patient's employment as a hair stylist.

3. J. L. is a 60-year-old male patient with prostate cancer. He is being assessed by a nurse in an oncology clinic with complaints of what the nurse suspects to be dyspnea. Based on her suspicion, the nurse's documentation might include which one of the following?
   A. He reports shortness of breath while taking a shower.
   B. He reports a past episode of anxiety 5 years ago.
   C. He uses two pillows to sleep.
   D. He has signs of clear, thin sputum production.

4. D. R. is a 62-year-old male patient who was admitted to an oncology unit for symptoms of dyspnea, and is undergoing work up for suspected lung cancer. The nurse caring for him knows the patient will be undergoing a PET scan, which measures the amount of which one of the following?
   A. air flow limitation
   B. disease involvement
   C. lung capacity
   D. air expulsion from their lungs

5. An oncology nurse is caring for a 59-year-old female patient with lung metastases who is complaining of shortness of breath. The nurse is preparing to educate the patient on measures that the she can take to increase the effectiveness of her breathing. Her teaching includes which one of the following?
   A. keeping the temperature warm in the house
   B. limiting activity to conserve energy
   C. decreasing the amount of fluid intake
   D. instructing the patient to use a walker

6. An oncology nurse is caring for a patient who develops immunotherapy-induced pulmonary toxicity. The oncology nurse is aware that this is caused by which one of the following?
   A. release of hormones into the vascular system
   B. the signaling of an antigen response
   C. equal amounts of dose and volume of drug administered
   D. an inflammatory process causing lung injury

7. A 52-year-old male patient with cancer is suspected of having pneumonitis. The oncology nurse caring for him is aware that the cardinal symptom of this condition when assessing the patient includes which one of the following?
   A. an elevated heart rate
   B. malaise
   C. dyspnea
   D. crepitus

8. T. S. is a 63-year-old patient on an oncology unit who has developed chemotherapy-induced pulmonary toxicity. The nurse is knowledgeable that the management of this condition includes which one of the following?
   A. The patient will be put on strict bedrest until resolution of symptoms.
   B. The patient might continue the chemotherapy at a reduced dose.
   C. Monitoring of electrocardiograms (ECGs) and echocardiogram (ECHO) will be required
   D. Serial arterial blood gas (ABG) will be required.

9. A nurse on an oncology unit is caring for a 61-year-old male patient with metastatic lung cancer. The nurse reviews the medical record of the patient and determines that he is at risk for shortness of breath due to which one of the following?
   A. metastases to the brain
   B. comorbidity of Crohn's disease
   C. advancing age
   D. 200 mL of IV fluids given over 24 hours

10. A nurse in an outpatient clinic is assessing a 54-year-old male patient who is being seen for signs of dyspnea and poor oxygenation. Which of the following findings could indicate chronic hypoxemia?
    A. A carotid artery pulse on palpation
    B. A perfusion index of 20%
    C. Upper-extremity swelling
    D. A ventilation rate 20/min

11. An oncology nurse is caring for a patient who has been admitted for dyspnea. The physician orders immediate-release oral opioids. The nurse knows the purpose of this is to:
    A. increase the physical and psychological demand to increase oxygen
    B. increase the release of histamines to increase permeability
    C. elevate the amount of carbon dioxide to reduce sighing
    D. decrease the central respiratory drive by reducing ventilatory demand

12. A nurse on the thoracic oncology floor is caring for a patient with a pleural effusion. The patient questions the nurse as to why this may have occurred. She responds that it is most likely due to the tumor causing:
    A. increased negative pressure in the pleural space
    B. development of spontaneous hemopericardium
    C. inflammation of the pleural space
    D. formation of pustules within the pleural space due to infection

13. On assessing a patient with a pleural effusion, on examination the nurse is most likely to find:
    A. rhonchi and rales
    B. tracheal shift to the left
    C. egophony
    D. resonance upon percussion

14. A nurse is caring for a patient with a pleural effusion. She is aware that the most efficacious, evidence-based treatment for this patient is:
    A. insertion of a peritoneal catheter to drain fluid
    B. wedge resection to remove a portion of pleural effusion
    C. immunotherapy to decrease the tumor
    D. therapeutic aspiration with an intrapleural chemical agent

15. In caring for patient who had a therapeutic aspiration for a pleural effusion, the nurse is aware of the need to continually monitor:
    A. the type of fluid draining from the catheter
    B. fluid build-up around the insertion site
    C. the rate of fluid re-accumulation
    D. magnesium levels after the procedure

16. Which one of the following chemotherapy or targeted therapy agents is associated with pulmonary and radiologic abnormalities and hemoptysis?
    A. Bortezomib
    B. Alpha-interferon
    C. Erlotinib
    D. Bevacizumab

17. Which one of the following chemotherapy or targeted therapy agents is associated with pulmonary and radiologic abnormalities most associated with acute pneumonitis?
    A. Sorafenib
    B. Busulfan
    C. Etoposide
    D. Doxorubicin

18. Which one of the following chemotherapy or targeted therapy agents is associated with pulmonary and radiologic abnormalities related to hypersensitivity reactions?
    A. Sorafenib
    B. L-asparaginase
    C. Carmustine
    D. Thalidomide

19. Abnormal accumulation of air within the pleural space is known as which one of the following?
    A. an empyema
    B. a pneumothorax
    C. parenchymal disease
    D. a pleural effusion

20. Which one of the following would a nurse anticipate for a patient with cancer who has just been given a diagnosis of empyema?
    A. Treatment will involve radiation therapy to the lung field(s)
    B. Systemic antibiotics will be used to treat the infection
    C. Subcutaneous epinephrine 1:100 solution will be used
    D. The patient will be placed in a semi-Fowler position and oxygen will be given at 30% face mask

21. J. D. is a 52-year-old male patient with cancer, who has been receiving a combination of radiation therapy and bleomycin (Blenoxane) chemotherapy. The oncology nurse caring for him knows that he will be at risk for which one of the following types of pulmonary toxicity?
    A. Hemothorax
    B. Pulmonary empyema
    C. Pneumonitis
    D. Pleural effusion

22. Which one of the following classes of pharmacologic agents is used to decrease the level of inflammation in a patient who has been diagnosed with dyspnea?
    A. Bronchodilators
    B. Glucocorticoids
    C. Antibiotics
    D. Diuretics

# 46 Sleep Disturbances

1. Which one of the following best describes sleep-wake disturbances?
   A. An active biobehavioral process that causes night-time anxiety.
   B. Actual or perceived interruption in sleep with resulting daytime impairment.
   C. Transient inability to initiate or maintain sleep.
   D. Circadian rhythm disorders.

2. G. K. is a 58-year-old male patient who complains to his nurse that he is feeling very tired secondary to issues with falling asleep. However, once fallen asleep, he sleeps soundly. Which one of the following class of medications would be best to assist this patient in falling asleep?
   A. Antihistamines
   B. Antipsychotics
   C. Alpha-adrenergic receptor blockers
   D. Antidepressants

3. Which one of the following interventions will help to promote sleep hygiene?
   A. Make sure the patient has their last cup of coffee in the early evening.
   B. Have the patient go to bed even if they are not sleepy.
   C. Encourage the patient to watch TV prior to falling asleep help calm down.
   D. Educate the patient to keep their room cool and dark.

4. F. J. is a 71-year-old male patient who tells the nurse caring for him that he has not been sleeping well. He reports that he wakes up every day at 6 am, and drinks a cup of coffee, he exercises each day, and then enjoys an afternoon nap. Which one of the following is the biggest risk factor for a sleep-wake disturbance in this patient?
   A. He wakes up at 6 am each morning.
   B. He drinks his coffee shortly after waking.
   C. He exercises each day.
   D. He enjoys an afternoon nap.

5. Which one of the following best describes the sleep-wake cycle?
   A. Non-rapid eye movement phase of sleep until, waking in the morning.
   B. Rapid eye movement, non-rapid eye movement and the awakening phase.
   C. Rapid eye movement phase and non-rapid-eye movement phase, with repeat cycles approximately every 90 minutes.
   D. Rapid eye movement phase and non-rapid eye movement phase, with repeat cycles lasting approximately every 180 minutes.

6. Which one of the following represents the best time to assess a patient's sleep cycle?
   A. At the initial patient assessment.
   B. After their first cycle of chemotherapy.
   C. At the beginning and end of all treatment.
   D. At regular intervals and with any changes in clinical status.

7. A patient with cancer reveals that he is awake often at night and relates this condition to job concerns, feelings of anxiousness, and fear of what the future holds. He also reports having pain in his hip. Of his concerns, which one of the following describes a physical stressor?
   A. Job concerns
   B. Feelings of anxiousness
   C. Fear of the future
   D. Pain in his hip

8. Which one of the following diagnostic tests is utilized to assess sleep?
   A. Electorencephalogram (EEG)
   B. Polysomnography
   C. NCCN Distrress Thermometer
   D. Assessment of sleep patterns including usual bedtime, bedtime routine, and usual time to sleep

# 47 Altered Body Image

1. Altered body image is defined as which one of the following?
   A. As a change in a patient's perception of how friends react to the change.
   B. As a change in a patient's perception of how they feel about themselves.
   C. As a change in a patient's perception of how other individuals view them.
   D. As a change in a patient's perception of how their children will respond or have responded to them.

2. Which one of the following nursing interventions is the most supportive in facilitating acceptance of a change in body image?
   A. Providing a time frame to grieve and then quickly moving on.
   B. Facilitating conversations between the patient and long-lost family members.
   C. Encouraging self-compassion and use of previously successful coping strategies.
   D. Educating family members pre-operatively regarding body image changes.

3. When assisting an oncology patient's reintegration into the workplace, the nurse should do which one of the following?
   A. Tell the patient it is going to be all right and it is time to get back to work.
   B. Go into the workplace and share information about the patient's treatment with his employer.
   C. Encourage them to take a lot of time off in order to regain emotional strength.
   D. Assist patients in verbalizing concerns, allow for dialogue and identify support.

4. When describing chemotherapy-induced alopecia, which one of the following statements should the nurse use as an explanation regarding the patient's condition?
   A. "Hair loss is total including eyebrows."
   B. "It typically starts 2 days after chemotherapy."
   C. "Hair regrowth is 2-4 weeks after treatment."
   D. "Hair regrowth may take more than 3 years."

5. When assessing for psychosocial adjustment, body image issues are most significantly reduced in cancer survivors who are which one of the following?
   A. females
   B. socially supported
   C. younger
   D. recently diagnosed

6. Which one of the following patient outcome behaviors represents the highest level of adaptation to body image changes?
   A. The patient dicusses plans to return to previous work role.
   B. The patient discusses changes in body structure and function.
   C. The patient serves as a volunteer in a client-to-client visitation program.
   D. The patient lists emergency resources to deal with self-destructive behavior.

7. J. C. is a 46-year-old female breast cancer survivor with altered body image. She asks her oncology nurse how she should help her 12-year-old daughter best adjust to the changes in her mother's body. Her oncology nurse informs the patient that she should do which one of the following?
   A. Have another family member discuss it with her.
   B. Keep a limited, structured communication style in place.
   C. Discuss the illness and treatment with her.
   D. Inform the daughter when the disease treatment is complete.

**99**

8. H. K. is a 39-year-old female patient with breast cancer who has undergone a mastectomy and is distressed over showing her body to her husband. Which one of the following statements by the patient's nurse is defined as an empathic approach to a nursing communication strategy with the patient?
    A. "Don't worry, you look great, your husband won't even notice after a while."
    B. "When you look in the mirror, what is it that you see?"
    C. "Have you talked about how you feel with your husband?"
    D. "This must be a huge adjustment for you."

9. J is a 50-year-old male patient who has been ordered to have a colostomy bag. He refuses to wear a bag, worried that the bag will be visible through his clothes, and his wife won't come near him. Which one of the following statements by the patient's nurse is defined as a typical approach to a nursing communication strategy with the patient?
    A. "Tell me more about why you are so concerned."
    B. "Have you talked over any of this with your wife."
    C. "If you don't get proper treatment, you will die."
    D. "I understand the thought of having a colostomy bag is difficult to accept, and you have a lot of concerns."

# 48 Caregiver Burden

1. Which one of the following statements is true regarding caregiver burden?
   A. Caregiver burden is a continuum of healthcare activities for someone unable to independently care for themselves.
   B. Caregiver burden is provision of services and support and health management for the well-being of another person.
   C. Caregiver burden is a time-sensitive, life-changing commitment and experience.
   D. Caregiver burden is influenced by multiple patient and caregiver co-morbidities and symptoms.

2. Which one of the following is true regarding the Caregiving, Advise, Record, and Enable (CARE) Act?
   A. CARE applies to the ambulatory setting
   B. CARE supports family caregivers who work
   C. CARE requires hospitals to record family caregiver name
   D. CARE oversees a tax credit for qualified expenses to help a loved one.

3. Which one of the following demographic features is associated with a higher level of caregiver burden distress?
   A. Male gender
   B. Holding a graduate degree
   C. Lives in a separate residence
   D. Younger in age

4. When assessing health risk factors of the caregiver, which one of the following would be a physiological factor?
   A. Cardiometabolic risk
   B. Weight gain
   C. Excessive sleep
   D. Social isolation

5. A nurse asks a caregiver, "What medical problems does your care recipient have?" The nurse is assessing the caregiver's perception of the patient's:
   A. cognitive status
   B. health status
   C. caregiving needs
   D. caregiver values

6. Caregiving has become a major public health concern due to which one of the following?
   A. an aging and growing population
   B. lack of formal caregiver training
   C. an economic burden
   D. impact on long standing relationships

7. The role of the caregiver is normally associated with which one of the following?
   A. compensated work
   B. time limited care
   C. assisting with daily care
   D. financial responsibility to cover medical care.

8. Which one of the following creates an environmental stressor that can cause depression in both the caregiver and recipient?
   A. Involvement of secondary caregiver
   B. Caregiver resilience
   C. Plan of care not documented
   D. Dependency

9. Therapeutic communication between the caregivers and healthcare team should occur:
   A. at onset of caregiving experience
   B. continuously
   C. at advance care planning appointment
   D. through the patient

10. Which one of the following caregiver clinical tools measures caregiver burden through such factors as employment, finances, physical, social, and time aspects, and includes 13 number of items?
    A. Caregiver Reaction Assessment
    B. Caregiver Strain Index
    C. Caregiver Burden Scale
    D. Zarit Burden Interview

11. The nurse is assessing the caregiver profile. Which of the following information would be included?
    A. Length of time in the caregiver role
    B. If the care recipient homebound
    C. Educational level of the caregiver
    D. Presence of additional paid caregivers

# 49 Cultural and Spiritual Care

1. Culture is defined as which one of the following?
   A. customary beliefs, social forms, material traits, and characteristic features of everyday existence shared by people of a racial, religious, or social group in a place or time
   B. a condition of being composed of differing elements, especially the inclusion of people of different races or cultures in a group
   C. a social construct based on expressed phenotype, in which people are categorized based on external, selective, and arbitrary physical features
   D. a heritage of historical, contextual, and geographic experiences of a specific community or population

2. Race and ethnicity differ from each other in which one of the following ways?
   A. Race is identified in social definitions, whereas ethnicity is identified by biological foundations.
   B. Race is based in cultural heritage, whereas ethnicity is based in social construct.
   C. Race is based on external, selective, arbitrary physical features and genetic make-up, whereas ethnicity is based on historical, cultural, contextual, and geographic experience of community.
   D. Race is based in the identity of wide racial diversity within shared characteristics based on geographic, historic, contextual, and cultural group of origin, whereas ethnicity is based on the phenotype of a culture that expresses observable characteristics such as skin tone, hair texture, and eye color.

3. Race may be defined by which one of the following?
   A. phenotype
   B. geographic experiences
   C. cultural heritage
   D. historical origins

4. As an oncology nurse, it is important to understand that cultural norms influence relationships between healthcare practitioners and patients or caregivers. When communicating with patients, an oncology nurse may consider avoiding which one of the following?
   A. folding hands in lap
   B. planting feet solidly on the floor while seated
   C. giving the "thumbs up" gesture
   D. standing at least 2 feet away from the patient or caregiver

5. Spiritual distress can result in a disconnect from which one of the following?
   A. religious practices
   B. sacred ties to a higher power
   C. cultural heritage
   D. a faith-based organization

6. Poverty may lead to late-stage diagnosis of cancer due to which one of the following?
   A. lack of quality healthcare despite adequate access to facilities
   B. necessity to prioritize basic needs over seeking cancer care
   C. higher exposure to poor nutrition, workplace carcinogens, and modifiable risk factors
   D. regular cancer screening

7. Modifiable risk factors that lead to a higher risk of cancer in poor people include which one of the following?
   A. smoking tobacco
   B. homelessness
   C. poor nutrition
   D. workplace carcinogens

8. Responses to a diagnosis of cancer varies widely based on a person's cultural norms and behaviors. Which one of the following factors may hinder a person's willingness to undergo cancer screening?
   A. Emphasis on traditional healers
   B. Fear of having to be in a clinical trial for treatment
   C. Ignorance of cancer treatment process
   D. Fatalistic view of a cancer diagnosis, with cancer being synonymous with certain death and the inability to change this

9. F. L. is a 58-year-old female who was admitted for hematopoietic stem cell transplantation. She divulges to her oncology nurse the healing impact that caring for her rose garden has had on her life, and that she will miss her weekly ritual once discharged after her transplant. The oncology nurse realizes that her relationship with nature is rooted in which one of the following?
   A. religion
   B. spirituality
   C. culture
   D. ethnicity

10. Which one of the following terms is defined as protected knowledge, typically bestowed by a higher power, that exists outside the parameters of an established faith?
    A. Religion
    B. Sacred
    C. Spirituality
    D. Belief

11. An oncology nurse may assess the level of spiritual support that a patient or caregiver needs by doing which one of the following?
    A. consulting pastoral services
    B. praying with the patient
    C. reading a passage from a holy scripture of the patient's religion
    D. deep listening

12. The nurse is caring for a patient with cancer from a different culture than other patients on the unit and from her own. When the nurse enters the patient's room, the patient maintains a downward gaze and avoids eye contact. Which one of the following represents an indication of the most likely cause of the patient's actions?
    A. The patient is not comfortable with cultural diversity and healthcare providers.
    B. The patient's culture may view direct eye contact as a sign of disrespect.
    C. The patient is dealing with depression related to her cancer diagnosis.
    D. The patient wants the nurse to avoid close physical contact.

13. Spirituality and religion are not mutually exclusive and are not interchangeable. Which one of the following statements is most accurate when describing the concepts of religion and spirituality?
    A. Religion describes organized systems of faith that follow regulated group practices.
    B. Spirituality applies to persons who practice the tenets of organized religion.
    C. A fatalistic view is seldom seen in an individual with strong spiritual or religious beliefs.
    D. The role of spirituality and religion will stay consistent across the stages of cancer.

# 50 Psychosocial Considerations

1. One of the primary treatment approaches for patients experiencing severe cancer related distress is the use of which one of the following?
   A. An antidepressant medication (SSRI) prescription and a referral to psychiatry
   B. an anti-anxiolytic every 4 hours and imagery
   C. psychotherapy and a benzodiazepine agent
   D. psychotropic medications and hydrotherapy

2. An oncology nurse is caring for a 60-year-old female patient with metastatic disease. She is on third-line therapy and has difficulty concentrating, frequently cancels appointments, and has had emotional outbursts with family and the medical team. There is no history of past mental illness or unusual behavior. The oncology nurse recognizes that the correct course of action is which one of the following?
   A. Discuss hospice with the healthcare team as the patient does not want to continue treatments.
   B. Ask to be removed from the patient's care because the patient refuses to cooperate with the medical team.
   C. Consider asking the healthcare team if the patient should be seen for a psychology evaluation.
   D. Her behavior is a normal symptom in patients receiving third-line treatment and the patient should be treated with an anti-anxiolytic.

3. Possibly non-psychiatric causes of depression may include which one of the following?
   A. well-controlled HTN
   B. hypocalcemia
   C. vitamin B12 deficiency
   D. hyperglycemia

4. An oncology nurse is teaching a patient with cancer about how to take their new antidepressant medication (SSRI). The oncology nurse knows that teaching has been successful when the patient verbalizes which one of the following?
   A. "If I do not feel differently after 2 weeks, I should stop my medication immediately and see my doctor at the first available visit."
   B. "It may take several weeks to months for this medication to work, and I need to keep taking it as prescribed, and see my therapist regularly."
   C. "This medication will work right away, and I will be able to get better sleep and wake up feeling refreshed."
   D. "This medication can have interactions with other drugs, and I should talk to my doctor before starting any new medications, but herbal supplements are okay to take."

5. When caring for a pediatric patient, which one of the following interventions will assist in preventing their loss of personal control while being treated for cancer? Pediatric patients should:
   A. be allowed to make decisions in their own care
   B. be distracted with books, toys, and TV
   C. defer to their parents serve as the decision-makers
   D. keep the patient out of the room when discussing treatment options

6. Practical and effective nursing strategies to address multiple aspects of psychological distress and impaired coping are to do which one of the following?
   A. Provide educational materials about the patient's diagnosis, treatment, and care plan.
   B. Automatically have all patients screened by a social worker before beginning treatment.
   C. Screen patients as needed only if they are displaying symptoms of psychological distress.
   D. Avoid asking questions about potentially sensitive subjects, because this will impair coping.

7. The best nursing intervention to identify cancer-related distress in the cancer patient is to do which one of the following?
   A. Screen for distress within the first several visits.
   B. Ask the family about the patient's distress during each clinic visit.
   C. Screen for distress when symptoms are identified.
   D. Observe the patient's behavior and screen as necessary.

8. A risk factor for complicated grief includes which one of the following?
   A. an expected death for a terminal condition
   B. a deep emotional relationship to the deceased
   C. a large multi-generational family
   D. an ambivalent relationship to the deceased

9. Which one of the following types of patients are at the highest risk for emotional distress?
   A. diagnosis of breast cancer, newly promoted to manager at work, history of anxiety
   B. diagnosis of lung cancer, employed for 35 years in same company, history of arthritis
   C. diagnosis of stage 1 breast cancer, recently retired and history of depression
   D. diagnosis of lung cancer, newly promoted to vice president of company, and poor pain control

**104**

10. A patient receiving which one of the following medications is at increased risk for experiencing anxiety?
    A. beta-adrenergic stimulants
    B. angiotension receptor blockers
    C. angiotensin-converting enzyme inhibitors
    D. beta blockers

11. Which one of the following statements is true regarding reactive depression?
    A. Reactive depression is more common in elderly persons.
    B. Reactive depression is a normal response to a precipitating event or situation.
    C. Reactive depression commonly occurs in people taking corticosteroids for cancer treatment.
    D. Reactive depression is more common in persons who have experienced domestic abuse.

12. A person experiencing loss of control might manifest in which one of the following?
    A. excessive house cleaning
    B. frequent outbursts
    C. frequent compliments to staff on care delivery
    D. reluctance to express emotions

13. Developmentally, a 6 year old might view the death of a parent as which one of the following?
    A. as a punishment for bad behavior
    B. as a temporary situation
    C. as a separation
    D. as a threat to independence

14. Symptoms of grief include which one of the following sets of terms?
    A. hyperactivity, distractibility, and avoidance
    B. intrusive thoughts, sleep disturbances, and occupational lapses
    C. preoccupation with loss, hyperactivity, and increased energy
    D. changing beliefs or views, increased energy, and rumination

15. J. W. is a 55-year-old male patient who is undergoing chemotherapy. He is experiencing problems with coping. To help, he decides to engage in a weekly support group and see a counselor. This is an example of which one of the following?
    A. problem-focused coping
    B. emotion-focused coping
    C. primary-appraisal coping
    D. meaning-focused coping

16. Symptoms of anxiety includes which one of the following sets of symptoms?
    A. feelings of suffocation, dizziness, fatigue or exhaustion
    B. palpitations, eating disturbances, feeling of worthlessness or guilt
    C. difficulty swallowing, crying easily, insomnia
    D. sense of impending doom, easily overwhelmed, psychomotor agitation

17. Symptoms of depression include which one of the following pairs of symptoms?
    A. easily overwhelmed, change of appetite
    B. unable to relax, insomnia
    C. sense of impending doom, hypersomnia
    D. decreased energy, recurrent thoughts of death or suicide

18. H. K. is a 49-year-old female who has been recently diagnosed with cancer. She has reported having trouble coping with her diagnosis and has said she feels "sad." Her oncology nurse is evaluating her patient's condition to determine if she is at risk for a diagnosis of a major depressive disorder. Which one of the following symptoms should the nurse recognize as a potential sign that her patient should be referred for further evaluation?
    A. H. K. is complaining of a sense of impending doom.
    B. H. K. is highly agitated and easily overwhelmed.
    C. H. K. is having trouble swallowing and often feels suffocated.
    D. H. K. is reporting that she'll sleep well into the afternoon on a regular basis.

19. H. K. – the 49-year-old female patient with cancer from the previous question – is being evaluated to determine if she is at risk for diagnosis of a major depressive disorder. As part of her evaluation, her nurse knows that H. K. will be evaluated for both subjective and objective symptoms. Which one of the following is an example of an objective symptom?
    A. Report of depressed mood
    B. Report of insomnia
    C. Measurement of weight loss or gain
    D. Report of feeling worthless or guilty

20. Which one of the following is a characteristic of the HADS assessment tool for distress?
    A. 0 (no distress) to 10 (severe distress) measurement, with accompanying simple questions identifying source of distress
    B. 14-item scale (7 questions: anxiety; 7 questions: depression)
    C. Recommendation that score of 4 or more triggers further physician or nurse evaluation, referral to psychosocial services, or both
    D. Score from 0 to 25 (0-5 per question) to evaluate anxiety or depression levels

**105**

21. Distress is a multidimensional construct that:
    A. is impacted by developmental stage, phase of disease, past coping skills, and available resources
    B. does not require routine screening, because patients will self-identify if they need help
    C. has a simple straightforward process for management
    D. is a normal response to a diagnosis of cancer and seldom needs additional intervention

22. The family of a patient who died 2 months ago is planning a visit to the cancer center to meet with staff. Which one of the following grief responses by the family would cause the nurse who had cared for the deceased patient the greatest concern?
    A. Crying, angry outbursts, and accusations
    B. Preoccupation with the deceased family member
    C. Somatic symptoms similar to the deceased
    D. Withdrawal or social isolation

# 51 Sexuality and Sexual Dysfunction

1. The PLISSIT model of sexual health communication stands for which one of the following?
   A. patient to discuss the topic, provide limited information, provide specific suggestions, request intensive therapy
   B. permission to discuss the topic, provide limited information, provide specific suggestions, refer for intensive therapy
   C. push to discuss the topic, provide written and detailed information, provide general suggestions, refer for intensive therapy
   D. permission to discuss the topic, provide detailed information, provide general suggestions, refer for intensive therapy if patient requests

2. Which one of the following is an example of a non-pharmacologic intervention for sexual concerns in cancer?
   A. Eros therapy for clitoral stimulation
   B. Lubricant oil
   C. Natural herbs
   D. Couple's counseling targeting communication and relationship dynamics

3. Nurses and physicians may hesitate to ask about sexuality because of which one of the following?
   A. Nurses and physicians may hold biased beliefs about the patient's age, prognosis or partner availability.
   B. Nurses and physicians know sexuality questions were already asked at the initial patient assessment.
   C. Nurses and physicians are aware that patients do not want to be asked questions about this topic.
   D. Nurses and physicians assume patients have access to internet information and do not need further information.

4. A sexual practice that can be safely practiced when immunocompromised or thrombocytopenic is which one of the following?
   A. stoma coitus
   B. vaginal stimulation without lubrication
   C. massage, caressing, kissing
   D. nipple or penile rings

5. Which one of the following is true regarding fertility preservation?
   A. Does not affect quality of life
   B. Does not affect sexual function
   C. Does constitute a key survivorship issue
   D. Does not affect treatment decision-making

6. J. M. is a 41-year-old female patient with breast cancer who is getting ready to begin chemotherapy. Her oncology nurse knows that the patient should be aware of which one of the following?
   A. She may be affected by menopausal changes.
   B. Her libido may be increased.
   C. She cannot engage in sexual intercourse.
   D. She may experience increased vaginal secretions and discharge

7. Which one of the following statements is true about anti-Müllerian hormone (AMH)?
   A. AMH is the most reliable strategy to assess ovarian reserve, but only in women under the age of 25 years.
   B. AMH is the most reliable strategy to assess ovarian reserve and predict onset of menopause, but only in women under the age of 25 years.
   C. AMH is the most reliable strategy to assess ovarian size, but only in women over the age of 25 years.
   D. AMH is the most reliable strategy to assess ovarian reserve and predict onset of menopause, but only in women over the age of 25 years.

8. Which one of the following is a fertility preservation option for males?
   A. Oophoropexy
   B. Spermatogonial diploid stem cells
   C. Oocyte cryopreservation
   D. Gonadotropin-releasing hormone agonist hormone

9. General recommendations suggest waiting at least which one of the following periods of time before attempting to conceive after cancer treatment is complete?
   A. 3-6 months
   B. 6-12 months
   C. 12 months
   D. 24-36 months

10. In the "5 A's" discussion model to enhance sexual health communication, which one of the following examples is the definition of the "advise" step?
    A. Bring the topic up
    B. Ask about sexual functioning
    C. Provide information and resources
    D. Normalize symptoms and acknowledge the problems

11. Which one of the following is a benefit of fertility preservation counseling?
    A. Decreased sense of control
    B. Decreased distrust of and resentment toward medical staff
    C. Decreased communication amongst couples
    D. Less realistic expectations about future planning

12. Which one of the following age groups is least likely to be given the opportunity to discuss their concerns about sexuality?
    A. Males of any age
    B. Females of any age
    C. Males between the ages of 25 and 50
    D. Males and females who are terminally ill

13. Which one of the following is a potential change that would affect sexuality or sexual functioning in a patient with cancer due to the treatment of steroids in either men or women?
    A. Alopecia to include the loss of pubic hair
    B. Peripheral neuropathy
    C. Infertility
    D. Reduced sexual function and decreased sexual desire

14. Which one of the following is a potential change that would affect sexuality or sexual functioning in a patient with cancer due to the treatment of pelvic radiation therapy for men?
    A. Vascular or nerve damage causing temporary or permanent erectile dysfunction
    B. Decreased or loss of libido
    C. Flu-like symptoms that could affect libido
    D. Mouth sores that could affect sexual behavior

15. Which one of the following is a potential change that would affect sexuality or sexual functioning in a patient with cancer due to the treatment of chemotherapy for women?
    A. Decreased vaginal elasticity/stenosis
    B. Diarrhea that affect sexual behavior
    C. Vaginal stomatitis
    D. Chest pain and shortness of breath that might affect sexual behavior

16. In the PLISSIT model for sexual counseling, the "P" in the model, which stands for "permission," conveys which one of the following messages?
    A. Any sexual activity is deemed as appropriate behavior.
    B. Dosage levels of treatments that are known to cause sterility in patients with cancer are similar in both males and females.
    C. About 95% of women older than 40 years of age will be sterile with 20 Gy over 5 to 6 weeks.
    D. Pelvic radiation in men at greater than 6 Gy causes temporary sterility.

17. C. K. is a 27-year-old female who has just been diagnosed with cancer. She asks if the diagnosis means that she will not be able to have children. She adds, "Will I even live long enough to see my first baby?" The response of the nurse caring for her would be guided by which one of the following?
    A. Awareness of the need to address preservation of fertility from a preventive model.
    B. Stressing to her patient at diagnosis the improvements that have been made in survival with cancer treatment and the need to focus on care
    C. Understanding that, at the patient's current age, there will be a variety of fertility options available to her in the future
    D. Providing the reassurance to her patient that when she survives the treatment, adoption will always be an option

18. H. W. is a 37-year-old woman who is undergoing chemotherapy for ovarian cancer. It is important for her oncology nurse to educate her on which one of the following?
    A. The patient may be affected by premature menopausal changes.
    B. The patient's libido will be increased.
    C. Intercourse for the patient will be impossible because of the pain.
    D. Side effects of chemotherapy will not interfere with sexual activity.

# 52 Metabolic Emergencies

1. The oncology nurse is caring for Mr. L., a 74-year-old male patient with advanced prostate cancer, who has been admitted to the hospital for workup of suspected disseminated intravascular coagulation (DIC). The oncology nurse explains to Mr. L. and his family that DIC is which one of the following?
   A. systemic disorder of coagulation resulting in the consumption of platelets and coagulation factors
   B. systemic disorder of hematopoiesis due to the lack of available hemoglobin
   C. systemic disorder of coagulation related to the overproduction of platelets and coagulation factors
   D. local disorder of coagulation leading to the consumption of platelets and coagulation factors within a single organ

2. The oncology nurse caring for Mr. L. should assess him for which set of signs and symptoms often associated with DIC?
   A. Bradycardia and dizziness
   B. Itching and flushing
   C. Diaphoresis and thirst
   D. Pallor and petechiae

3. Knowledge of the sequence of events that triggers the development of DIC helps the oncology nurse understand that successful treatment of Mr. L's DIC is aimed at which one of the following?
   A. identifying and treating the underlying cause
   B. administering platelet transfusions as the only source of treatment
   C. identifying the precipitating genetic mutations
   D. administering prophylactic anticoagulants to prevent clots

4. The oncology nurse should focus on which one of the following non-pharmacological measures in the management of Mr. L's DIC?
   A. transfusing platelets and fresh frozen plasma until normal laboratory values are reached
   B. educating the patient and caregiver to use a straight edge razor when shaving
   C. applying pressure to bleeding sites as appropriate
   D. teaching the patient and caregiver to use non-steroidal anti-inflammatory drugs for pain

5. Thrombotic thrombocytopenic purpura (TTP) is a blood disorder characterized by widespread clotting in small blood vessels of the body, resulting in which one of these laboratory values?
   A. low platelet count and microangiopathic hemolytic anemia
   B. high platelet count and microangiopathic hemolytic anemia
   C. low platelet count and macroangiopathic hemolytic anemia
   D. high platelet count and macroangiopathic hemolytic anemia

6. The etiology of thrombotic thrombocytopenic purpura (TTP) is not well understood but the condition is commonly associated with which one of the following?
   A. an increase in ADAMTS 13 (a disintegrin and metalloproteinase with thrombospondin type I motif, 13)
   B. the presence of a Philadelphia chromosome
   C. a decrease of ADAMTS 13
   D. microsatellite instability that is seen on pathology exam

7. A patient on the oncology unit is experiencing mucosal bleeding. Laboratory test results reveal a decreased hemoglobin level and a decreased platelet count. Schistocytes are present on peripheral blood smears. The oncology nurse is aware that these changes may be signs that the patient is experiencing which one of the following?
   A. superior vena cava syndrome
   B. syndrome of inappropriate anti-diuretic hormone
   C. anaphylaxis
   D. thrombotic thrombocytopenic purpura

8. In the medical management of a patient experiencing thrombotic thrombocytopenic purpura (TTP), the oncology nurse would expect to receive an order for which of these interventions?
   A. Administer plasma exchange with fresh-frozen plasma.
   B. Withhold blood products.
   C. Initiate macrolide antibiotics for prophylaxis.
   D. Restrict fluids.

9. Syndrome of inappropriate antidiuretic hormone (SIADH) that develops in patients with cancer occurs when secretion of antidiuretic hormone (ADH), known as arginine vasopressin (AVP) in its active form, becomes dysregulated. Release of AVP is:
   A. appropriately triggered in the presence of normal or increased fluid balance
   B. inappropriately triggered despite the presence of normal or increased fluid balance
   C. inappropriately triggered in the presence of decreased fluid balance
   D. appropriately triggered in the presence of decreased fluid balance

10. Syndrome of inappropriate antidiuretic hormone (SIADH) can be caused by a variety of malignant and non-malignant conditions. The condition with the highest risk of SIADH is which one of the following?
    A. small cell lung cancer
    B. anti-tumor antibiotics
    C. congestive heart failure
    D. breast cancer

11. The nurse caring for a patient with SIADH should monitor for all of these signs and symptoms of SIADH **except**:
    A. Decreased serum sodium
    B. Normal serum potassium
    C. Increased urine output
    D. Decreased mentation

12. The oncology nurse caring for a patient with SIADH should expect that the patient's management will include which one of the following?
    A. initiation of a hypertonic saline infusion, 3% hypertonic saline infusion
    B. administration of a rapid infusion of hypertonic saline, 3% hypertonic saline infusion
    C. decreased oral intake of soy sauce and salty foods
    D. increased fluid intake to 2 L per day

13. Hypersensitivity reactions in cancer care are often associated with which one of the following?
    A. chemotherapy
    B. herbal remedies
    C. radiation therapy
    D. environmental toxins

14. Initial symptoms of a hypersensitivity reaction may include which one of the following?
    A. peripheral edema
    B. arrhythmia
    C. stridor
    D. flushing or rash

15. Which one of these conditions occurs because the patient's immune system was previously sensitized to a particular allergen and produces severe symptoms when the patient is re-exposed to the same allergen?
    A. Thrombotic thrombocytopenic purpura (TTP)
    B. Anaphylaxis
    C. Disseminated intravascular coagulation (DIC)
    D. Sepsis

16. A patient is demonstrating signs of anaphylaxis minutes after the second cycle of paclitaxel is initiated. The chemotherapy nurse immediately stops the infusion and gets ready to administer which one of the following agents used for first line pharmacologic management of anaphylaxis?
    A. epinephrine
    B. inhaled alpha agonist
    C. IV antibiotics
    D. H2 receptor agonists

17. A nurse in the oncology clinic examines Ms. A., a 77-year-old female patient who has chemotherapy-induced neutropenia. The oncology nurse is aware that Ms. A is at increased risk for sepsis and notes that which one of the following findings may be an early sign of sepsis in this patient?
    A. hypertension
    B. thrombocytopenia
    C. tachycardia
    D. fever

18. The oncology nurse sends Ms. A. to have blood drawn and monitors the laboratory results. The nurse focuses on which one of the following laboratory values that may indicate that Ms. A. is experiencing sepsis?
    A. white blood cell (WBC) count with a left shift
    B. increased platelets
    C. normal prothrombin time (PT)/international normalized ratio (INR)
    D. hypoglycemia

19. Patients at increased risk of tumor lysis syndrome (TLS) are those with malignancies associated with a high burden of rapidly proliferating cells, such as the leukemias. TLS is an oncologic emergency that occurs when cytotoxic treatment causes the rapid destruction of large numbers of tumor cells. Diagnosis of TLS is typically based on the results of which one of the following tests?
A. complete blood count
B. PT/INR
C. electrolytes
D. glucose

20. Prevention of Tumor Lysis Syndrome (TLS) in patients at high risk of the complication following initiation of antineoplastic therapies includes administration of which one of the following?
A. IV hydration 24-48 hours prior to treatment initiation
B. potassium supplementation 24 hours prior to first infusion
C. antibiotics if WBC less than 4000
D. allopurinol beginning after initial chemotherapy cycle

21. Which one of the following is an example of the most commonly seen oncologic emergency?
A. Disseminated intravascular coagulation (DIC)
B. Syndrome of inappropriate antidiuretic hormone (SIADH)
C. Hypercalcemia
D. Tumor lysis syndrome (TLS)

22. Tumors associated with hypercalcemia include which one of the following?
A. prostate, breast, and lung
B. multiple myeloma, colon, and prostate
C. colon, breast, and leukemia
D. breast, thyroid, and pheochromoctyoma

23. Symptoms of severe hypercalcemia include which one of the following?
A. increased appetite, fatigue, and frequent urination
B. nausea/vomiting, coma, and polydipsia
C. hyperactivity, nocturia, and anorexia
D. lethargy, frequent urination, and hypertension

24. Which one of the following medications could be used in the treatment of hypercalcemia of malignancy in a patient with renal insufficiency?
A. Bevacizumab
B. Infliximab
C. Denosumab
D. Pembrolizumab

25. G. H. is a 71-year-old woman with a diagnosis of breast cancer. She was admitted to the hospital this afternoon with mental status changes. In reviewing the laboratory reports, the nurse caring for G. H. notes that the patient's serum calcium is 14 mg/dL, her potassium is 3.0 mEq/L, and her phosphorus is 7 mg/dL. Which one of the following metabolic emergencies should the nurse be most concerned about based on the laboratory values?
A. Hypercalcemia
B. Tumor lysis syndrome (TLS)
C. Disseminated intravascular coagulation (DIC)
D. Syndrome of inappropriate antidiuretic hormone (SIADH)

26. Treatment of hypercalcemia may include all of the following therapies **except**:
A. vasopressors
B. calcitonin
C. diuretic medications
D. bisphosphonates

27. Signs and symptoms of anaphylaxis include which one of the following?
A. fatigue
B. urticaria
C. pain around an intravenous insertion site
D. itching around an intravenous insertion site

# 53 Structural Emergencies

1. An oncology nurse is caring for a patient with breast cancer and brain metastases who has recently been admitted to the ICU for management of increased intracranial pressure. The cause of the increased intracranial pressure in this patient is most likely due to which one of the following?
   A. vitamin deficiency related to increased metabolic needs of tumor cells
   B. increased brain tissue volume related to expanding tumor
   C. head injury resulting in increased cerebral blood flow
   D. increased hormone production by the brain cancer cells

2. A nurse is caring for a patient on a hematology/oncology unit. A factor that may put the patient at risk for increased intracranial pressure (ICP) is which one of the following?
   A. history of cervical spine surgery
   B. patient's recent diagnosis of multiple myeloma
   C. recent treatment with high dose cytosine arabinoside
   D. history of degenerative disc disease

3. A nurse is assessing H. C., a 68-year-old-female patient with lung cancer who has received cranial radiation therapy as prophylaxis for lung cancer metastases to the brain. The patient reports that she is suffering from headaches, which are worse on awakening, nausea, vomiting, and weakness. The nurse caring for her suspects that the patient is exhibiting signs of which one of the following?
   A. delirium
   B. dehydration
   C. seizures
   D. increased ICP

4. H. C. is admitted to the oncology unit for work up of possible increased intracranial pressure (ICP). The nurse explains to the patient and her caregivers that the most reliable method to diagnose ICP is which one of the following?
   A. positron emission tomography (PET) with CT scan
   B. bone marrow biopsy
   C. labs to evaluate glucose and protein
   D. epidural ICP monitoring

5. H. C. is diagnosed with elevated intracranial pressure and is transferred to the ICU for immediate treatment to rapidly decrease the ICP. The oncology nurse caring for the patient should anticipate an order for which one of the following?
   A. radiation therapy to the head
   B. administration of systemic biotherapy agents
   C. intubation and hyperventilation
   D. injection of steroids into the cervical spine

6. Which of these nursing measures should be included in the management of H.C.'s increased intracranial pressure?
   A. Monitoring for decreased cardiac output, including decreased urine output
   B. Assisting patient to lay on their stomach to relieve pressure on the head
   C. Keeping the patient's head of bed low to prevent headaches
   D. Frequent suctioning to prevent aspiration of saliva

7. A patient with multiple myeloma presents to the oncology clinic with signs and symptoms of spinal cord compression. The nurse knows that spinal cord compression is an oncologic emergency that may have developed in this patient due to which one of the following?
   A. hypertrophy of vertebral bone due to disease involvement
   B. regeneration of bone marrow cells in the vertebrae
   C. compression of the spinal cord
   D. misalignment of the vertebrae because of improvement in the size of the tumor

8. An oncology nurse is assigned to care for Mr. P., a 75-year-old male patient who has just arrived on the unit for work up of suspected spinal cord compression. The oncology nurse understands that which one of the following is the diagnostic procedure of choice for assessing the extent of Mr. P.'s spinal cord involvement?
   A. Computerized tomography of the spine
   B. Positron emission tomography of the whole body
   C. Diagnostic radiology films of the thoracic spine
   D. Magnetic resonance imaging of the entire spine

9. A nurse is instructing the patient regarding management of his spinal cord compression. Education might include which one of the following?
   A. moderate exercise to improve motor function
   B. assessment for and reporting of sensory and sexual changes
   C. incontinence of stool, as it is likely and should be expected
   D. urinary hesitancy as the patient may have extended periods without urine output

10. A nurse on the oncology unit is caring for a male patient diagnosed with lung cancer in the right lung. When assessing the patient, the nurse notes distended jugular veins and facial swelling. The nurse is aware that, based on his cancer history, this patient is at increased risk for which one of the following?
    A. plaque deposition in the carotid vein
    B. pulmonary embolism
    C. obstruction of the superior vena cava
    D. myocardial infarction

11. A patient with non-small lung cancer arrives at the oncology clinic for a follow-up visit. The patient reports that he has dyspnea, feelings of fullness in his head, dysphagia, and nasal stuffiness upon awakening, but improves throughout the day. The nurse suspects the patient is experiencing signs of which one of the following?
    A. sinusitis
    B. pneumonia
    C. Churg-Strauss syndrome
    D. superior vena cava syndrome

12. An oncology nurse makes a post-discharge phone call to a patient who recently had a colon resection. The patient reports nausea and vomiting of orange-brown material with a fecal odor. The nurse recognizes that the symptoms the patient is describing may be due to an obstruction of which one of the following?
    A. proximal small intestine
    B. distal small intestine
    C. small bowel
    D. gastric outlet

13. While caring for a patient with mesothelioma who has been admitted for cardiac tamponade, the nurse is aware that the fluid accumulation in the pericardial sac may be a result of which one of the following?
    A. comorbid coronary artery disease
    B. confirmed accurate insertion of a new triple lumen central line
    C. increased capillary permeability secondary to chemotherapy
    D. leakage of fluid into the chest from a pneumothorax

14. A patient with a history of colon cancer has been admitted to the oncology unit for treatment of a bowel obstruction. The oncology nurse anticipates an order to prepare the patient for which one of the following interventions?
    A. removal of the colon with anastomosis
    B. administration of hyperosmolar agents to stimulate the bowel
    C. insertion of a biliary stent to bypass the obstruction
    D. injection of methylnaltrexone to relieve constipation

15. The nurse in the oncology clinic is assessing a patient who has developed pneumonitis while undergoing therapy for advanced kidney cancer. The nurse should recognize that the pneumonitis has most likely been caused by which of the following types of therapy?
    A. systemic hyperthermia
    B. issels immunotherapy vaccine
    C. dendritic cell treatment
    D. checkpoint inhibitor immunotherapy

16. A nurse is caring for a patient who recently had a colon resection. The patient is having new onset severe pain in the abdomen and states that the pain was initially manageable, but then has gotten much worse. The oncology nurse reports to the physician that she believes the patient has developed which one of the following?
    A. constipation
    B. post-surgical ileus
    C. bowel perforation
    D. addiction to pain medication

17. The oncology nurse is assessing a patient who has just been admitted to the unit. The nurse should recognize that a history of which one of the following factors would increase the patient's risk of developing compression of the spinal cord?
    A. Vertebral compression fracture
    B. Chronic myelogenous leukemia
    C. Osteomyelitis
    D. Childhood scoliosis

18. A 66-year-old male with SCLC is emergently admitted to the ICU with significant upper torso and facial swelling and severe shortness of breath. The oncology nurse should recognize that the most effective initial treatment for this patient is which one of the following?
    A. radiation therapy
    B. chemotherapy
    C. percutaneous stent placement
    D. surgical resection

19. A 57-year-old female presents for her check-up eight weeks after completing chest radiation and multi-modality combination therapy for lymphoma. She reports that she is unable to take in a full breath, has chest pain, and a low-grade fever. Her oncology nurse recognizes these symptoms may be due to which one of the following?
    A. superior vena cava syndrome
    B. myocardial effusion
    C. cardiac tamponade
    D. pneumonitis

20. A 78-year-old patient with a history of mesothelioma is admitted to the medicine unit with complaints of dyspnea upon exertion, tachycardia, and chest pain that intensifies when lying down. The patient has comorbid heart disease and has been treated for mesothelioma with doxorubicin and more than 4000 cGy of radiation to the chest. Based on the data provided, the nurse is aware that the patient is most likely experiencing which one of the following?
    A. superior vena cava syndrome
    B. cardiac tamponade
    C. costochondritis
    D. cardiomyopathy

21. A new oncology nurse is reviewing her assignment. She knows that the patient at highest risk for cardiac tamponade is:
    A. the 76-year-old male with mesothelioma
    B. the 42-year-old female with colon cancer
    C. the 62-year-old female with multiple myeloma
    D. the 62-year-old male with prostate cancer

22. In providing education to new nurses on the oncology unit, the experienced nurse should explain that superior vena cava syndrome occurs when:
    A. excess fluid collects in the pericardial space
    B. excess fluid collects in the pleural cavity
    C. extrinsic compression causes an obstruction of the superior vena cava
    D. excess fluid accumulates and causes intrinsic pressure within the vessel

23. The oncology nurse is reviewing the list of patients for the outpatient clinic scheduled for the next day. The nurse knows that which condition is most commonly associated with development of superior vena cava syndrome (SVCS)?
    A. Nonhodgkin lymphoma
    B. Thyroid cancer
    C. Metastatic breast cancer
    D. Multiple myeloma

24. A nurse on the oncology unit is caring for a male patient diagnosed with lung cancer in the right lung. When assessing the patient, the nurse notes distended jugular veins and facial swelling. The nurse is aware that, based on his cancer history, this patient is at increased risk for which one of the following?
    A. plaque deposition in the carotid vein
    B. pulmonary embolism
    C. obstruction of the superior vena cava
    D. myocardial infarction

25. J. L. is a 64-year-old female patient who has leukemia with a new diagnosis of leptomeningeal metastases. The oncology nurse should understand that the patient has metastatic disease located in which one of the following locations?
    A. lymph nodes
    B. spleen
    C. cerebrospinal fluid
    D. liver

26. J. L., the patient with leptomeningeal metastases, according to her daughter, has been mentally "off" for the past several weeks. The oncology nurse should assess the patient for the presence of which one of the following?
    A. bradycardia, respiratory distress, and hypertension
    B. constipation, increased appetite, and esophageal spasm
    C. euphoria, labile emotions, and manic episodes
    D. reduced urination and painful urination

27. Early detection of spinal cord compression (SCC) is essential for prompt intervention and preventing loss of function. The most common presenting symptom of SCC in patients with cancer is which one of the following?
    A. motor weakness and motor loss
    B. sensory loss
    C. neck and back pain
    D. bowel or bladder incontinence

28. Which one of the following are examples of early signs of SVCS?
    A. Muffled heart rate of 100 beats/min, abdominal distention, and fever
    B. Hypertension, bradycardia, widening of pulse pressure, and abnormal respirations
    C. Jugular vein distention and edema of the face, periorbital area, back, neck, upper thorax, breasts, and upper extremities
    D. Hypotension and Cheyne-Stoke respirations

# 54 Standards of Practice

1. To best understand the standards for professional practice in various oncology settings, the nurse should refer to which one of the following?
   A. Standards of Oncology Nursing Education: Generalist and Advanced Practice Levels
   B. Oncology Nursing Scope and Standards of Practice
   C. American Society of Clinical Oncology (ASCO)/ Oncology Nursing Society (ONS) Chemotherapy Administration Safety Standards
   D. a nurse recruiter at a Commission on Cancer Accredited Cancer Center

2. An oncology nurse unit educator is updating a policy. In this role she is responsible for which one of the following?
   A. her own self-assessment to guide professional growth
   B. integrating evidence-based science into practice
   C. determining if staff affected by the policies are in agreement with changes
   D. supporting continuing education programs

3. The ASCO/ONS Chemotherapy Administration Safety Standards are recognized by oncology nurses as which one of the following?
   A. a two-tiered system for nurses and physicians to report unsafe practices
   B. an evidence-based resource for locating current clinical trials
   C. interprofessional standards outlining best practices for reducing errors in administration
   D. a document for patients to better understand efficacy and side effects of antineoplastic therapy

4. An oncology nurse is caring for a young woman experiencing severe hot flashes related to treatment for her breast cancer. The nurse consults the Oncology Nursing Society Symptom Interventions. Which of the following statements is true about this resource?
   A. Oncology Nursing Society Symptom Interventions is a standard for professional oncology nursing practice.
   B. Oncology Nursing Society Symptom Interventions is a clinical practice guideline.
   C. Oncology Nursing Society Symptom Interventions is an evidence-based protocol.
   D. Oncology Nursing Society Symptom Interventions is a standard for multidisciplinary oncology practice.

5. An effective way for institutions to evaluate the required documentation of oncology care is to perform which one of the following?
   A. Survey the staff about ease in locating the policies related to documentation of care
   B. Hire a compliance consultant to review documentation policies
   C. Send all documents to the compliance department for review
   D. Do a side-by-side comparison of standards to current processes.

6. Standards of Oncology Practice include which one of the following set of components?
   A. Planning, coordination of care, ethics, and outcomes identification
   B. Assessment, diagnosis, coordination of care, health teaching, and health promotion
   C. Communication, collaboration, leadership, quality of practice
   D. Coordination of care, health teaching and health promotion, resource utilization, ethics

**115**

7. Which one of the following is a definition for standards for professional nursing practice?
   A. Statements that include recommendations for optimal patient care.
   B. Authoritative statements of the duties that subspecialties of nurses are expected to perform with competence.
   C. Authoritative statements of the duties that all registered nurses are expected to perform with competence.
   D. Recommendations of the duties that all registered nurses are expected to perform with competence.

8. Which one of the following statements is a definition of the education component in the Standards of Professional Performance?
   A. The oncology nurse partners with the patient and family, the interprofessional team, and community resources to optimize cancer care.
   B. The oncology nurse seeks and expands personal knowledge and competence that reflect the current evidence-based state of cancer care and oncology nursing.
   C. The oncology nurse identifies clinical dilemmas and problems appropriate for study while supporting research efforts.
   D. The oncology nurse considers factors related to safety, efficiency, effectiveness, and cost in planning and delivering care to patients.

# 55 Evidence-Based Practice

1. Which one of the following statements accurately describe evidence-based practice (EBP)?
   A. EBP has been implemented throughout the United States consistently.
   B. EBP contradicts pay-for-performance programs.
   C. Evolution of evidence is limited.
   D. Nonpayment for complications model exists when EBP is not followed.

2. Which one of the following statements accurately describes an element of the PICOT format?
   A. P = Patient
   B. I = Improvement
   C. O = Opportunity
   D. T = Theory

3. The highest level of evidence is which one of the following levels?
   A. Level 1
   B. Level 2
   C. Level 5
   D. Level 7

4. To ensure feasibility and sustainability, practice changes in a clinical setting should first be which one of the following?
   A. incorporated into policy
   B. published
   C. piloted
   D. reviewed by the Institutional Review Board (IRB)

5. EBP is most valuable when which one of the following occurs?
   A. outcomes are disseminated
   B. clinical practice changes
   C. incorporated into EBP grand rounds
   D. presented at a national conference

6. A characteristic of qualitative research is which one of the following?
   A. focus on outcome
   B. focus on objective
   C. focus on generalizable results
   D. focus on process

7. Which one of the following represents the highest level of evidence in a quantitative study?
   A. Single-site randomized control studies (RCT) studies
   B. Case or cohort studies
   C. Single descriptive study
   D. Systemic review of RCTs

8. An oncology nurse is interested in creating a culture of evidence-based practice (EBP) at her workplace and begins a journal club with her colleagues. Which one of the following is a journal club in the multistep process of using evidence to support clinical practice?
   A. Identifying a problem or trigger
   B. Searching and critiquing the literature for relevant studies
   C. Identifying information and stakeholders needed to solve the problem
   D. Creating a sense of inquiry and create an EBP culture

# 56 Principles of Education and Learning

1. Before development of a targeted program or material, a focus group is appropriate when assessing which one of the following populations?
   A. Individuals
   B. Caregivers
   C. Survivors
   D. Community

2. The SMART methodology for writing objectives includes which one of the following components?
   A. S = Survey
   B. M = Measurable
   C. A = Action
   D. R = Results

3. Which one of the following nutritional goals are focused on an objective outcome?
   A. Understand nutritional impact on the body
   B. Prepare low-fat foods
   C. Maintain adequate sodium intake
   D. List four vegetables with high-fiber content

4. Diagnostic methods are frequently used as an assessment for which one of the following groups?
   A. Staff
   B. Patient
   C. Caregiver
   D. Community

5. Performance analysis is helpful with which one of the following phases of staff education?
   A. Development of the teaching plan
   B. Determination of teaching objectives
   C. Evaluation
   D. Content identification

6. Learning that takes place by watching and imitating others is based on which one of the following learning theories?
   A. Social
   B. Cognitive
   C. Behavioral
   D. Humanistic

7. H. R. is a 50-year-old male who has recently been diagnosed with prostate cancer. To learn more about his disease, he conducts an internet search prior to his next appointment. A patient performing an independent internet search for their specific cancer diagnosis is an example of which one of the following learning theories?
   A. Operant conditioning
   B. Motivational
   C. Adult learning
   D. Pedagogic learning

8. Learning that is activated through internal and external cues is based on which one of the following learning theories?
   A. Social
   B. Cognitive
   C. Motivational
   D. Humanistic

# 57 Legal Issues

1. The enforcement of Nurse Practice Acts to guide nursing practice is regulated by which one of the following?
   A. National Council of State Boards of Nursing (NCSBN)
   B. Nurse Practice Acts
   C. State Boards of Nursing (BoN)
   D. National Council Licensure for Registered Nurses (NCLEX)

2. The Affordable Care Act advocates for patient's rights in the healthcare environment to include which one of the following?
   A. Requiring insurers to provide coverage to dependent children if enrolled in college
   B. Providing coverage to patients with a history of cancer
   C. Placing annual limits on coverage provided
   D. Placing limits on lifetime coverage

3. Which one of the following is a national oncology-specific accreditation program?
   A. The Joint Commission (TJC)
   B. National Institutes of Health (NIH)
   C. Centers for Medicare and Medicaid (CMS)
   D. Quality Oncology Practice Initiative (QOPI)

4. Legal issues for individuals with cancer include which one of the following?
   A. ensuring insurance coverage for a bone marrow transplant
   B. obtaining reimbursement for prescribed oral chemotherapy
   C. bankruptcy
   D. accepting a promotion at work because they are a cancer survivor

5. Breach of duty is best defined as which one of the following?
   A. deviation from a professional standard of care
   B. failure to meet an acceptable standard of care
   C. deviation from the acceptable standard of care that a reasonable person would use in a specific situation
   D. a cause that directly produces an event and without which the event would not have occurred

6. Reasons for litigation against nurses include which one of the following?
   A. following established standards of care and hospital policies and procedures
   B. performing a patient assessment and reporting the findings to a physician
   C. advocating for a patient's right to refuse treatment
   D. witnessing an informed consent when the nurse didn't hear what was explained to the patient

7. Nurses can utilize strategies for minimizing risk of malpractice or disciplinary action. Which one of the following strategies involves the development of skills in interpersonal communication?
   A. Attending relevant continuing education programs
   B. Obtaining specialty certifications
   C. Becoming involved in patient advocacy programs and listening to patient concerns
   D. Communicating clearly when educating patients and families

8. Which one of the following legal terms is defined by the "deviation from the acceptable standard of care that a reasonable person would use in a specific situation?"
   A. Malpractice
   B. Negligence
   C. Defamation
   D. Breach of duty

9. Which one of the following legal terms is defined by the "deviation from a professional standard of care?"
   A. Negligence
   B. Slander
   C. Malpractice
   D. Duty

# 58 Ethical Issues

1. A patient who has recently undergone a bone marrow transplant is in the intensive care unit (ICU) receiving aggressive treatment. A source of moral distress in the nurse caring for the patient may include which one of the following?
   A. availability of technology that may result in overtreatment
   B. collaboration between physician and nurse about treatment
   C. a request by the patient to continue treatment
   D. actively helping the patient to complete an advance directive

2. A nurse is about to administer a clinical trial drug and asks the patient if he has signed an informed consent and if he understands the treatment. By doing so, the nurse is requesting of the patient which one of the following?
   A. That he must complete the entire treatment plan and follow up
   B. That he acknowledges that no harm will become him during treatment
   C. That he understands the risks, benefits, and consequences of treatment
   D. That he understands that the treatment will ultimately cure him of his disease

3. According to the American Nurses Association Code of Ethics, which of the following is a provision that represents nursing's core values, duties, and accountabilities? An oncology nurse who:
   A. calls a physician for additional medications for a patient in pain
   B. joins a research group to study the effects of pain medication
   C. decides to go back to school to study palliative care
   D. arrives on time for work and completes tasks when due

4. An oncology nurse working on a bone marrow transplant unit is caring for Mr. R, a 75-year-old patient who had an allogenic transplant. The nurse questions why they are treating a patient of his age group. This statement by the nurse is an example of the ethical theory of which one of the following?
   A. utilitarianism
   B. ethical egoism
   C. deontology
   D. divisability

5. G. R. is a 39-year-old male who has been newly diagnosed patient with leukemia. During his office visit, he discusses treatment options for therapy with the physician. The oncology nurse understands that this type of decision making is an example of which one of the following?
   A. informed consent
   B. shared decision-making
   C. power of attorney
   D. combined decision-making

6. Which one of the following ethical principles is defined by the duty to not harm others?
   A. Beneficence
   B. Autonomy
   C. Justice
   D. Nonmaleficence

7. Which one of the following is an example or a definition of the ethical principle of justice?
   A. Ensuring the benefits of a patient's treatment outweighs the harm.
   B. Showing compassion toward a patient in a nurse's care.
   C. Respect for a person's right to choose their own destiny, or, in medical terms, their own plan of care.
   D. Allocating the same resources to each patient, no matter their socioeconomic status, race, religion, or moral standing.

8. Which one of the following is the third step in identifying ethical concerns?
   A. Explore practical alternatives.
   B. Analyze the problem using ethical theories.
   C. Gather the information from key participants and obtain the facts.
   D. Evaluate the process and outcome.

# 59 Professional Issues

1. Collaborative partnerships are critical in optimizing the care of oncology patients. Which one of the following is an example of an obstacle to building a collaborative relationship?
   A. Interdisciplinary team meetings involving doctors, nurses, social workers, and leadership
   B. Lack of recognition of the knowledge and expertise of the oncology nurse
   C. Relationship building with team members other than the physician
   D. Initiation of change of shift reporting guidelines

2. Oncology patients experience health care in many different ways. Beliefs and values surrounding the concepts of suffering, pain, and end-of-life care are unique to every individual. Ensuring that these views are respected and observed through care is an example of which one of the following?
   A. human advocacy
   B. paternalistic advocacy
   C. simplistic advocacy
   D. existential advocacy

3. Certification in oncology nursing is critical for which one of the following examples?
   A. Obtaining higher pay
   B. Mandated for relicensure
   C. Representation of the knowledge and qualifications unique to oncology
   D. Required by the Board of Registered Nursing (BRN) by 2020

4. Strategies to Stop Colon Cancer in Priority Populations is an example of _____; a model for _____
   A. PICOT; primary care
   B. PDSA; protocol standardization
   C. PDSA; quality improvement
   D. PICOT; tertiary care

5. Medical errors have significant financial and nonfinancial costs to the healthcare system. Which one of the following represents an opportunity for the oncology nurse to minimize this risk?
   A. Obtain certification
   B. Recognize and remove faulty equipment
   C. Participate on an evidence-based care committee
   D. Read journals in their specialty area regularly

6. Which one of the following types of advocacy is exemplified when the nurse provides education about a chemotherapy agent and a hormonal treatment to a woman recently diagnosed with metastatic breast cancer?
   A. Human advocacy
   B. Paternalistic advocacy
   C. Simplistic advocacy
   D. Consumer advocacy

7. Which one of the following best describes the Individual Mandate as framed as part of the Affordable Care Act?
   A. Individuals must undergo health screenings annually.
   B. Individuals must participate in wellness programs offered by their health insurance.
   C. Individuals must participate in prevention education for diseases such as diabetes and cancer.
   D. Individuals must sign up for health insurance.

# 60 Compassion Fatigue

1. An oncology nurse's coworker has been exhibiting increased behaviors of emotional distress after several patient deaths. The oncology nurse is concerned that these symptoms may be signs of which one of the following?
   A. chronic job stress
   B. compassion fatigue
   C. moral distress
   D. hyperactivity

2. An oncology nurse working on a bone marrow transplant unit may be at risk for developing compassion fatigue. A factor that may increase her risk includes which one of the following?
   A. being married with children
   B. overconfidence in caring for patients
   C. caring for high-acuity patients over a long period of time
   D. having more than 10 years oncology nursing experience

3. Suggested activities for an oncology nurse displaying symptoms of compassion fatigue might include which one of the following?
   A. going out for drinks and staying out late with friends
   B. scheduling a day at a spa for a massage and facial
   C. avoid talking with anyone about issues with work
   D. frequent resting in bed when not at work

4. An oncology nurse is concerned about a long-time coworker on her nursing unit because she has become distant and distracted. When questioned, the coworker states that she is just overwhelmed and exhausted. The coworker may be experiencing which one of the following?
   A. chronic fatigue syndrome
   B. compassion fatigue
   C. burnout
   D. a cognitive disorder

5. An oncology nurse working on a unit where there is a heavy caseload and high levels of stress may best be assessed for secondary distress disorders through use of which one of the following?
   A. Montreal Cognitive Assessment Scale
   B. Mini Mental Status Exam
   C. Professional Quality of Life Scale (ProQOL)
   D. Maslach Burnout Inventory—Human Services Survey MBI-HSS

6. Which one of the following is an example of a self-reflection exercise that a nurse could try as part of self-care management?
   A. Indulging in a massage
   B. Exercise (recommend three to four times weekly for 20-30 minutes)
   C. Enjoying a hobby, listening to music, humor, and enjoying nature
   D. Making time for prayer and meditation

7. Which one of the following is an example of managing self-care through grief counseling and support?
   A. Nutrition and eating well
   B. Send cards to the family, reminisce about time spent with patients, sometimes attend the funeral of patients with whom there has been a close bond
   C. Activities that focus a person's attention on the present experience, becoming more aware of one's physical, mental, and emotional condition, in a way that is nonjudgmental.
   D. Schedule preventive and medical care appointments

# Answer Key

1. **Answer:** C

   **Rationale:** Cancer epidemiology is defined as the study of the distribution and determinants of cancer in population groups. The rates of cancer occurrence in a population indicates the incidence of cancer, usually reported for a given period of time. Number of deaths is the mortality rates for cancers over a given period of time.

2. **Answer:** D

   **Rationale:** Cancer incidence rates have been decreasing or stable from 2005 to 2014 for cancers of the breast, ovary, lung, prostate, stomach, and larynx. However, during this timeframe, annual cancer incidence has been increasing for cancers of the kidney and pancreas, as well as for melanoma, and cancers of the thyroid, liver, and bile duct.

3. **Answer:** A

   **Rationale:** According to the American Cancer Society, as of January 1, 2016, 59% of cancer survivors are 65 years of age or older. African Americans do not have higher relative survival rates than whites; they have higher death rates for most cancers. Five-year survival rates have not increased for lung cancer; it is among the cancers with the lowest survival rates (18%), along with liver cancer (18%), and cancer of the pancreas (5%). Relative survival rates for patients with chronic myeloid leukemia have not decreased, rather they have increased from 22% in the mid-1970s to 68% in 2013.

4. **Answer:** B

   **Rationale:** For prostate cancer, African American men have the highest incidence and mortality rates as compared with other ethnic groups in the U.S and are more than twice as likely as white men to die from prostate cancer. Asians/Pacific Islanders have the highest incidence and death rates of all groups for cancers of the liver and stomach, not kidney cancer. While white women have had the highest incidence rate for breast cancer, African American women have the highest mortality rate from breast cancer. Hispanic/Latina women have the highest incidence rate for cervical cancer, but the highest mortality rate is seen among African American women.

5. **Answer:** C

   **Rationale:** Tobacco use is the single largest preventable cause of disease and premature death in the U.S and is associated with approximately 480,000 premature deaths each year. Smokeless tobacco is not a safe alternative to cigarettes. It is associated with increased risk of oral, pancreatic, and esophageal cancers. Adults without a high school degree are two to four times more likely to be current smokers than those with a college degree. Daily smoker prevalence has not increased but has decreased between 2005 to 2015.

6. **Answer:** B

   **Rationale:** Cancers of the gastrointestinal system (i.e., those of the esophagus, liver, stomach, pancreas, gallbladder, and colorectum) are among cancers linked to overweight and obesity. Lung cancer risk is not elevated in obesity. Overweight and/or obesity contribute to an estimated 20% of all deaths due to cancer. African American women have the highest rates of obesity (58%) compared with non-Hispanic white women (38%).

7. **Answer:** D

   **Rationale:** Vaccination against HPV is recommended for all children aged 11 or 12 years given in two doses separated by at least 6 months. HPV vaccine is not reserved for female children only and can be given in males and females as early as age 9 and as late as age 26. Over age 15, a three-dose series is recommended.

8. **Answer:** A

   **Rationale:** Tamoxifen and raloxifene are FDA-approved for use as chemoprevention agents to reduce risk of breast cancer. These agents have been shown to reduce breast cancer incidence by up to 50% among high-risk women The other drugs are not indicated for chemoprevention of breast cancer. In the past, diethylstilbestrol use during pregnancy has been associated with cancer of the vagina in female offspring. Anabolic steroids may be associated with liver cancer. Menotropins are fertility drugs that may increase the risk of ovarian cancer.

9. **Answer:** D

   **Rationale:** When accessing Ms. P for motivation for preventative behavior as per the health belief model, she should be asked the question, "How difficult do you think it will be to decrease your risk for cancer by quitting your smoking habit?" Since Ms. P as a smoker, her healthcare provider would have recognized that smoking is an unhealthy behavior that could lead to a diagnosis of cancer. Under the health belief model, her healthcare provider would want to know what barriers exist in her overcoming harmful habits. Asking about current medical conditions and medications, her own and her family's history cancer diagnoses, and previous treatments, such as chemotherapy, radiation therapy, and immunotherapy would all be asked during earlier medical history and physical examinations.

10. **Answer:** C

    **Rationale:** According to the American Cancer Society, a fact that is true regarding cancer mortality in populations with low socioeconomic status is that there is a higher rate of advanced disease is found at diagnosis among poorer populations and those who live in rural regions than in the rest of the U.S. population. The other answers are all false. Instead of high socioeconomic status being associated with increased risk of lung cancer, cervical cancer, stomach cancer, and cancer of the head and neck, it is low socioeconomic status that is a contributor. The use of alcohol is not a leading cause of cancer mortality in poorer populations, but tobacco use is and is increasing in persons from lower socioeconomic status. High socioeconomic status is associated with increased risk of breast, prostate, and colon cancers.

11. *Answer:* A

*Rationale:* As of 2016, more than 2 million middle and high school age students were identified as e-cigarette users, with a variety of appealing flavors cited as the primary reason for use. This increase in use of teens and young adolescents has given rise to parental warnings of school-age students over the use of e-cigarettes and a restriction on the types of flavors that can be manufactured sold to minors. The other responses are incorrect. As of 2016, the U.S. Food and Drug Administration (FDA) has not approved e-cigarettes as a cessation aid. Nicotine is found in e-cigarettes, in which the inhaled vapor is produced from cartridges that contain flavoring and other chemicals. Use of e-cigarettes has been linked to leading non-smokers and children to begin smoking.

# CHAPTER 2

1. *Answer:* C

*Rationale:* Sensitivity of a test measures the test's ability to correctly identify individuals with the disease comparing the results to those obtained from a gold standard. Reliability of a test is the level of agreement between measurements taken at different times. Negative predictive value is the percentage of persons who screen negative and who do not have the disease. Specificity of a test measures the test's ability to correctly identify individuals who do not have the disease comparing the results to those obtained from a gold standard. Both sensitivity and specificity can show how accurate the results are, but they do not measure reliability.

2. *Answer:* B

*Rationale:* This screening modification is recommended in individuals with a family history of colorectal cancer or colorectal polyps in a first-degree relative due to the increased risk of adenomas or cancer. From the genetics perspective, first-degree relatives (siblings, parents, and offspring) should be considered to be at increased risk. Therefore, it is recommended for these individuals to get a colonoscopy starting at age 40, or 10 years younger than age at diagnosis of the youngest affected relative, whichever is earlier. Observational studies have shown that the average time required for a polyp to develop into an invasive malignancy is 10 years. Colonoscopy is to occur every 5 years in those who have a first-degree relative with colorectal cancer or adenomatous polyps. In an individual considered to be at an average risk, colonoscopy is recommended every 10 years, beginning at age 50.

3. *Answer:* A

*Rationale:* Between ages 21-29, cytology (Pap test, also known as a Pap smear) is needed every 3 years. It is the principle screening tool for cervical cancer. Yearly screening is no longer recommended because it generally takes 10-20 years for cervical cancer to develop. HPV testing in this age group is only needed after an abnormal Pap result and it not recommended as a routine screening test. Those who are between the ages of 30-65, it is preferred to do an HPV with Pap test every 5 years. However, a Pap test alone every 3 years is also acceptable in this age group. In women who are 65 and older, and have undergone regular cervical cancer testing with normal results, screening is not recommended. For women who have had a hysterectomy, cervical cancer screening is also not needed unless the surgery was done to remove cervical cancer or a precancerous lesion.

4. *Answer:* A

*Rationale:* The goal of primary prevention is to reduce the risk factors of cancer or increase an individuals' resistance to them. This is considered to be the most effective management for cancer. Secondary prevention prevents disease progression by the early detection and treatment of cancer. Tertiary prevention is the application of effective therapy to improve the outcomes and disease morbidity and mortality in affected individuals. Quaternary prevention refers to avoiding consequences of unnecessary or excessive interventions.

5. *Answer:* D

*Rationale:* Average risk for breast cancer is defined as those with no personal history of breast cancer, a strong family history, or a genetic mutation known to increase the risk. In average-risk women aged 45-54 years of age, an annual clinical breast exam with an annual mammography is recommended. For those who are 55 years of age and older with an average risk, they have the option to switch to mammography every other year or choose to continue yearly mammogram. High-risk women are considered to be those with a greater than 20% lifetime risk, *BRCA1* or *BRCA2* gene mutation, or a first-degree relative, an annual mammography should start at age 30, along with an MRI screening, clinical breast exams every 6-12 months, and consideration of risk reduction strategies such as bilateral salpingo-oophorectomy, or chemoprevention with tamoxifen, raloxifene, or exemestane.

6. *Answer:* C

*Rationale:* This woman is considered to be at an increased risk for breast cancer as she has had a history of thoracic radiation therapy between the ages of 10 and 30 years for her childhood leukemia. Therefore, the screening guidelines will be different for her in comparison to someone who is at an average risk for breast cancer. For women under 25 years of age, a clinical breast exam is recommended every 12 months beginning 8-10 years after radiation therapy. For women who are 25 years of age and older, a clinical breast exam is recommended every 6-12 months, along with an annual breast MRI, and an annual mammogram to begin 8-10 years after radiation therapy, but not prior to age 25.

7. **Answer:** B

**Rationale:** According to the American Cancer Society, screening for prostate cancer includes prostate-specific antigen (PSA) blood test and a digital rectal exam (DRE). Discussion about screening should take place at age 50 for men with average risk. In men with a high risk, such as being African American, having a first-degree relative diagnosed with prostate cancer before the age of 65, the discussion for screening should begin at age 45. In men with an even higher risk, such having more than one first-degree relative who had prostate cancer at an early age, the discussion for screening should come at age 40.

8. **Answer:** A

**Rationale:** Individuals who are over the age of 50 with greater than 20-pack year history of smoking are considered to be at a moderate risk. Lung cancer screening is not recommended for the general population. Screening is to be considered for those between 55 and 80 years of age with at least a 30-pack-year smoking history and those who continue to smoke or have quit less than 15 years ago. In these individuals LDCT is recommended as it is the most sensitive test available, resulting in a 20% reduction in lung cancer mortality versus a plain chest X-ray.

9. **Answer:** C

**Rationale:** Screening tests are used to detect early stages of cancer in people who are otherwise healthy without any symptoms. They also help to detect risk factors that could later develop into a disease. Diagnostic tests are usually done to find out what is causing certain symptoms that have already become noticeable. Many of the screening tests are used to detect abnormalities first, which can then be looked at more closely in other tests. However, not all screening tests are safe as there are some which may expose the body to radiation and others can potentially be invasive. Therefore, it is always important to outweigh the risk and benefits of a screening test.

10. **Answer:** A

**Rationale:** A positive predictive value (PPV) identifies the percentage of persons who screen positive who actually have the disease. Negative predictive value (NPV) is the percentage of persons who screen negative who do not have the disease. The higher the prevalence of a disease, the higher the PPV and lower the NPV. Sensitivity measures a tests ability to recognize persons who have the disease, also referred to as true positives. In other words, it does not miss any people who are ill. Specificity measures a tests ability to recognize persons who do not have the disease, also referred to as true negatives. This means the test is not precise as it only captures persons who already have the disease.

11. **Answer:** B

**Rationale:** BRCA1 and BRCA2 mutations are rare in the general population, therefore genetic testing for these mutations is not recommended unless there is an individual or family history suggesting a possible presence of the mutation. Individuals who have an increased likelihood of having a BRCA1 or BRCA2 mutation are those who have a family history of breast cancer diagnosed before the age of 50, multiple breast cancers in the family, breast and ovarian cancer in either woman herself or in the family, cancer in both breasts in the woman herself, two or more primary types of BRCA1 or BRCA2 related cancers in a single-family member, and Ashkenazi Jewish ethnicity. BRCA1 and BRCA2 gene mutations are responsible for approximately 20-25% of hereditary breast cancers.

12. **Answer:** B

**Rationale:** Assessing key characteristics can help identify which screening tests are needed for individuals. This involves reviewing their demographics for age, gender, race, and occupation. It also involves reviewing a personal medical history such as previous state of health, previous cancer and cancer treatment, chronic illnesses, vaccinations, and hospitalizations. Reviewing a family history for medical and cancer history in relatives is also important to identify which cancer-oriented screening exams are needed. Medication history, allergies, sleep habits, and exercise are components of a health history but they do not generally guide screening recommendations.

13. **Answer:** A

**Rationale:** Fatigue, malaise, recent weight gain or weight loss are considered to be constitutional symptoms which can affect many different systems of the body. Other symptoms can also include fever, chronic pain, dyspnea, night sweats, cough, and decreased appetite. These are nonspecific symptoms which can present in many diseases, but can present in some primary lung malignancies. Therefore, when assessing a patient, it is important to do a thorough physical exam, and review of cancer-related symptoms.

14. **Answer:** C

**Rationale:** For men ages 45-75, the NCCN recommends to repeat testing at 1-2 year intervals for a PSA between 1-3 ng/mL. If the PSA is less than 1.0 ng/mL, testing should be repeated at 2-4 year intervals. If the PSA greater than 3 ng/mL or the DRE is suspicious, then the PSA should be repeated, Providers should also consider performing a percent free PSA Prostate Health Index (phi) score. Phi is a mathematical formula that provides a probability of prostate cancer (PCa) by combining three tests (prostate-specific antigen [PSA], free PSA, and p2PSA) into a single score. p2PSA) into a single score. Phi is intended to fill the diagnostic "gap" between PSA screening and a prostate biopsy. The higher specificity of phi means a greater probability of identifying those patients who actually need a biopsy. A transrectal ultrasound (TRUS) guided biopsy should be considered if needed. Follow-up should be done in 6-12 months with a PSA and DRE.

15. **Correct answer:** B

**Rationale:** The correct answer is B, a screening mammogram. This woman is asymptomatic. If a problem is detected on physical examination or on the screening mammogram, a diagnostic mammogram will be ordered. Women who have a known symptom of breast cancer (lump, nipple discharge, nipple deviation, skin changes, bulge, or puckering), women with a personal history of

**125**

breast cancer, or women with breast implants will need a diagnostic mammogram. Screening mammography is recommended for women age 40 and over. Breast tomosynthesis, which is also referred to as three-dimensional (3-D) mammography, is a form of mammography that uses a low-dose X-ray system and computer reconstructions to create three-dimensional images of the breasts. In two-dimensional (2-D) mammography two X-ray images are taken, one from the top and a second from the side. Both 3-D and 2-D mammography can be used for either screening or diagnostic mammograms.

16. *Correct answer:* C

*Rationale:* The correct answer is C, the Gail model. The Gail model is a multivariable statistical model that has been developed to help estimate a woman's personal breast cancer risk. The Gail model incorporates characteristics and risk factors of the woman including age of menarche, age at first live birth, number of first-degree relatives with breast cancer (mother and sisters), number of previous benign breast biopsies, atypical hyperplasia in a previous breast biopsy, and race) to assess 5-year and lifetime risks of developing breast cancer. It is appropriate to use in women 35 and older. It does not include maternal second and third-degree relatives (grandmother or aunt) paternal family history of breast cancer, height, weight, or family history of ovarian cancer, so it will underestimate breast cancer risk for some women. The PREMM model is a clinical prediction model that estimates the probability of an individual carrying a germline mutation in the MLH1, MSH2, MSH6, PMS2, or EPCAM genes. Mutations in these genes cause Lynch syndrome, an inherited cancer predisposition syndrome associated with elevated risks of developing colon, uterine, ovarian and other cancers. The Penn II model can be used to predict the pre-test probability that a person has a BRCA1 or BRCA2 mutation. The Penn II model does not predict breast cancer risk. It focuses only on the chance that an individual has inherited a mutation in BRCA1 or BRCA2. BRCAPRO is a statistical model used for assessing the probability that an individual carries a germline mutation in the BRCA1 and BRCA2 genes, based on family history of breast and ovarian cancer, based on his or her family's history of breast and ovarian cancer, including male breast cancer and bilateral breast cancer.

17. *Correct answer:* D

*Rationale:* The correct answer is D. An effective, ideal screening test has the ability to discriminate between those who have the cancer being screened for and those who do not have a current diagnosis of cancer. Screening tools must be safe, reliable, valid, and cost-effective. The potential benefit of the test should outweigh the results. The interval for screening depends on the natural history of the malignancy. Some cancers develop more quickly than others and some have a slower doubling time and do not require annual screening such as colorectal cancer. The location where the screening occurs depends on what is needed for the test. Taking a screening program into the community may actually make the screening more accessible than in a hospital such as mobile mammography or a skin screening event. It does not necessarily have to be available in the hospital. Negative predictive value refers the probability that persons with a negative screening test truly do not have the disease. A high, not low negative predictive value would be desirable.

18. *Correct answer:* C

*Rationale:* The correct answer is C. Components of the history include demographic information such as age, gender, race, ethnicity, and occupation. Other components of the history include past medical history and family history of malignancy. Assessment of social habits that potentially increase risk for cancer should also be considered such a smoking, alcohol, illicit drug use, sexual habits, dietary habits, and amount of regular exercise. Assessment of pain and stiffness in the bones and joints, cranial nerves, and skin surfaces are all part of the physical examination in cancer assessment.

## CHAPTER 3

1. *Answer:* A

*Rationale:* A cancer diagnosis impacts not only the affected individual, but also family and friends who may experience challenges in dealing with the illness and its sequalae. The National Comprehensive Cancer Network (NCCN) states that the term "survivorship" applies to all disease stages and may be used starting at the time of diagnosis. Survivorship does not extend to family and children of patients with cancer, nor is survivorship limited to an early-stage cancer diagnosis. In addition, a time frame is not placed upon survivorship so identifying someone who is greater than 5 years from a cancer diagnosis as a survivor is also an incorrect response.

2. *Answer:* C

*Rationale:* Late effects are absent or subclinical during treatment and occur months or years later, requiring focused follow-up care and monitoring. Long-term effects do not begin at least one year after treatment completion. In fact, long-term effects begin during treatment, persist throughout treatment, and may continue long after treatment has been completed, so answer A is inaccurate. The first year after treatment has no impact on treatment for sequelae development and is not the most critical period of time. A patient who is of a younger age at the time of diagnosis – such as an adolescent or a young adult– does place the patient at higher risk for significant late effects, such as cardiomyopathy, where the cumulative incidence increases over time.

3. *Answer:* B

The Americans with Disabilities Act (ADA) prohibits discrimination based on disability and is not limited to survivors with prosthetic devices. It is true that changes in roles and relationships can cause feelings of isolation, depression, and may contribute to survivors of any age experiencing difficulty finding a new 'normal' in the post treatment setting. Cancer survivors are known to experience higher rates of unemployment and struggle returning to the full-time work force. Unemployment can also lead to financial problems, further exacerbating the plight of some cancer survivors.

4. *Answer:* B

*Rationale:* Female survivors who have received chest radiation prior to age 30 should have annual breast imaging including mammography, breast MRI or both starting at age 25 or at least 8 years after radiation, whichever occurs last. Lifestyle and age do contribute to risk for second malignancy and should be considered in planning second malignancy screening and health promotion counseling. PET scans are not routinely ordered in female breast survivors who have received chest radiation prior to age 30.

5. *Answer:* C

*Rationale:* Essential components of survivorship care include surveillance for recurrence, monitoring for late treatment effects, health promotion, and communication with other healthcare providers. As the oncology workforce shrinks, other healthcare providers such as urologists, primary care physicians, and nurse practitioners will increasingly assume the care of cancer survivors. To promote care coordination, survivorship care plans should be provided to the patient and non-oncology providers after treatment completion. This provision should be automatic and not require a patient request.

6. *Answer:* A

*Rationale:* Obtaining a comprehensive patient history is an important component of any survivorship visit, and should include comorbidities, family history, genetic history (if available), healthy behaviors, and preventive health services. Insurance information is not essential, although patients may experience limitations in access to healthcare based on coverage or lack thereof. Cancer survivors tend to have a higher unemployment rate, which can lead to problems obtaining insurance.

7. *Answer:* C

*Rationale:* Cancer survivors may experience a range of psychosocial challenges, making assessment an important component of follow-up care. Past coping skills, social support, and social history also help to guide the assessment. Fatigue, insomnia, and pain may be contributing factors to risk for depression, anxiety, and fear of recurrence. Reliable and valid screening tools such as the HADS and PHQ-9 should be considered for anxiety and depression assessment, and, instead of being avoided, should be utilized regularly. Frequent changes in occupation and living arrangements should not be considered as a positive sign and could be seen as sign that a person is having a difficult time adapting to life as a cancer survivor. While personal questions can be difficult for both the patient and the healthcare provider, they should not be avoided, as learning details about a patient's personal life can assist a healthcare provider in accessing how a person is coping with their life as a survivor.

8. *Answer:* D

*Rationale:* Rehabilitation services are underutilized, despite the growing number of survivors and significant rates of cancer-related physical impairments. Investing time in rehabilitation results in an improved ability to work, decreased sick time, and reduced rates of lost productivity. With the positive benefits of rehabilitation centers in mind, the nurse should consider partnering with a rehabilitation center as worthwhile, and, when providing feedback, should encourage such a partnership with her healthcare center.

9. *Answer:* B

*Rationale:* Patients should be encouraged to remain or become physically active as soon as possible and to avoid sedentary behaviors so rest would be discouraged, as in answer D. Stretching is recommended for muscle health. Two to three weekly sessions of strength training that involves major muscle groups and tendons is recommended. Physically inactive survivors should begin with one to three light to moderate-intensity exercises, 20-minute sessions per week, with progression based on tolerance. Since Mr. S. had led a previously active lifestyle, the recommendation should be for 150 minutes of moderate-intensity or 75 minutes of vigorous-intensity exercise per week, should be recommended for him. The correct answer, then, is B.

10. *Answer:* D

*Rationale:* Achieving and maintaining a healthy weight requires healthy eating habits, including portion control and a plant-based diet. Routine weight checks are helpful in assessing progress and should not be discouraged. Fast food, fried foods, and red meat consumption should be limited or avoided altogether, even once a healthy goal weight has been achieved.

11. *Answer:* C

*Rationale:* Survivorship care plans are customized for each patient, and should include a summary of cancer diagnosis, stage, and treatment, as well as recommendations for follow-up care, including potential long-term and late effects, healthy behaviors, and surveillance for recurrence. However, screening for high-risk siblings is not included in a typical cancer survivorship care plan.

12. *Answer:* C

*Rationale:* Adolescent and young adult survivors are at higher risk for physical and psychosocial sequelae including limited access to follow-up care and insurance, as well as increased reports of medication nonadherence due to cost and limited financial resources. Special attention should be paid to survivors that are of school age so that cognitive issues such as altered attention, concentration, and processing speed are addressed.

13. *Answer:* B

*Rationale:* General health recommendations, such as those adapted from the American Cancer Society, are important for all survivors and should be reviewed or provided in writing to survivors to promote optimal health, even if unrelated to cancer history and treatment exposures. These include sun protection, safe sex, tobacco prevention and abstinence, as well as information on vaping, bone health, and immunizations.

14. *Answer:* B

*Rationale:* The number of cancer survivors will continue to increase, and the majority, an estimated 60%, are age 64 and older. Deficits in the oncology workforce are anticipated by the year 2020 and are not expected to match the growing survivor population needs.

15. *Answer:* D

*Rationale:* Treatment with anthracyclines may cause late cardiac effects months to years after treatment. Being at a younger age at the time of treatment increases the risk for late physical sequalae, including cardiomyopathy, congestive heart failure, carotid artery disease, valvular heart disease, arrhythmias, and pericardial disease. Prompt evaluation and a plan for long-term management are indicated.

16. *Answer:* B

*Rationale:* Fear of recurrence and anxiety are common around testing/surveillance appointments. It is important to encourage patients to keep their regularly scheduled follow-up appointments and let them know feelings of anxiety and fear are not unusual. Symptoms should be reported if they are occurring with greater frequency or intensity as they may negatively impact quality of life and adherence to follow-up recommendations. Worsening symptoms may also be sign of other factors, such as pain or insomnia.

## CHAPTER 4

1. *Answer:* A

*Rationale:* Palliative care is the concept that includes delivering ancillary therapy to treat side effects of treatment and the disease so that quality of life (QOL) is improved. It is defined as patient and family-centered care that optimizes QOL by anticipating, preventing, and treating suffering as well as addressing physical, intellectual, emotional, social, and spiritual needs. The goal of palliative care is to facilitate patient autonomy, access to information, and choice with respect to treatment and symptom management throughout the continuum of illness. Palliative care is a structured approach that improves the QOL of patients and their families facing the problem associated with life-threatening illness, through the prevention and relief of suffering by means of early identification and focused assessment and treatment of pain and other physical, psychosocial, and spiritual problems Key components of palliative care include patient and family-centered care across the serious illness trajectory. Articulating goals of care and shared decision making are essential elements of the palliative care approach.

B is incorrect because palliative care is not focused on the actual treatment of the cancer, but on the other issues surrounding it. C is not correct because palliative care is most commonly delivered by an interdisciplinary team of providers and ancillary staff. D is incorrect because palliative care can be instituted at the time of diagnosis; it is not reserved only for use during end of life care.

2. *Answer:* B

*Rationale:* Although many other people may become involved in the palliative care of a cancer patient, a pain management specialist, a chaplain, and a social worker are the most common staff included. Typical members of a palliative care team include a physician and/or nurse

(with expertise in pain and symptom management), social worker, spiritual care provider, and other healthcare professionals as needed whose approach to care is to identify and meet the needs of patients and caregivers. Other people in the patient's life, including the providers mentioned in C, may also assist. D is incorrect as not all patients utilize integrative therapy.

3. *Answer:* C

*Rationale:* Although other insurance plans may have different parameters, Medicare maintains a parameter of 6 months life expectancy as a requirement for patients to access Medicare hospice benefits. Eligibility criteria should not be confused with length of service; patients can receive hospice care for as long as they meet eligibility criteria.

4. *Answer:* B

*Rationale:* Cost savings is not something that is usually focused on in cancer care. However, studies have shown that patients who have early appropriate referral to palliative care have increased acceptance of their disease trajectory and make decisions that often reflect in decreased costs both for inpatient and for outpatient care. Decreased burden of care to the primary team may occur tangentially because the palliative care team is addressing symptoms and improving quality of life, but the main improvement is in cost savings. Palliative care involvement rarely includes increased chemotherapy administration or extended disease survival, as those are not the focus of palliative care models.

5. *Answer:* D

*Rationale:* Tertiary care is the highest level of palliative care, usually carried out by a well-coordinated and developed team at a designated cancer center with a Joint Commission care certification, where guidelines, research, and organized care conferences are utilized to provide multifaceted services to the patient and family. Primary palliative care includes basic palliative care skills, advance care planning, symptom assessment and management, communication among healthcare provider, patient, and family caregivers, as well as, support for the patient and family caregiver. Primary palliative care can be offered by all oncology healthcare providers as well as primary care providers to patients and family caregivers. Secondary palliative care is a bridge between primary and tertiary palliative care. Secondary palliative care is offered by healthcare professionals and organizations who provide specialty palliative care and consultation. Secondary palliative care is accessed in community or rural settings, where needs often exceed the skill of primary care providers and access to palliative care experts is scarce.

6. *Answer:* B

*Rationale:* Telehealth connectivity allows providers in rural community settings access to extended services such as consultation with pain management, extensive case review by a palliative care team to provide recommendations, and coordination of care when a patient is able to get to a tertiary center. Social work, local emergency services, and home health may all play a role in rural palliative care, but telehealth is what connects these services together for the patient in a rural setting.

7. *Answer:* C

*Rationale:* Two physicians must certify that the patient is terminally ill. This typically includes the referring provider and the hospice medical director. This is made after independent assessment of the patient and based on the best judgment of the two physicians.

8. *Answer:* C

*Rationale:* Patients must agree to cessation of aggressive therapy in order to enroll in hospice care. Accessing a second opinion, intubation for respiratory distress, and chemotherapy are not included in a hospice care plan.

9. *Answer:* A

*Rationale:* Providers tend to be optimistic and usually estimate the patient's survival as four times longer than the patient actually survives.

10. *Answer:* D

*Rationale:* Patients live on average 17 days after admission to hospice, with a large percentage (35%) of deaths occurring within 7 days of admission.

11. *Answer:* C

*Rationale:* While it may be appropriate to evaluate the needs of family members separately from the patient to get a clear picture of the needs of the whole person and milieu, it would not be appropriate to do such an evaluation without the knowledge of the patient. Nor would it be appropriate to only conduct one evaluation of the hospice patient or to do a physical examination of a family member of a hospice patient.

12. *Answer:* A

*Rationale:* The first modern hospice, St. Christopher, was founded in 1967 in England, and based on the work of Dame Cicely Saunders, whose work with terminally ill, starting in 1948, is credited as starting the modern hospice movement. The first hospice program in the United States was opened in 1974 in Branford, Connecticut, and was founded by Dr. Florence Wald, Yale School of Nursing dean, and an early pioneer in the hospice movement in the U.S. The Medicare hospice benefit was approved by Congress in 1982 after demonstration projects demonstrated that interdisciplinary team care focusing on quality of life and addressing symptom burden of terminal illness improved outcomes and cost less than usual care. The Medicare benefit became permanent in 1986, which provided a stable source of payment for hospice care and resulted in a steady growth of hospice programs throughout the U.S.

13. *Answer:* D

*Rationale:* Grief benefits are offered to the family of hospice patients after the death of the patient so that they do not have to rely on only other family members, clergy, or therapists. Grief counseling is a large part of hospice care, is the responsibility of the entire interdisciplinary team, and support groups should be offered to all family members whenever possible.

14. *Answer:* B

*Rationale:* SWAT or the Social Work Assessment Tool is the tool most commonly used by social workers to evaluate the patient/family environment and assessment their sociocultural needs. Examples of what is assessed during a SWAT include safe and affordable housing, public safety, and access to local emergency and health services. NCCN stands for the National Comprehensive Cancer Network, ECOG is the abbreviation for the Eastern Cooperative Oncology Group, and EQOL is the abbreviation for an evaluation of the quality of life of the patient.

15. *Answer:* D

*Rationale:* Studies have demonstrated that patients who die in the hospital experience more physical and emotional distress prior to death as compared to patients who die at home. One third of all patients die at home. Dying at home is associated with greater caregiver, satisfaction, less aggressive care at the end of life, higher quality of death as assessed by family members, and lower overall caregiver burden. Persons receiving hospice care have an impending expected death and family members may experience more support both as they care for the patient and through bereavement care.

16. *Answer:* B

*Rationale:* Elevation of the head of the bed can often decrease the noise and distress caused by secretions pooling in the back of the oropharynx. These can also be alleviated by anticholinergic drugs and suctioning, but these interventions are more invasive. Cool wash cloths do not help terminal secretions.

17. *Answer:* C

*Rationale:* If the score of the Distress Screening tool is lower than a 4, then the tool suggests that the primary oncologist and their staff can manage the distress. If the score is higher than a 4, the patient should be referred to specialty services such as psychiatrist, support group, clergy, or palliative care team.

18. *Answer:* C

*Rationale:* Describing the quality of Cheyne-Stoke breathing to the patient's family can help them recognize this as one of the signs of impending death. Other clinical signs of impending death which families should be aware of include pulselessness of the radial artery, respiration with mandibular movement, decreased urine output, terminal secretions, nonreactive pupils, and a decreased response to visual stimuli. Rapid breathing, restless movements, and bounding pulse are less likely to be signs of eminent death, though restless movement may precede the more terminal phases.

19. *Answer:* C

*Rationale:* Artificial nutrition and hydration (ANH) is not known to reduce the sensation of thirst or dry mouth. According to the Hospice and Palliative Nurses Association, many patients experience the sensation of dry mouth but this symptom is associated with other factors besides lack of fluids, and, as a result, the introduction of parenteral fluids is unlikely to alleviate thirst. On the other hand, answers A, B, and D are all factors and potential complications associated with the use of ANH. The use of ANH may increase the likelihood of aspiration and ANH given through a feeding tube is associated with an increased chance of infection and fluid overload. Finally, a Cochrane review has found that there is no clinical difference on quality of life was found in artificial hydration versus a placebo.

20. *Answer:* D

*Rationale:* The answer D is not an element of Shared Decision Making. Advance care planning is often confused with goals of care and Shared Decision Making but the element of advance care planning is not part of the goals of care. Answers A, B, and C, however, all go into the goals of care for the palliative care team. In planning out goals of care, the plans are meant to be based upon the shared beliefs of patients, families, and caregivers; the plans are meant to be flexible and may change over the course of the illness, and are enacted in an intentional and structured way, so that the patient and the palliative care team can plot out the best way for a patient to move through this phase of their disease course.

21. *Answer:* D

*Rationale:* According to the NCCN's standards of palliative care in oncology, symptom burden from disease or treatment is anticipated, prevented, and skillfully managed. This standard is best exemplified in how the palliative care team treated G.T's symptom of pain and is reflected in Answer D. Answer A is incorrect because developing a treatment plan for cancer is not a standard of palliative care, even though respecting the autonomy of the patient is a standard. Answer B is also incorrect. A standard of palliative care in oncology is treating psychosocial and spiritual distress with the same importance as a physical condition, but, in this example, the palliative care team was dealing with the symptom of pain, making B an incorrect response. Answer C is also incorrect. End-of-life care is not a standard of palliative care identified by the NCCN.

## CHAPTER 5

1. *Answer:* A

*Rationale:* Created by Dr. Harold Freeman in New York City in 1990, the first patient navigation program targeted women with breast cancer. Fifty percent of these women were uninsured. Many of these women were black. Today navigators work with oncology patients with a variety of diagnoses.

2. *Answer:* A

*Rationale:* The goals are to: serve as a patient's advocate, identify and resolve barriers to care, provide education about treatment plan that empowers patients to actively engage in decision-making and self-care, provide education on symptom and side effect management to reduce early and late treatment associated complications, reduce distress, and provide psychosocial support. This care can occur throughout the cancer trajectory and can be in person or by other communication methods. Only answer A represents a goal of care.

3. *Answer:* D

*Rationale:* The ONN Core Competencies describe the role of the navigator in five categories: coordination of care, communication, education, professional role, and oncology nurse navigator and core competencies. In 2016, a second RDS identified differences between a clinical oncology nurse and an ONN. Navigators help assure screening guidelines are implemented but do not change the guidelines. The same is true of guidelines for protective equipment. While navigators might support improved staffing rations, they are not responsible for implementing them.

4. *Answer:* A

*Rationale:* The Cancer Care Continuum Model has created navigator definitions to describe differences based on job description, certification/schooling, and other skills. Other definitions of navigator include novice ONN and expert ONN. Lay navigators do not have a professional degree, medical licensure, or credentials, and education at or below a bachelor's degree. Allied health navigators have professional backgrounds (i.e. medical assistants), educational degrees higher than bachelor's degree but not clinically focused. Nurse navigators have a two-year or BSN or RN, APN, NP, and other nursing backgrounds. Social work navigators have education with at least a BS in social work and may have an MS in counseling. The ONN facilitates the appropriate and efficient delivery of healthcare services, both within and across systems, and serves as the key contact to promote optimal outcomes while delivering patient-centered care. The expert ONN is proficient in the role and has the education, knowledge, and experience to use critical thinking and decision-making skills pertaining to the evolution of the ONN role and process improvement in the navigation processes. Both the novice and expert ONN roles are professional roles. There is no community clinic navigator.

5. *Answer:* C

*Rationale:* There was a significant increase in 5 year survival rates by 39% to 70%. The goal of the program was to reduce cancer mortality by improving access quality care.

6. *Answer:* C

*Rationale:* The AONN+ was incorporated in 2009.

7. *Answer:* D

*Rationale:* The CoC program standards established a foundation for patient-centered care. The standards cover the entire health continuum – from prevention to survivorship care.

8. *Answer:* A

*Rationale:* A PNRP study showed that delays in diagnosing cancer can be overcome with patient navigation, addressing unemployment, housing type, and marital status.

9. *Answer:* C

*Rationale:* Provider, patient, and family satisfaction scores directly assess ONN value. Other measures of value include timeliness of care/access to care, management and monitoring of the plan of care, clinical trial accrual, and reduced hospital readmissions. The other answers are the responsibility of inpatient nurses.

10. *Answer:* A

*Rationale:* Regardless of the patient's past history of depression, the nurse navigator should assess the patient's psychosocial distress during each clinic visit. A psychologist does not need to be present to assess for psychosocial distress. While patients might experience psychosocial distress at the end stage of disease, patients can experience psychosocial distress at any time during the cancer continuum.

11. *Answer:* C

*Rationale:* The limitations to determine effectiveness are associated with studies with relatively small sample sizes, poor response rates to questionnaires, not using valid instruments to gather data, and lack of data about patients who have used navigation services. Additionally, there is a limited amount of published research about nurse navigation program to establish a foundation for research inquiry.

12. *Answer:* A

*Rationale:* This is a transportation barrier because the patient does not have the capability or resources to reach the facility for appointments and treatment. These are many different types of barriers to care. There is no indication that there is a cultural or language barrier, or a lack of family support.

13. *Answer:* B

*Rationale:* Navigators can communicate with a financial assistance team or designated financial assistance experts to help decrease the financial burden to patients. There are options to offer patients: medication assistance programs, charity care, copay assistance programs, as well as assistance with transportation and lodging expenses. This is not a transportation barrier. It is not realistic for the treating facility's staff to pay for medications and patients cannot donate medications to other patients.

14. *Answer:* D

*Rationale:* AONN+ offers the ONN-Certified Generalist and Certified Generalist Thoracic certifications, as well as the Oncology Patient Navigator-Certified Generalist. ONS offers certifications but they are not designated as certifications in nurse navigation. ONC stands for Oncology Certified Nurse and is not specific to patient navigation. ACOS stands for American College of Surgeons and although they require navigation for credentialing and certification of an institution they do not offer individual certification for nurse navigators.

15. *Answer:* B

*Rationale:* While there are different Models of Care, this model describes the Planetree Model. Other models include the cancer care continuum model, transitional care model, and the ONN care model. The transitional care model focuses on continuity of care, especially for high-risk patients and for hospitalized patients and has a goal to reduce patient complications and readmissions. The ONN care model focuses on continuity of care and coordination of care, based on providers in the community, and includes cultural traditions in the community and survivorship. The survivorship model focuses on initiating and maintaining surveillance programs and screening for late and long-term side effects, recurrent disease, and secondary malignancies.

16. *Answer:* D

*Rationale:* Allied health patient navigators require a professional background, with an educational degree higher than bachelor's, but a requirement is that an allied health patient navigator does not necessarily need to be clinically focused. Lay navigators need no professional degree, medical licensure, or credentials; education at or below a bachelor's degree. Nurse navigators require a two-year or BSN or RN, APN, NP, and other nursing backgrounds, while social work/counselors need education with at least a BS in social work, MS in counseling, and are required to be licensed mental health counselors

17. *Answer:* B

*Rationale:* The answer is B. The statement "The ONN provides appropriate and timely education to patients, families, and caregivers to facilitate understanding and support informed decision making" is part of the education competency category. The other statements – identifying potential and realized barrier to care, applying knowledge of clinical guidelines and specialty resources throughout the cancer continuum, and facilitates timely scheduling of appointments – are all part of coordination of care category.

18. *Answer:* B

*Rational:* Care planning begins as soon as the patient is diagnosed with cancer, as the plan for the entire continuum of care needs to be addressed from the beginning. At the treatment and survivorship stages, the time for care planning has passed, and, at the screening stage, it is too soon.

## CHAPTER 6

1. *Answer:* C

*Rationale:* Charles, Gafni and Whelan (1997) described Shared Decision Making as a model of care delivery that requires collaboration between the patient and the clinician.

2. *Answer:* C

*Rationale:* Step 1 of AHRQ's Shared Decision Making process requires the clinician to inform the patient of choices as well as explicitly invite and involve the patient in the decision-making process. Step 2: Assist your patient in comparing and evaluating treatment options by discussing the risks and benefits of each option. Step 3: Assess your patient's goals, values, and priorities and incorporate what matters most to your patient. Step 4: Make a decision with your patient. Step 5: Evaluate the treatment decision: plan to follow-up and revisit the decision, monitor progress, and revise as needed.

3. *Answer:* D

*Rationale:* Key elements of shared decision making include at least two participants: clinician and patient; both parties share information and take steps to build consensus about preferred treatment, weighing risks and benefits. Mutual agreement should be reached between patient and clinician on treatment approach (verbal and/or written). Choices a, b, and c all suggest collaboration among families or among healthcare providers not patient and healthcare provider.

4. *Answer:* C

*Rationale:* Options A, B, and D are all long-term benefits of Shared Decision Making. C is a short-term benefit. Short-term benefits include increased confidence in treatment decisions, higher satisfaction with treatment decisions, enhanced trust with providers, improved self-efficacy, and less stress and anxiety related to treatment decision making. Long-term benefits relate to adherence to treatment, improved quality of life, and remission.

5. *Answer:* C

*Rationale:* Oncology nurses reported scope of practice, limited time, limited resources devoted to Shared Decision Making education and training, and lack of leadership support for Shared Decision Making as barriers to Shared Decision Making implementation.

6. *Answer:* D

*Rationale:* Older adults with cancer reported that convenience, trust with their physician, and their recommendation were influential in their treatment decisions. Access to patient decision aids has not been reported as an influential factor for treatment decisions in older adults with cancer.

7. *Answer:* B

*Rationale:* Two published systematic reviews on preferred and actual preferences for patient participation in decision making found that the Control Preferences Scale was the most frequently used instrument to measure the patient's preferences for participation in decision making.

8. *Answer:* C

*Rationale:* Understanding the cancer diagnosis is the #1 information needs of patients diagnosed with cancer. Knowing how much longer they are going to live is ranked #2 and knowing the treatment options for their cancer diagnosis is ranked #3. In older adults with cancer, knowing how they can maintain independence and continue self-care is ranked #3 and knowing the treatment options is ranked #4.

9. *Answer:* B

*Rationale:* The clinician's awareness of personal locus of control, socioemotional approach to communication, and empathy to patients were found to be strong determinants of quality patient and clinician communication.

10. *Answer:* D

*Rationale:* A reflects the advocacy role, B reflects the patient education role, and C reflects the information sharing to multidisciplinary team role of the oncology nurse during the treatment decision-making process. D is the correct answer because it addresses uncertainty and the complexity of a diagnosis.

11. *Answer:* B

*Rationale:* The correct answer is B. The signing into law of the Affordable Care Act (ACA) was not a factor in the emergence of Shared Decision Making. Though the ACA has had a wide-reaching impact on cancer care and,

healthcare, in general, it did not affect SDM. SDM, however, was affected greatly by the desire for patient autonomy and active participation in their own healthcare. The rapid change and general explosion of healthcare options also had patients wishing to gain more control over the decision-making process and, also, consumerism in countries such as Canada and the U.S, as well as in Australia and Europe, made patients more discerning consumers, thus increasing demand for them to have a say in their healthcare.

12. *Answer:* A

*Rationale:* The oncology nurse meeting with Mrs. S provided both patient education material and psychosocial support for her patient. In the future, she might provide advocacy for the patient, but, at this time in their nurse and patient relationship, she is offering up patient education and psychosocial support. She did not complete a patient needs assessment, nor did she perform an outcome evaluation, so answers B through D are incorrect.

## CHAPTER 7

1. *Answer:* C

*Rationale:* Proto-oncogenes that are mutated, such as Ras, can enable a cancer cell to be self-sufficient in growth, and are common in pancreatic and colorectal cancers. In chromosome translocations, one chromosome moves to another as the cell divides, thereby activating an oncogene, such as occurs in CML where the BCR gene on chromosome 9 is fused to the Abl gene on chromosome 22, making a protein called tyrosine kinase, which proliferates myeloid cells. Missense mutation changes a DNA base pair that results in the substitution of one amino acid for another in the protein made by a gene and is typically the cause of sickle cell disease. An insertion mutation is the addition of one or more nucleotide base pairs into a DNA sequence, such as occurs in Huntington's disease or fragile X syndrome.

2. *Answer:* B

*Rationale:* Epidermal growth factor receptors participate in colon cancer development and play a role in some colon cancer metastases. Vascular endothelial growth factors may cause tumor cells to spread to regional lymph nodes. Nerve growth factors are primarily involved in the regulation of growth, maintenance, proliferation, and survival of certain target neurons, especially those that transmit pain, temperature, and touch sensations. There is no medial growth factor.

3. *Answer:* A

*Rationale:* Clonal evolution describes the process of cells within a tumor accumulating genetic changes over time that are different from once cell to the next, A tumor may be varied and consist of cells that rose from the same mother cell that are genotypically different from one another, and arise from the survival of the fittest collection of cancer cells. Convergent evolution and changes and coevolution are two of the six important patterns of macroevolution, which are not involved in the development of carcinogenesis. Perseverance is a term to indicate steadfastness and does not relate to the process of carcinogenesis.

4. ***Answer:*** D

***Rationale:*** Angiogenesis is the creation of new blood vessels from existing ones to provide nutrients and remove waste products. Carcinogenesis is the formation of a cancer where normal cells are transformed into cancer cells. Glycolysis is the breakdown of glucose by enzymes, releasing energy and pyruvic acid and is not involved in metastases. Pathogenesis of a disease is the biological mechanism that leads to the disease state, and can describe the origin and development of the disease.

5. ***Answer:*** B

***Rationale:*** "Skip metastasis" is an example tumor cell dissemination throughout the lymphatic system. "Skip metastasis" occurs when cells bypass the first lymph node and reach more distant sites. Tumors bypassing one organ and metastasizing in another is not an example of a pathway in which tumor cells disseminate. Tumor cells spreading through pulmonary capillary beds or pulmonary arteriovenous (AV) shunts is an example of arterial spread. Arteries have thick walls, and are not able to be penetrated as veins are.

6. ***Answer:*** A

***Rationale:*** Non-small cell lung cancer (NSCLC) accounts for 85% of lung cancer diagnoses and is also the most common primary tumor metastasizing to brain, with about 9% of patients with NSCLC developing brain metastases. Prostate cancer commonly metastasizes to the adrenal gland, bone, liver, and lung. Liver cancer is often the site of metastatic cancer. Colorectal cancer typically metastasizes to the liver, lung, and peritoneum.

7. ***Answer:*** C

***Rationale:*** A history of sunburns and tanning parlor use is a key association and cause of cancer. Too much fiber in a person's daily diet is not identified as key association and cause of cancer rather lack of fiber is identified as a cause for cancer. Other key association and causes of cancer include lack of exercise and daily intake of processed red meat. Five to nine servings of fruits and vegetables are recommended daily. Lack or limited intake of fruits and vegetables is a key association and cause of cancer.

8. ***Answer:*** A

***Rationale:*** The acquisition of cancer hallmarks is classified as the third phase of the process of cell mutation. A tumor is formed from a single precursor cell with genetic alterations that undergoes clonal expansion. Clonal evolution is the process of cells within a tumor accumulating genetic changes over time that are different from one cell to the next. Initiating mutation is considered the first step in the process, acquisition of genetic instability is next, and, finally, the cell undergoes further genetic mutation.

9. ***Answer:*** B

***Rationale:*** During carcinogenesis, normal cells are transferred into cancer cells through a complex and dynamic process that starts with mutations in regulatory cells and is promoted by genomic instability, inflammation, and interactions within the tumor microen-vironment. Angiogenesis is the creation of new blood vessels from existing ones to provide nutrients and remove waste products. Normal cells have a developmental regulatory program called epithelial mesenchymal transition (EMT). This process causes epithelial cells to lose cell polarity and cell–cell adhesion and have invasive properties so that they can become mesenchymal cells. This process is involved in mesoderm formation and neural tube formation during embryogenesis. It has also been found to play a role in wound healing and organ fibrosis Epigenetics describes a mechanism that may change the activity of a gene without changing the sequence of DNA.

## CHAPTER 8

1. ***Answer:*** C

***Rationale:*** The elimination phase represents ongoing immune surveillance where the host is cancer free. In the situation above, the patient has relapsed. The equilibrium phase is a phase by which a rare tumor clone mutates to avoid elimination by the innate immune system. There is no evidence of clinically measurable disease in this phase. This does not apply to patient situation, as he/she has new lesions. The escape phase correlates with mutated tumor clones which have evaded the innate and adaptive immune systems, resulting in clinically measurable disease, as seen in this example. Progression is not a phase of the proposed tumor suppression mechanism.

2. ***Answer:*** A

***Rationale:*** Innate and adaptive immunity is the elimination phase of extrinsic tumor suppression mechanism, where the host's immune system responds to microscopic invasion by destroying circulating tumor cells. This is a homeostatic process ongoing in host's with an intact immune system. B is an example of the equilibrium phase of tumor suppression where the first line of defense with natural barriers and inflammatory response have been overcome. Humoral and cell-mediated immunity mechanisms are now holding tumor growth in check. C is incorrect as the equilibrium phase occurs once resistant tumor clones escape immune surveillance and innate immunity has been overcome. D is incorrect as the mechanism of action with chemotherapeutic agents is cell death through cytotoxic cellular processes that inhibit mitosis. Immunotherapy agents function to increase immune surveillance through modification of the adaptive immune system.

3. ***Answer:*** A

***Rationale:*** Only the adaptive immune system has memory. The innate immune system is a rapid cellular response to invasion of pathogens and/or tissue damage and does not rely on previous exposure to initiate an immune response. Humoral immunity uses antibodies produced by B lymphocytes, which respond to a specific antigen. Cell-mediated immunity uses T lymphocytes to active immune responses. Inflammatory response is controlled by the innate immune system, not adaptive immune system. Nonspecific processes for immune defense is related to innate immunity. The adaptive immune system uses processes to create antibodies and T lymphocyte activation to respond to specific antigens.

4. *Answer:* B

*Rationale:* Chemotherapy resistance occurs as a result of changes in tumor biology, such as drug inactivation, drug target alteration, drug efflux, DNA damage repair, and cell death inhibition. These are changes that occur with the tumor's interaction with the chemotherapeutic agent and not with the host's immune system. Response B reflects one of many examples of how persistent tumor clones have acquired the ability to "hide" from the immune system, leading to continued reproduction and cancer progression. By promoting T cells to increase PD1/PDL1 on their surface, tumor cells are decreasing T-cell immune surveillance and reproduction, which allows for continued growth of the tumor. Recently developed immunotherapeutic medications, called checkpoint inhibitors, use this known concept of tumor biology to block tumor cells from promoting hosts' T-cell exhaustion, which stimulates the adaptive immune system. The innate immune system is the body's first line of defense against host invaders and works with the adaptive immune system in tumor surveillance. When the innate immune system can no longer keep the tumor in check (equilibrium phase), the adaptive immune system can function independently to perform ongoing immune surveillance. Another method of immune system evasion is decreasing or losing antigens, not increasing, on the tumor's surface. When this occurs, the adaptive immune system can no longer recognize the tumor cell. This leads to ongoing progression/reproduction of cancer.

5. *Answer:* D

*Rationale:* Antigen presentation refers to the process of activating T cells, which is called cell-mediated immunity. T lymphocytes activation by APCs leads to T-cell multiplication immune surveillance/ response. T lymphocytes are involved in cell-mediated immunity as part of the adaptive immune system. Neutrophils are a part of the innate immune system, not adaptive immune system. Humoral immunity involves antibodies produced by B lymphocytes. Each B cell reproduces and differentiates to become either a memory B cell or plasma cell. Plasma cells then circulate and bind to specific antigens, which starts a cascade of cytokine reactions to attract macrophages and NK cells.

6. *Answer:* A

*Rationale:* Cytokines are proteins that assist in communication between cells of the immune system to aid in rapid response. Macrophages are immune cells of the innate immune system that release cytokines to produce inflammatory response and present antigens to T cells. Plasma cells are differentiated B cells, which produce one specific antibody against a specific antigen as part of the humoral immune response. Erythrocytes or red blood cells develop in the bone marrow and transport oxygen to the body's tissues.

7. *Answer:* C

*Rationale:* The bone marrow functions as both a primary and secondary lymphoid tissue. The thymus is a primary lymphoid organ and allows for the maturation of the lymphocytes. The spleen, lymph nodes, and tonsils/adenoids are examples of secondary lymphoid tissue. The spleen responds to bloodborne antigens, while the lymph nodes initiate immune responses to antigens circulating in the lymph, skin, or mucosal surfaces.

8. *Answer:* C

*Rationale:* The T cells migrate to the thymus gland for maturation and are integral to immune surveillance and response. NK cells are large granular cells that release cytokines, migrate rapidly to the site of the inflammation, and directly kill tumor or viral-infected cells without previous antigen exposure. Cytotoxic T cells play a role in autoimmunity and allogenic organ rejection and destroy viral infections and cancers. B cells develop in the bone marrow and include memory B cells and plasma cells.

9. *Answer:* A

Granulocytes have granules in cytoplasm with enzymes that aid in digestion of foreign particles (phagocytosis) and cause inflammation. Neutrophils are the most abundant granulocytes, but they only live about 6 hours. Neutrophils cause inflammatory response due to engulfing and destroying foreign particles and debris. Basophils have IgE receptors that are involved in allergic responses and cause release of histamine and prostaglandins. Eosinophils attack parasites and secrete cytokines that cause inflammation during allergic responses. Macrophages rapidly recognize, ingest, and kill microbes; macrophages are not granulocytes.

## CHAPTER 9

1. *Answer:* B

*Rationale:* Precision medicine is the use of specific information about a person's genes, proteins, and environment to prevent, diagnose, and treat disease. Tumor size, treatment history, and laboratory values may affect response but are not the primary consideration when applying precision medicine. PD-L1 expression is an example of using genomic information from the tumor and impacts treatment decisions in head and neck squamous cell, Hodgkin lymphoma, Merkel cell carcinoma, urothelial carcinomas. Targeted therapies that might be utilized in those with high PD-L1 expression include atezolizumab, avelumab, durvalumab, nivolumab, and pemrolizuma

2. *Answer:* D

*Rationale:* Risk assessment tools estimate a person's risk of developing cancer over set period of years (next five years) or over a lifetime. There are tools readily available to provide estimates of the likelihood of developing cancers of the breast, colon, malignant melanoma, prostate, and lung cancers. These risk assessment models combine demographic variables such as age, gender, and ethnicity, medical history such as prior surgeries, presence of colon polyps and reproductive history, family history of malignancy, and lifestyle factors such as tobacco use, diet, and sun exposure. Tumor stage means the patient has already been diagnosed with cancer and can be a factor considered when determining prognostic information and treatment.

3. *Answer:* A

*Rationale:* Biomarkers can determine disease severity and outcomes and aids in treatment planning. A biomarker is a molecule found in blood, tissues, or other body fluids that signals the presence of a condition or disease; can be used to evaluate response to treatment. Predictive biomarkers provide information on the effect of a therapeutic intervention. A prognostic biomarker biomarker provides information about the patient's overall cancer outcome, regardless of therapy. Biomarkers are not generally used to determine if a patient is a candidate for surgery. A germline mutation may suggest the need for risk reducing surgery.

4. *Answer:* C

*Rationale:* ER/PR/Her-2 Neu are examples of biomarkers used to guide treatment decisions. Germline genetic testing might confirm the presence of a hereditary cancer predisposition syndrome. ER/PR/Her2 Neu status does not alter the dose of the drug but it might alter the choice of agent. Adjuvant chemotherapy decisions might also be based on tools that assess a combination of genes on a tumor to determine the potential efficacy of chemotherapy (e.g. Mammaprint, Endopredict, or Oncotype). Er/PR/Her2Neu status might be one criteria utilized to determine if a patient is eligible for a clinical trial but it will not be the sole criteria.

5. *Answer:* D

*Rationale:* Pharmacogenomics is the integration of pharmacology and genomics in developing safe and effective medications. Pharmacogenomics can determine safe doses based on genomic data. It can help reduce the use of drugs with serious or toxic side effects thereby increasing rates of adherence to therapy. It does not necessarily decrease the cost of medications or increase enrollment in clinical trials.

6. *Answer:* C

*Rationale:* Clinically relevant biomarkers are associated with specific cancers; ideal targets are present in cancer cells but not in normal cells. Targeted therapy has adverse reactions, albeit different from traditional chemotherapy. Targeted therapies can be classified as hazardous drugs, and can be delivered orally (small molecule drugs) or parenterally (Monoclonal Abs).

7. *Answer:* A

*Rationale:* Genetic testing results may take up to 8 weeks and cause waiting-related patient anxiety when treatment is dependent on results. Germline genetic testing has implications for both the patient and family members. It can be expensive and insurance preauthorization is often required. Informed consent issues include how privacy will be maintained and use of the specimen after testing is completed

8. *Answer:* C

*Rationale:* The correct answer is C. Gene amplification is defined as the increase in the number of copies of a gene that may cause cancer cell growth or resistance to anticancer drugs. The loss of all or part of a gene found in cancer and other genetic diseases is defined as gene deletion (answer A). Answer B is epigenetic alteration, which is defined as a heritable change that does not alter the DNA sequence but changes gene expression. And, finally, the increase in the copies of a protein made from a gene that may play a role in cancer development is gene overexpression (answer D).

9. *Answer:* B

*Rationale:* The correct answer is B. Gene deletion is defined as the loss of all or part of a gene found in cancer and other genetic diseases is defined. Answer A is epigenetic alteration, which is defined as a heritable change that does not alter the DNA sequence but changes gene expression. Gene overexpression (answer C) is the increase in the copies of a protein made from a gene that may play a role in cancer development. Answer D is gene amplification, which is defined as the increase in the number of copies of a gene that may cause cancer cell growth or resistance to anticancer drugs.

10. *Answer:* B

*Rationale:* The correct answer is B. Pharmacokinetics examines how the individual will affect the drug. This is contrary to pharmacodynamics, which is how the drug will affect the individual (Answer A). Pharmacogenomics (Answer C) is the study of how a patient's genomes affect responses to medications. And genetics is the study of heredity and the variation of inherited characteristics.

11. *Answer:* D

*Rationale:* The correct answer is D. Patients provide biospecimens for biorepository and research purposes in addition to use in clinical decision making, and an ethical consideration for a patient undergoing treatment with precision medicine is whether or not their personal information is safe and secure from cyber crime as well as intrusions from the government. Adverse events and side effects are clinical concerns and not necessarily ethical considerations, and, while financial toxicity is a major concern for patients and families undergoing expensive treatments, the cost of treatment may not be an ethical concern, especially if costs were explained before treatment begins.

## CHAPTER 10

1. *Answer:* B

*Rationale:* "DNA makes RNA and RNA makes protein," explains the production of protein for all body functions". This knowledge aids in the education of patients and families about their inherited genetic testing results. A is incorrect because, while this is an accurate statement, it is not necessary information for oncology nursing practice. D is also false as "DNA makes RNA and RNA makes protein" directs the protein production in the body. C is also false as RNA contains Uracil instead of the Thymine contained in DNA.

2. *Answer:* D

*Rationale:* Epigenetics is defined as switching genes on and off with a variety of "chemical tails" attached to the DNA structure, without changing the DNA sequence. DNA transcription is controlled by opening or closing the tightly wound histone structure. This occurs by opening (allowing transcription) and closing the histone structure to alter the "DNA to RNA to protein" outcome. A is incorrect as this statement is incomplete and therefore incorrect. B is also a FALSE statement because any of the environmental effects noted can be positively (prevention) or negatively (causative) associated with development of cancer. C is a FALSE statement. Most cancers are the result of environmentally caused mutations in single cells over the lifetime of an individual.

3. *Answer:* B

*Rationale:* HBOC is associated with ovarian cancer especially when it occurs before age 50. HBOC is also associated with early onset breast cancer (before age 50) especially when there are multiple family members diagnosed with breast cancer, triple negative breast cancer diagnosed before age 60 or a family history of pancreatic cancer or metastatic prostate cancer. A is incorrect because these individuals are each from both maternal and paternal lineages. C is also incorrect, because even though her brother is young, testicular cancer is not associated with HBOC and testicular cancer is usually diagnosed in younger men. D is incorrect because childhood leukemia is not associated with HBOC.

4. *Answer:* C

*Rationale:* Germline mutations occur in the reproductive cells of a person with an inherited predisposition to cancer. A is incorrect because single nucleotide polymorphism (SNPs) occur in both germline or somatic cells. A SNP is a change in a nucleotide of a gene causing variation in the DNA sequence that affects 1% of population. B is incorrect as both males and females develop mutations in their somatic cells over a lifetime. Only females have a monthly reproductive cycle. D is incorrect as somatic mutations occur in body cells (except the gametes) after conception and are acquired over a lifetime.

5. *Answer:* A

*Rationale:* A malignant tumor is derived from genetic instability and genetic mutations in genes that control cell growth and proliferation. B is incorrect as proto-oncogenes are normal genes essential for normal cell growth and proliferation. Mutations occurring in proto-oncogenes convert to oncogene activation to cause uncontrolled cell division. C is incorrect because driver mutations offer a selective growth advantage to cancerous cells, while passenger mutations do not. D is incorrect as mutations in DNA repair genes may be inherited from a parent or acquired over time due to aging or impact of carcinogens from the environment.

6. *Answer:* C

*Rationale:* Most hereditary cancer syndromes are inherited in an autosomal dominant fashion. A is incorrect because in most cases the altered gene is passed from one side of the family. B is incorrect as there are deleterious germline mutations in cancer susceptibility genes that are suggestive of risk for hereditary cancer. D is incorrect as cancer types are similar in multiple generations,

usually from one side of the family, with a risk for hereditary cancer.

7. *Answer:* D.

*Rationale:* Any individual with a diagnosis of cancer should provide information about treatments, age at onset, and other pertinent medical history that might explain the diagnosis of cancer such as risk factor exposures. A is an incorrect answer as only three generations of cancer information for both lineages is required. B is incorrect as females are designated as circles while males are designated as squares. C is incorrect as race, ethnicity, and age of individuals should be included for all of the individuals in a 3. Identification of a germline mutation in a cancer susceptibility gene may not be possible because of the limited sensitivity of the techniques used generation pedigree.

8. *Answer:* C

*Rationale:* When an individual is tested for a known family mutation, they did not inherit the risk associated with the mutation from the side of the family with the known mutation. The history from the other side can also influence risk. A negative test result in a family with a known mutation implies at least population risk for developing malignancy and if there is risk from the other side of the family risk could be increased. A is incorrect as identification of a germline mutation in a cancer susceptibility gene also may not be possible because of the limited sensitivity of the techniques used and this can occur with both a known family mutation and when there is no known family mutation. B and D are incorrect as this can be found with a "no known family genetic mutation," and may offer a reasonable explanation as to why a mutation was not detected in a family with suspected genetic risk.

9. *Answer:* B

*Rationale:* A VUS is a change in the genetic material for which there is not enough data to determine if it is a harmful or harmless change in the genetic material. A is incorrect as a VUS is identified when a cancer risk has NOT been established. C is also incorrect as a VUS label can change to pathogenic or benign based on information identified in new types of genetic testing. D is incorrect as a VUS can be a fairly common finding.

10. *Answer:* A

*Rationale:* This test includes only the three *BRCA1/2* (selected variants) mutations most common in persons of Ashkenazi descent. These are the most common out of thousands of mutations which are *not* included in the direct-to-consumer test. B is incorrect as it is FDA approved. C is incorrect as it is not FDA approved for diagnosis or clinical decision making in breast cancer. D is incorrect as Only 23 and ME is FDA approved but there are other types of direct to consumer genetic testing.

11. *Answer:* A

*Rationale:* Cytogenetic reports include modal number of chromosomes, sex chromosome designation; abnormality abbreviation - first chromosome separated with a semicolon from the second chromosome, then the arm and band number B is incorrect as this detects sequence changes in regions being analyzed. Sanger sequencing is a form of gene sequencing that determines the sequence of a gene being tested and detects sequence changes in regions being analyzed. A limitation of this testing is that it may miss mutations outside the coding region or mutations that are large genomic rearrangements or large deletions The GWAS sequencing reviews for changes with specific disease (cancer type) versus people without the cancer. D is incorrect as microarrays are used for mutation detection and gene expression.

12. *Answer:* C

*Rationale:* A de novo mutation is change in a gene and is present for the first time in one family member due to mutation in a germ cell (egg or sperm) of one of the parents or in the fertilized egg. A is incorrect as a germ-line mutation is passed from generation to generation. B is incorrect as germline mutations are present in the reproductive cells (the eggs and sperm). D is incorrect as it only occurs in the gametes: eggs and sperm.

13. *Answer:* C

*Rationale:* Heightened anxiety may result when patients learn that they are at a substantially increased risk for developing cancer or another primary lesion. A is incorrect as, although there can be depression, a sense of relief has not been reported; in fact they experience more anxiety. B is incorrect as this relates to family members versus the patient as it occurs when family members pass on the genetic mutation to one of their offspring. D is incorrect as you see this type of guilt in persons who have not inherited the genetic mutation present in other close family members.

14. *Answer:* A

*Rationale:* The Genetic Information Nondiscrimination Act (GINA), federal legislation enacted in 2008, applies to health insurance and employment discrimination based on genetic information. GINA does not apply to active duty military personnel, Veterans Administration, or Native American Health Service because the laws amended for GINA do not apply to these groups. Health insurance protections with GINA include protections against accessing an individual's genomic information, requirements for an individual to undergo a genetic or genomic test, and using genomic information against a person during medical underwriting. Employment protections include prohibiting employers from accessing an individual's genetic information, use of genomic information to deny employment, or collecting genomic information without consent. GINA does not supersede state legislation that provides for more extensive protections.

15. *Answer:* D

*Rationale:* Genetic testing cannot determine longevity of life so it is not part of the informed consent process. Answers A, B, and C are parts of the informed consent. Elements of informed consent include discussion of the purpose of the test, motivation for testing, risks and benefits of testing, potential limitations of testing, risk of misidentified paternity, inheritance pattern of the gene and likelihood of a mutation being detection, accuracy of the test, potential outcomes of testing, how confidentiality

will be maintained, the possibility of discrimination, alternatives to testing, how testing will influence health care decision making, costs of testing and considerations for testing in children.

16. *Answer:* A

*Rationale:* All the listed are genetic diseases, but the only one that is not associated with risk of developing brain cancer is Huntington's disease. Neurofibromatosis type 1 is associated with malignant peripheral nerve sheath tumors, optic gliomas, meningiomas, hamartomatous intestinal polyps other gliomas, and leukemias. Li Fraumeni syndrome is associated with soft tissue sarcoma, osteosarcoma, pre-menopausal breast cancer, brain tumors, adrenocortical carcinoma (ACC), and leukemias. Von Hippel Lindau disease is associated with renal cancers, pancreatic neuroendocrine tumors, hemangioblastomas, and pheochromocytomas.

17. *Answer:* B

*Rationale:* The small arm is known as the petite arm and is labeled as "p". The long arm is labeled as "q" because "q" comes after "p" in the alphabet. There is no "o" or "s" arm.

18. *Answer:* A

*Rationale:* Exons are protein-coding segments of a gene. Introns are non–protein-coding segments, the sequence-interrupting piece of a gene. A codon is a sequence of three mRNA nucleotides (e.g., ACG) yielding one (threonine) of the 20 amino acids. An autosome is any chromosome that is not a sex chromosome.

19. *Answer:* B

*Rationale:* MUTYH-associated polyposis (MAP) is an autosomal recessive hereditary cancer syndrome and is associated with colon cancer and duodenal cancer, as well as colon, duodenal, and gastric fundic gland polyps, osteomas, sebaceous gland adenomas, and pilomatricomas. Polyp counts range from a few to >1000 with biallelic MUTYH mutations. Hereditary retinoblastoma, hereditary diffuse gastric cancer, and multiple endocrine neoplasia are all inherited in an autosomal dominant fashion. Hereditary diffuse gastric cancer found on the CDH1 gene is associated with diffuse gastric cancer, lobular breast cancer, adenocarcinoma and epithelial ovarian cancer, prostate and signet ring colon cancer. Hereditary retinoblastoma is found on the RBI gene and is associated with malignant tumors of the retina, usually occurring before age 5. A family history of retinoblastoma, bilateral retinal tumors, and multifocal tumors have the highest chance to have hereditary retinoblastoma. Individuals with hereditary retinoblastoma also have an increased risk for pinealoblastoma, osteosarcomas, sarcoma, and melanoma. Multiple endocrine neoplasia type 1 (MEN1) is found on the MEN1 gene. It is associated with endocrine and nonendocrine tumors, including tumors of the parathyroid glands, pituitary gland, and the pancreas.

20. *Answer:* B

*Rationale:* Lynch syndrome, which was previously known as hereditary nonpolyposis colorectal cancer [HNPCC]), is associated with mutations in the following genes: MLH1, MSH2 (including methylation due to

EPCAM deletion), MSH6 and PMS2. Lynch syndrome is characterized by microsatellite instability (MSI) due to defective mismatch repair. Cancers associated with Lynch syndrome include cancers of the colon, rectum, stomach, small intestine, esophagus, biliary tract, brain, endometrium, and ovary. Other cancers at elevated risk are transitional cell carcinoma of the ureters and renal pelvis and pancreatic cancer. Lynch syndrome is not typically associated with cancers of the lung or thyroid or sarcomas.

## CHAPTER 11

1. *Answer:* D

*Rationale:* In an observational study, participants are not assigned to a specific intervention and health care outcomes are assessed. In an experimental study, participants receive specific interventions and each type is designed to answer different research questions. An interventional study is another name for experimental as described above. Expanded access occurs when a clinical research study provides a means for patients to receive an investigational drug outside of a designated clinical trial. In expanded access, the investigational agent is restricted to patients with a serious condition or disease who no longer have satisfactory medical options available and who may benefit from the investigational therapy.

2. *Answer:* A

*Rationale:* A screening trial evaluates the effectiveness of new techniques for early detection of cancer in the general population. A diagnostic trial evaluates tests or procedures that may better identify cancer in symptomatic individuals. A quality of life trial explores pharmacologic or non-pharmacologic therapies to minimize cancer related toxicities. A prevention trial evaluates the safety and efficacy of various risk reduction strategies such as chemoprevention or actions such as increasing fruit and vegetable intake, adding exercise, avoiding tobacco, or limiting alcohol use.

3. *Answer:* A

*Rationale:* Expanded access provides a means for patients and their physicians to use an investigational drug outside of a designated clinical trial. Off label use of a drug is not a characteristic of expanded access. Expanded access is restricted to patients with a serious condition or disease who no longer have satisfactory medical options available. In compassionate use, not expanded access, approval from FDA may be obtained within 24 hours in emergency situations.

4. *Answer:* C

*Rationale:* The "3+3" Phase I trial designed to determine maximum tolerated dose is an adaptive design. Adaptive design allows investigators to change trial design without compromising the integrity and validity of the trial. In a 3+3 trial, three patients start the trial at a given dose and, if no dose-limiting toxicities are observed, three more patients are added at a higher dose until the first instance of limiting toxicity is observed, then three more patients will be added at the same dose.

Dose limiting toxicity in two or all three patients will identify the next lower dose as the maximum tolerated dose. Factorial design allows for multiple factors to be studied simultaneously. Parallel design randomizes participants to one of several treatment groups. Basket trials enroll patients with any cancer type sharing a specific target.

5. *Answer:* B

*Rationale:* The principal investigator ensures the ethical conduct of the research study. The study coordinator, statisticians, and data managers are all important members of the research team, but not responsible for the research study as a whole. The responsibilities of these other research members may vary from study to study.

6. *Answer:* D

*Rationale:* The Belmont Report focused primarily on beneficence, respect for persons, and justice. The Nuremberg Code focused on voluntary consent. The Declaration of Helsinki focused on informed consent, therapeutic versus non-therapeutic research, and surrogate decision making. The Common Rule, also known as the Protection of Human Research Subjects, focused on informed consent and institutional review boards.

7. *Answer:* B

*Rationale:* Eligibility criteria are characteristics that potential participants must meet to be enrolled into the trial and includes demographic, disease-specific, and treatment-related variables. These include inclusion and exclusion criteria. Common inclusion criteria that must be satisfied before an oncology patient can enter a trial includes performance status using indicators such as laboratory values, Eastern Cooperative Oncology Group (ECOG) or Karnofsky Performance Status. Other common inclusion criteria include stage and/or status of tumor, presence of measurable disease, and presence or absence of biomarkers. Geography or place of residence is not usually an eligibility criteria, although proximity to the trial may make participation easier. Some studies may not allow previous research participation; this can vary from study to study. The number of children a potential study participant has is seldom an eligibility criteria.

8. *Answer:* B

*Rationale:* On average, 20 to 100 subjects are needed for a Phase I study. Phase I studies often include subjects with many cancer types (e.g., solid tumors), subjects with tumors refractory to standard therapy, and subjects with adequate organ function, specifically bone marrow, liver, and kidney function. Pediatric Phase I studies are conducted after a safety and toxicity evaluation in adults. Ten to twelve subjects are needed for a Phase 0 study, while 80-300 subjects are needed for a Phase II study on average. In contrast, hundreds to thousands of subjects are needed for Phase III and IV studies, on average.

9. *Answer:* C

*Rationale:* The definition of overall survival is the time from randomization until the time of death. Disease free survival is the time from randomization until recurrence of tumor or death from any cause. The objective response rate refers to the proportion of patients with a reduction of tumor size of a predetermined amount and for a minimum time period. The definition of the time to progression is the time from randomization until objective tumor progression, excluding death.

10. **Correct answer D**

**Rationale:** The example of "A, B, A and B, placebo" represents a factorial design. Factorial design allows for multiple factors, such as multiple treatments, to be studied simultaneously. The example of "A or B" represents a parallel design. In parallel design, a participant is randomized to one of several treatment groups. The example of "A→outcome→B" represents a crossover design. A crossover design allows participants to receive more than one treatment. A, B, A and B requires placebo (neither A nor B) to be added to represent a factorial design.

11. **Correct Answer: C**

**Rationale:** A clinical trial study where subjects who have no reported outcomes or conditions are followed and compared based on exposure is a cohort study.

In an experimental or interventional study, participants receive specific interventions. Each type of clinical trial in an experimental or interventional study is designed to answer a different research question. Studies defined as outcomes research explore the results of healthcare practices and interventions, and feature patient-based outcomes, as well as the study of populations and different healthcare delivery methods.

12. **Correct Answer: B**

**Rationale:** Outcomes research explore the results of healthcare practices and interventions, and feature patient-based outcomes, as well as the study of populations and different healthcare delivery methods. The clinical trials in experimental studies are designed to answer a different research question. Cohort studies are defined as clinical trial studies where subjects who have no reported outcomes or conditions are followed and compared, based on exposure. In a cross-sectional study, described is the association between a condition and other characteristics that may exist in a specific group.

13. **Correct Answer: C**

**Rationale:** J. L. is participating in a quality of life study. This type of clinical trial explores pharmacologic or nonpharmacologic treatments to minimize toxicities related to cancer and cancer treatments. In contrast, screening trials are meant to evaluate the effectiveness of new techniques for early detection of cancer in the general populous. Diagnostic trials evaluate types of procedures or tests that may better help identify cancer in individuals who present with symptoms of the disease. Treatment or therapeutic trials evaluate the safety of new drugs, vaccines, biological agents, approaches to surgery or radiation therapy, treatment combinations, or other interventions. Even though J. L. is enrolled in a study exploring drug treatments, his trial explores treatments to minimize cancer-related toxicities, rather than exploring the safety and efficacy of new drugs or treatments.

## CHAPTER 12

1. **Answer: A**

**Rationale:** Metastatic tumors spread to the bone from primary solid tumors. Common tumors include lung, breast, kidney, thyroid, and prostate cancers. Primary cancers that do not spread to the bone include brain cancer, leukemia, and melanoma.

2. **Answer: B**

**Rationale:** For EFTs, 50% of patients diagnosed are adolescents. Approximately 50% of patients diagnosed are adolescents. EFTs are associated with retinoblastoma and skeletal anomalies. They tend to be highly malignant (approximately 25% with metastases at time of diagnosis to lungs, lymph nodes, other bones). The five-year disease-free survival rate is approximately 73% because of effective multimodality therapies, and precision in surgery. EFTs are characterized as local or regional to the bone. EFTs, a type of bone cancer, are not associated with hormonal therapy.

3. **Answer: C**

**Rationale:** Bone pain is described as dull and aching, increasing at night and increasing over time. Prickly and sharp pain describes pain that involves the nervous system. Bone pain is steady pain, not intermittent pain.

4. **Answer: C**

**Rationale:** A possible bone or soft tissue mass may or may not be visible or palpable. The mass may be firm, nontender, and warm. Its size should be compared bilaterally to the other fibia. This type of mass is not described as pus-filed or pock-marked. Anemia is a condition related to the patient's blood, not the bone or soft tissue mass.

5. **Answer: C**

**Rationale:** The goals of surgical treatment include the following: survival, removal of the tumor, and preserving functionality. Amputation may be the chosen treatment, but it is not the goal of treatment. Removing the malignancy's blood supply is not a surgical goal of treatment.

6. **Answer: D**

**Rationale:** Issues of reconstruction include post-surgery union of non-malignant tissue, infections, healing, and functional concerns (especially with limb salvage). Thrombocytopenia is a condition of decreased platelets (clotting blood cells). Pruritis is an allergic reaction to topical or systemic treatment. For some targeted systematic treatments, cytokine response is when cytokines and other inflammatory mediators are released.

7. **Answer: D**

**Rationale:** Soft tissue tumors can be radiosensitive and radioresponsive. So, adjuvant radiotherapy can be a component of treatment before or after surgery, when the tumor is localized or after the tumor has been surgically debulked or removed. Radiotherapy is not a treatment for distant metastatic spread of disease. For soft tissue tumors, radiotherapy is an additional modality of treatment and not the primary treatment or considered a standard of care.

8. *Answer:* C

*Rationale:* Phantom limb pain or sensation can occur one to four weeks postoperatively. This type of pain can resolve in a few months or can be chronic. The patient may describe phantom limb pain as itching, pressure, tingling, severe cramping, throbbing, and/or a burning pain. Phantom limb pain occurs over a period of time and not just when the patient intermittently stands.

9. *Answer:* A

*Rationale:* Sarcomas of the blood vessels include hemangiosarcoma and Kaposi Sarcoma. Liposarcoma is a sarcoma that starts in the fat cells. Rhabdomyosarcoma and leiomyosarcoma are sarcomas that originate in muscle cells.

10. *Answer:* D

*Rationale:* Chondrosarcoma originates in the cartilage and typically occurs in the pelvis, upper legs, and shoulders. Chondrosarcoma is commonly diagnosed in patients who are 50 to 60 years old, and it is not considered a pediatric disease. Lymphangiosarcoma originates from the lymph nodes. Osteosarcoma originates from osteoid tissue.

11. *Answer:* C

*Rationale:* With complaints of worsening abdominal pain and potential blood in his stools, R. J. is presenting with possible signs of a possible soft tissue sarcoma. There may be worsening abdominal pain due to a retroperitoneal mass. When conducting her examination, the nurse may discover that the mass may or may not be visible, is firm to the touch, nontender, and possibly warm. Many soft tissue lesions can be benign. Chondrosarcoma is a cartilaginous tissue, commonly affecting the pelvis, femur, and shoulder. Kaposi sarcoma usually appears first as legions on the skin and is in the same family as Epstein-Barr virus. Osteosarcoma is commonly found in adolescents and young adults.

12. *Answer:* A

*Rationale:* According to the American Cancer Society and the National Cancer Institute, exposure to radiation is an identified risk factor for developing cancer of the soft tissue. A damaged immune system is not a risk factor, but a damaged lymph system is an example of a risk factor. Food allergies and exposure to viruses have not been identified as risk factors in developing soft tissue cancers. However, exposure to certain types of chemicals and particular types of family cancer syndromes are examples of risk factors that have been identified.

13. *Answer:* C

*Rationale:* Based on statistics reported by the National Cancer Institute (NCI) in 2018, between 1975 and 2010, childhood osteosarcoma mortality decreased by more than 50%. In adolescents ages 15 to 19 years old, the 5-year survival rate was reported to have increased 56% to approximately 66%, so those percentage values do not equal the decrease in mortality. Forty percent is incorrect.

## CHAPTER 13

1. *Answer:* A

*Rationale:* There are multiple risk factors for developing breast cancer. Breast cancer is 100 times more common in woman than men. The incidence of breast cancer is higher with aging, only 5% of women before the age of 40 develop breast cancer, but 60% of breast cancer cases occur after age 60 years or older. Breast cancer is 100 more times more common in women than in men. A person's family history also increases risk. Approximately 10% of all breast cancers are due to genetic susceptibility. Pregnancy after the age of 30 or nulliparity is associated with an increased risk.

2. *Answer:* B

*Rationale:* Family history of a first-degree relative having breast cancer is a consideration for genetic evaluation. This is especially important in women with a first degree or second-degree relative with breast cancer diagnosed before the age of 50, multiple family members with breast cancer, or a family history of ovarian cancer. Breast biopsy, reproductive factors such as nulliparity or age at menarche, first pregnancy or menopause are personal, not hereditary, risk factors for developing breast cancer.

3. *Answer:* A

*Rationale:* Male breast cancer is an indication for referral for genetic evaluation. Women diagnosed with breast cancer at age 50 or under should be given consideration for genetic evaluation, as well as women age 60 and under with triple negative breast cancer. Answers B, C, and D reflect on women with average or older age of onset. These women would not be considered for referral for genetic evaluation unless there was a family history of breast, ovarian, melanoma, pancreatic, prostate, or colon cancer, or possibly a diagnosis of two primary breast cancers.

4. *Answer:* C

*Rationale:* Aromatase inhibitors can prevent a new breast cancer from developing and are appropriate to utilize in women who are known to be postmenopausal. Premenopausal and postmenopausal women can also consider utilizing tamoxifen to reduce the risk of developing breast cancer. Metformin, retinoids, and cox-2 inhibitors are under investigation to determine if they are effective for the primary prevention of breast cancer.

5. *Answer:* C

*Rationale:* Basal cancers, known as triple negative breast cancer, tend to have a worse prognosis. Luminal A tumors have a high ER/PR expression and tend to respond well to endocrine therapy and are often associated with a better prognosis. The prognosis of lobular carcinoma is similar to that of ductal carcinoma. A poorer prognosis is associated with lymph node involvement

6. *Answer:* A

*Rationale:* WBRT is indicated when there are 4 or more brain metastases and the goal of therapy is palliative (to reduce symptoms and promote comfort care). WBRT is not curative. While pain management and improved or stabilizing neurologic status may be a potential benefit of WBRT, these both fall under the palliative intent of therapy. Adjuvant therapy in breast cancer usually refers to treatment given after surgery to remove the breast cancer. Neoadjuvant therapy is therapy given prior to breast surgery.

7. **Answer:** B

**Rationale:** The patient has received trastuzumab, which can lead to a decreased left ejection fraction or pulmonary problems. An anthracycline can also lead to cardiac toxicity. Breast cancer often metastasizes to the lung. Breast cancer also metastasizes to the brain and liver, but her symptoms are not suggestive of metastasis to these organs.

8. **Answer:** C

**Rationale:** Diagnostic modalities for breast cancer include core needle biopsy, stereotactic vacuum-assisted breast biopsy, fine-needle aspiration (FNA), incisional biopsy, or excisional biopsy. Imaging with mammography, breast MRI, or breast ultrasound may be used to localize the site to be biopsied.

9. **Answer:** A

**Rationale:** Prevention of lymphedema is far easier than treatment. Prevention measures include measuring the arm for increase in diameter postoperatively as compared to preoperatively. Other prevention measures include avoiding constriction to the arm from tourniquets and blood pressure cuffs as well as trauma or injuries that could lead to infection. Exercise should be supervised and gradually be added into the patient's daily routine. A temperature of greater than 100.5°F could be suggestive of a postoperative infection. Sodium intake has not been shown to impact lymphedema risk.

10. **Answer:** C

**Rationale:** The Oncotype test is a 21-gene assay used to predict the effectiveness of chemotherapy and estimate the chance of recurrence in women with early-stage ER/PR-positive breast cancer. The recurrence score is calculated from gene expression. There is no category of no risk. Low risk is a score of 0 to 17, and the addition of chemotherapy may not be effective. A score of 18 to 31 is considered as an intermediate risk and patients need to consider other factors such as age and comorbidities when deciding whether or not to take chemotherapy. A score of higher than 31 suggests a higher risk of a recurrence, and chemotherapy is usually recommended. The Oncotype test reflects risk of recurrence based on genetic characteristics of the tumor. This female patient may have an extensive family history of cancer and possibly hereditary risk. Oncotype does not provide information about this risk.

11. **Answer:** A

**Rationale:** T. K, a 27-year-old white woman, has a 1 in 8 chance that she will develop breast cancer in her lifetime. J.L., who is Hispanic, has a lower rate than the other races. Breast cancer is 100 more times likely in woman than in men, so D.C. has the smallest chances of the four choices. Finally, B.R., a 37-year-old African American woman, has a 1 in 10 chance of developing cancer. However, more African American women are diagnosed with breast cancer before the age of 45.

12. **Answer:** A

**Rationale:** The terminal duct lobular units (TDLUs) produce breast milk. Adipose tissue becomes more prominent after menopause. Sebaceous tissues are microscopic glands in the skin that secrete an oily substance known as sebum. There are no primary duct units.

13. **Answer** C

**Rationale:** Mutations in the CDH1 gene are associated with a 45% lifetime risk of developing lobular breast cancer, as well as an increased risk for developing diffuse gastric cancer. MUTYH mutations are associated with an autosomal recessive condition that places the individual at increased risk for colon polyposis. BRCA 2 mutations are associated with an increased risk for developing breast cancer, but not necessarily lobular breast cancer. PMS2 mutations are part of Lynch syndrome. Individuals with Lynch syndrome are at particularly high risk for developing colon, uterine, ovarian, and other gastrointestinal cancers.

14. **Answer:** A

**Rationale:** Luminal A tumors have the highest levels of ER expression: ER-positive and/or PR-positive, these tumors tend to be low grade, are most likely to respond to endocrine therapy, are responsive to chemotherapy, and have a favorable prognosis. Luminal B tumors are typically ER-positive, PR- negative, HER2-positive, and may have an unfavorable subset with aggressive behavior that can be tamoxifen resistant. Basal tumors are negative for ER, PR, and HER2 (triple-negative). They tend to be high grade and often have a poor prognosis; therefore, these tumors will likely benefit from chemotherapy

15. **Answer** B

**Rationale:** In the Bloom-Richardson system or Nottingham grading system, Grade 1 reflects a low grade or well-differentiated breast cancer. Grade 2 represents an intermediate grade and moderately differentiated breast cancer. Grade 3 represents a high grade and poorly differentiated breast cancer.

## CHAPTER 14

1. **Answer:** B

**Rationale:** Esophagogastroduodenoscopy (EGD) is an endoscopy examination to examine the lining of the esophagus, stomach, and first part of the small intestine. Biopsies may be taken to evaluate for the presence of malignancy. Colonoscopy is a screening test for colorectal cancer. An MRI of the brain and abdominal ultrasound are not part of a routine work-up for esophageal cancer. Other diagnostic modalities for esophageal cancer include a CT or a PET scan of the chest and abdomen, endoscopic ultrasound, and bronchoscopy.

2. **Answer:** A

**Rationale:** Modifiable risk factors are those within the control of the individual. For example, alcohol use is considered a modifiable risk factor. Individuals cannot

**141**

control their family history nor can they control a history of genetic risk, such as Lynch syndrome. Exposure to the Epstein-Barr virus is also considered nonmodifiable.

3. *Answer:* D

*Rationale:* A CT of the abdomen, abdominal ultrasound, and a CT of the pelvis are all staging and diagnostic procedures used in the evaluation of colon cancer, often following a positive biopsy. Screening tests for colon cancer include guaiac-based stool testing, fecal immunochemical test, immunochemical fecal occult blood test (iFOBT), barium enema, flexible sigmoidoscopy, colonoscopy, or CT colonography.

4. *Answer:* B

*Rationale:* Molecular classification in colon cancer includes KRAS/NRAS (in patients with metastatic disease), BRAF (in patients with metastatic disease), and MMR or MSI. PDL-1 and EGFR are used in the molecular classification of lung cancer. ER/PR (estrogen/progesterone) are used in the molecular classification of breast cancer.

5. *Answer:* C

*Rationale:* Risk factors for anal cancer include human papillomavirus infection (HPV) infections, human immunodeficiency virus (HIV) infection, anal sex, and lowered immunity. Hepatitis B (HBV) is associated with liver cancer. EBV is associated with nasopharyngeal cancer. Human herpes virus (HHV-8) is associated with Kaposi sarcoma.

6. *Answer:* A

*Rationale:* Risk factors for hepatocellular cancer include hepatitis C virus (HCV), hepatitis B virus (HBV), cirrhosis, diabetes, and obesity. Influenza is not a known risk factor for malignancy. Human papillomavirus infection (HPV) and human immunodeficiency virus (HIV) are risk factors for anal cancer.

7. *Answer:* D

*Rationale:* Local-regional therapies include RFA, TACE, DEB-TACE, and TARE. Nivolumab and Sorafenib are palliative therapies. Liver transplant is a potentially curative option for early-stage HCC.

8. *Answer:* A

*Rationale:* Pancreatic adenocarcinoma is the most common form of pancreatic cancer. It accounts for almost 95% of cases and arises from the exocrine pancreas. Pancreatic neuroendocrine tumors are less common but tend to have a better prognosis.

9. *Answer:* A

*Rationale:* Systemic therapies used in adjuvant and advanced settings include fluoropyridamine-based or gemcitabine-based therapies. Pembrolizumab for patients with MSI-H/dMMR for second-line therapy and third-line therapy for patients PD-L1 positive. Cytoxan is not used in the treatment of colon cancer.

10. *Answer:* A

*Rationale:* FOLFOX is a chemotherapy regimen used for colon cancer in both the adjuvant and metastatic settings. CAPEOX, capecitabine, and 5-FU/leucovorin are also often used in the adjuvant setting. Carboplatin/paclitaxel is not a chemotherapy regimen used for colon cancer, but is considered a common chemotherapy regimen used in ovarian and lung cancers. Cetuximab and FOLFIRI are used in the metastatic colorectal cancer setting.

11. *Answer:* C

*Rationale:* Gastroesophageal reflux disease (GERD) is a risk factor for adenocarcinoma of the esophagus. A somatic BRCA1/2 mutation is a potential mutation found in a tumor cell and is not a risk factor. Smoking and alcohol use are risk factors for squamous cell carcinoma of esophagus, not adenocarcinoma.

12. *Answer:* D

*Rationale:* The nurse should recommend to T. J. that he should limit alcohol intake to fewer than two drinks per/day as a course of action to prevent colorectal cancer. The recommendation is two drinks per/day for a male, and one drink/per day for a female. Treating *H. pylori*, gastric ulcers is a recommendation for the prevention of stomach cancer. Treating GERD and/or Barret's esophagitis is a prevention recommendation for esophageal cancer, while it is recommended to limit exposure to cancer-causing chemicals for prevention of hepatocellular cancer. Other recommendations for the prevention of colorectal cancer include maintaining a healthy weight, limiting red and processed meats while introducing more fruits and vegetables into a daily diet, and avoiding tobacco.

13. *Answer:* A

*Rationale:* Diets which are high in salted and smoked foods, and low in fruit and vegetable consumption is known as a modifiable risk factor for stomach cancer. Gastric polyps are considered a nonmodifiable risk, as is previous gastric surgery, and a family history of the disease. Other modifiable risks include alcohol intake of more than four drinks per day, smoking, and gastric ulcers. Obesity is also associated with gastric cardia cancer.

14. *Answer:* B

*Rationale:* Routine screening for pancreatic cancer is not recommended for individuals who are not presenting symptoms. EUS or MRI/magnetic resonance cholangiopancreatography (MRCP), however, may be used as a screening technique for individuals with genetic mutations such as HBOC, Lynch syndrome, or PJS. Ultrasound every 6 months is recommended as screening for high-risk individuals of developing hepatocellular cancer, which include patients with all types of cirrhosis and hepatitis B virus (HBV) carriers without cirrhosis. No screening methods have yet to be identified for cholangiocarcinomas – a rare cancer that encompasses all tumors originating from the epithelium of the bile duct.

## CHAPTER 15

1. *Answer:* D

*Rationale:* Clear cell carcinoma is a common type of kidney cancer because it comprises 70% to 80% of all kidney cancer cases. Clear cell carcinoma is thought to arise in the proximal renal tubule and is not a tumor of the renal pelvis, which are considered to be very rare. Clear cell carcinoma does not have the worst prognosis among types of kidney cancers; rather collecting duct carcinomas are aggressive tumors that are associated with rapid metastasis.

2. **Answer:** A

**Rationale:** Having a history of non-Hodgkin lymphoma and being overweight is the correct answer. The other choices are not correct because they are not known risk factors for kidney cancer, which include lifestyle risk factors such as tobacco use, obesity, and occupational exposure to petroleum products or heavy metals. Dietary risk factors include diets high in fats and protein. Finally, a history of non-Hodgkin lymphoma or sickle cell disease is also considered a risk factor.

3. **Answer:** C

**Rationale:** Intravenous pyelogram is the correct answer. This diagnostic test is commonly used to evaluate patients presenting with hematuria. Colonoscopy visualizes the colon, and is not used to determine the cause of hematuria. The kidney is not biopsied to determine the cause of hematuria, and blood chemistry results would not be diagnostic for hematuria.

4. **Answer:** A

**Rationale:** Partial nephrectomy is the preferred treatment whenever feasible, especially in patients with limited renal function, bilateral tumors, or a solitary kidney. Cytoreductive nephrectomy is a procedure that may be performed in patients with surgically resectable primary tumor and multiple metastatic sites prior to systemic therapy. Renal cell cancers are unresponsive to radiation therapy. Chemotherapy has not been shown to improve survival in kidney cancer.

5. **Answer:** D

**Rationale:** The correct answer is immunotherapy agents. These agents, such as interleukin-2 and interferon-alpha, have produced response rates of 10% to 15% when used as single agents for treating cancer of the kidney. Systemic radiation therapy, in which radioactive drugs are delivered either orally or intravenously, is not used to treat renal cell cancers which are not radiation sensitive. Antibody-drug conjugates, in which an antibody is linked to a cytotoxic agent, are not used to treat kidney cancer because the malignant cells do not express specific antigens that would be the target of antibodies. Cytotoxic chemotherapy has not been shown to improve survival.

6. **Answer:** B

**Rationale:** Urothelial carcinoma of the bladder is the most common type of bladder cancer and comprises about 95% of bladder tumors. In 70% to 80% of cases, this type of tumor is generally diagnosed before it has become invasive and invaded the muscle wall of the bladder. Urothelial tumors are not associated with changes to *chromosome 9*, which are associated with papillary bladder cancers.

7. **Answer:** B

**Rationale:** Tobacco use is the most significant risk factor, accounting for 50% to 66% of all bladder tumors in men and 25% in women. Weight loss is not a risk factor; rather a high BMI may increase risk, and contribute to risk of disease recurrence. Excessive fluid intake does not increase bladder cancer risk but not drinking enough fluids is reported to be a risk factor. Consuming a diet low in processed meats may be somewhat protective for bladder cancer.

8. **Answer:** C

**Rationale:** The correct answer is that UAU guidelines indicate that PSA screening between ages 55 to 69 years provides the greatest benefit. Therefore, it is not correct that results of PSA screenings are not useful for men at any age. Routine screening in men 40 to 54 years at average risk is not recommended. Men who decide to initiate PSA screening should have repeat screenings at intervals of 2 or more years.

9. **Answer:** B

**Rationale:** The Gleason Score is based on microscopic examination of the prostate tumor tissue specimen. The pathologist determines the most common cell grade seen in the largest portion of the specimen (the primary cell grade) and in the second largest portion (the secondary cell grade). The two grades are then added together to determine the Gleason score. This score provides information about the aggressiveness of the disease in the prostate and serves as a guide for treatment strategies. Imaging tests using MRI or CT provide information about the extent of the disease but are not part of the process for determining the Gleason score, which is based on characteristics of the malignant tumor cells. PSA levels are not used for computing the Gleason Score but may be useful as a marker for disease progression. Bone marrow aspiration is not used as a screening or diagnostic measure for prostate cancer.

10. **Answer:** B

**Rationale:** Hormonal manipulation is the accepted standard for treating patients with metastatic prostate cancer. The other options listed - radical prostatectomy, brachytherapy with radioactive seed placement into the prostate, and cryosurgery - are used to treat patients with early-stage prostate cancer.

11. **Answer:** C

**Rationale:** Impotence is the correct answer. Some form of impotence has been seen in 6% to 61% of men following brachytherapy to treat prostate cancer. Diarrhea, rather than constipation, is associated with both radiation therapy and brachytherapy. Anemia is not a side effect of brachytherapy because little bone marrow is exposed to radiation with this treatment.

12. **Answer:** B

**Rationale:** A recommendation to maximize patient safety postoperatively is monitoring vital signs, hemoglobin, hematocrit, kidney function tests, and urine output. These are critical measures when determining a patient's condition after surgery. Teaching a patient to manage and identify symptoms, including providing recommendations on when to report symptoms, occurs during patient education regarding follow-up care and surveillance, and not as a safety measure after surgery. Teaching patients how to perform coping skills to control anxiety and fear

**143**

is also not a safety measure; however, nurses do teach patients about pulmonary hygiene, including how to perform coughing and deep breathing exercises. Finally, monitoring patients for signs of distress is not a safety measure, though nurses must monitor a patient's pain level after surgery in order to provide adequate pharmacologic and nonpharmacologic pain relief measures.

13. *Answer:* B

*Rationale:* For a radiographic examination of the kidneys, ureter, and bladder (KUB), the nurse should instruct the patient to let flat on the examination table. Accessing the patient for a history of allergies to iodine dyes or contact media before testing is a nursing intervention instruction for an excretory urography test. For a retrograde urography diagnostic test, nurses are instructed to observe the patient for a reaction to anesthetic or analgesic, and monitor for bleeding, symptoms of a urinary tract infection, dysuria, or difficulty voiding after the test has been completed.

14. *Answer:* A

*Rationale:* Radical cystectomy is currently considered the primary treatment modality for bladder preservation but, due to the nature of the procedure, some patients either cannot tolerate the procedure or decline the treatment altogether. Alternatives to radical cystectomy include external beam radiation therapy, radiation therapy, and trimodality therapy—transurethral resection (TUR). Each of these treatments are considered as bladder preservation strategies, though the baseline therapy is currently radical cystectomy.

## CHAPTER 16

1. *Answer:* B

*Rationale:* Head and neck cancers include cancers of the oral cavity, oropharynx, nasal cavity, paranasal sinuses, nasopharynx, larynx, hypopharynx, and salivary glands; as well as cancers of the thyroid and parathyroid. The category of head and neck cancers does not include cancers of the esophagus, brain, or bone.

2. *Answer:* A

*Rationale:* Known risk factors for head and neck cancer include the following: tobacco use, excessive alcohol, indigestion, the human papillomavirus (HPV), gastroesophageal reflux, history of neck radiation, and environmental exposure (wood, dust, asbestos). In men, 81% of all HPV associated cancers are oropharynx cancers. In women, 15% of all HPV-associated cancers are oropharynx cancers. Diabetes, menopause, and dental implants are not known risk factors.

3. *Answer:* D

*Rationale:* To establish a treatment plan for head and neck cancer, hereditary testing is not the first step of the plan. Family history is important to assess, but it is not directly related to the treatment plan. After the patient has a treatment plan of care and it may include chemotherapy, a neutrophil count may be calculated. To establish a treatment plan for head and neck cancer, the tumor needs to be biopsied, then evaluated by a pathologist to provide information about histology, molecular, and other pathological factors.

4. *Answer:* B

*Rationale:* Radiologic studies for head and neck cancer include computed tomography (CT) and magnetic resonance imaging (MRI). Positron emission tomography (PET) with CT (PET-CT) is useful in determining specific areas for biopsy, lymph node involvement and the extent of disease to aid in treatment planning. CT is used to assist in determining the extent of the primary tumor and to identify metastasis to the cervical lymph nodes. MRI is superior to CT in staging nasopharyngeal primaries. PET is ordered to document metastatic spread of tumor cells. When providers order diagnostic radiologic studies, they do not order only chest X-ray or ultrasound. Intravenous Pyelogram is used to evaluate kidneys, ureters, and bladder. A gallium scan is useful in evaluating patients with potential lymphoma, infection, osteomyelitis, or pulmonary problems.

5. *Answer:* B

*Rationale:* Focused nursing care of head and neck cancer patients includes respiration, speech, swallowing, trismus (restriction in the opening of the mouth), and hormone regulation. Depending on the patient's overall health maintenance, nursing care can also include attention to neutropenia, skin care, and lymphedema. However, those conditions are not the specific focus of nursing care for patients with head and neck cancer.

6. *Answer:* D

*Rationale:* For head and neck cancer patients, preoperative teaching covers discussion of the disease, treatment, side effects, and anticipated postoperative changes. It also includes instruction about equipment (tracheostomy tube, drains, nasogastric tube, tonsil-tip suction catheter). Before surgery, the patient should have established ways to communicate post-surgery using paper and pencil, magic slate, picture board, nonverbal cues, electronic communication board, or device. Specific for laryngectomy, the focus of preoperative teaching does not include ambulation, endurance, or opioid addiction.

7. *Answer:* A

*Rationale:* After a patient undergoes head and neck surgery that includes skin or muscle grafts to cover the removed tumor site, postoperative wound care assessment is every 3 to 4 hours, noting color (pink versus cyanotic), temperature, and capillary refill after blanching of the skin and muscle. Flap perfusion and viability is maintained by avoiding excess pressure to the flap; the wound is assessed for infection and fistula formation. Nursing assessment of surgical grafts does not include range of motion, necrotic tissue removal, or regular lavage.

8. *Answer:* B

*Rationale:* During neck dissection, the patient's spinal accessory nerve and the sternocleidomastoid muscles may be resected. For the patient to regain range of motion and strength, the patient is referred to physical therapy. The patient is not likely to have significant pain issues by time of discharge nor do they require a gastroenterology consult as a routine referral. Occupational therapy is not a typical referral for neck dissection patients. Speech therapists play an integral role both preoperative and postoperatively to assist with issues in speech and swallowing.

9. *Answer:* C

*Rationale:* Since the structures above the false vocal cords are resected during a supraglottic laryngectomy, the patient is at risk for aspiration until the patient learns swallowing techniques to protect the airway. Postoperative care of any patient includes risk of falling, maintaining hydration, and somnolence, but these are not the primary concern of nurses caring for postop supraglottic laryngectomy.

10. *Answer:* B

*Rationale:* Signs and symptoms of head and neck cancer include a lump or sore that does not heal in the mouth, lip, throat or jaw; a sore throat that does not go away; a change or hoarseness in the voice that does not resolve; difficulty chewing, swallowing, or moving the jaw or tongue; and a pain in one ear without hearing loss. A temperature of > 100°F does not suggest a sign or symptom of head and neck cancer.

11. *Answer:* B

*Rationale:* The oropharynx extends from the circumvallate papillae below and hard palate above to the level of the hyoid bone. Structures of the oropharynx include the base of the tongue (posterior one third), soft palate, the tonsils, and posterior pharyngeal wall. The oral cavity extends from the lips to the hard palate above and the circumvallate papillae below, with structures including the lips, buccal mucosa, floor of the mouth, and upper and lower alveoli. The nasopharynx is located below the base of the skull and behind the nasal cavity and continuous with the posterior pharyngeal wall. Finally, the larynx extends from the epiglottis to the cricoid cartilage and protected by the thyroid cartilage.

12. *Answer:* B

*Rationale:* A hemilaryngectomy involves a vertical excision of one true and one false cord and the underlying cartilage. This procedure can give the patient a hoarse voice but leads to minimal to no swallowing problems. A laser has the least implications of any of these procedures, with little to no physical alterations and minimal bleeding. A maxillectomy involves partial or total en-bloc resection of the cavity. This procedure may include the ethmoid sinus, lateral nasal wall, palate, and floor of the orbit. Nursing implications include, postoperatively, maxillofacial prosthodontist making a dental obturator to fill the large surgical defect and to facilitate swallowing. Requires daily care to cavity and placement of obturator. A craniofacial or skull base resection is a surgical treatment to inaccessible midfacial and extensive paranasal sinus and nasopharyngeal lesions. This treatment may have facial defects and cranial nerve (III, IV, V) deficits.

13. *Answer:* C

*Rationale:* The hypopharynx extends from the hyoid bone to the lower border of the cricoid cartilage, and structures include the pyriform sinuses, the postcricoid region, and the lower posterior pharyngeal wall. The oropharynx extends from the circumvallate papillae below and hard palate above to the level of the hyoid bone; and structures include the base of the tongue (posterior one third), soft palate, and the posterior pharyngeal wall. The supraglottis is located below the base of the tongue, extending to but not including the true vocal cord, and includes the epiglottis, the aryepiglottic folds, the arytenoid cartilages, and the false vocal cords. Finally, the nasal cavity and paranasal sinuses include the nasal vestibule; paired maxillary, ethmoid, and frontal sinuses; and a single sphenoid sinus.

14. *Answer:* A

Treatment for nasopharyngeal cancer is primarily radiation. Surgery for this type of cancer is recommended to be avoided because the area is too close to vital structures of the brain. Select patients who do not respond to radiation therapy are treated with base-of-skull resection of tumor procedure. Preoperative radiation or permanently placed iodine-125 seeds are the primary treatment in debulking large or unresectable lesions. Brachytherapy is a treatment for lesions of the anterior and posterior tongue, the floor of mouth, and the nasal vestibule. According to the National Comprehensive Cancer Network (NCCN), a low dose of radioactive iodine given after surgery for thyroid cancer destroys (ablated) residual thyroid tissue as effectively as a higher dose, but with fewer side effects and less exposure to radiation.

## CHAPTER 17

1. *Answer:* A

*Rationale:* The average time from infection to active AIDS is approximately 10 years, not 15 years. It can be shorter in older adults and children. The average time from human immunodeficiency virus (HIV) infection to symptomatic disease depends on inoculation method, exposure, pre-existing health, and prompt initiation of treatment for antiretroviral disease, so A would be the best representative answer. The average time of infection is not dependent on the patient's age at time of exposure nor is it dependent on the number of sexual partners.

2. *Answer:* C

*Rationale:* Acute infection occurs, then proceeds to a chronic/progressive infection before manifesting into AIDS. During the chronic/progressive infection stage, qualitative and quantitative T4-lymphocyte dysfunction occurs, with resultant defects in both cellular and humoral immunity as immunoregulatory function of T4 cells is gradually impaired. The order in answer A of chronic/progressive disease, AIDS, and acute infection is incorrect since acute infection would come before either of the two steps. B is also incorrect. While acute infection occurs first in the progression of the disease, contracting AIDS is the final step and does not come prior to chronic/progress infection. Finally, D is also incorrect, and also incomplete, as the answer omits the final stage of AIDS.

3. *Answer:* B

*Rationale:* Lifestyle factors including nutritional status, overall health, and tobacco use may influence the course of infection. These lifestyle factors neither slow

**145**

nor do they hasten the disease progression, as it is difficult to distinguish between comorbid infection and a true causal relationship. There is an increased risk of infection in uncircumcised males related to dendritic cells on the foreskin. Other factors that might influence the progression of the disease might include the presence of cytomegalovirus (CMV), Epstein-Barr virus (EBV), hepatitis C virus, human papillomavirus (HPV), herpes simplex 6 (HSV- 6), herpes simplex 8 (HSV-8), and other viruses.

Approximately 67% of cases in gay, bisexual, and other men who have sex with men comprises half of newly infected HIV infection and half of people living with the disease, and not the 37% of cases listed in answer D, making that answer incorrect as well.

4. *Answer:* D

*Rationale:* Increases in the incidence of HIV-positive adults over 50 years of age are attributable to prolonged survival with disease, age-related physiologic changes enhancing risk of transmission, and propensity to engage in unprotected sex. Incidence among African Americans/white gay males has remained stable and not increased, while diagnoses among young Hispanic/Latino gay and bisexual men have increased, and not decreased. Heterosexual contact with HIV-infected individuals accounts for about 24% of new HIV diagnoses, and not 34% as is listed incorrectly in answer C.

5. *Answer:* D

*Rationale:* Both B-cell lymphoma (NHL) and Burkitt lymphoma are AIDS-defining malignancies, as well as Kaposi sarcoma and cervical cancer. AIDS-defining malignancies are malignancies related specifically to HIV infection and the subsequently altered immune system. Non-AIDS defining malignancies include oral, esophageal, prostate, anal, breast, and ovarian cancers.

6. *Answer:* C

*Rationale:* HIV-infected women are at an increased risk for cervical dysplasia that rapidly progresses to cervical cancer. AIDS-defining cancers include non-Hodgkin lymphoma (NHL), Burkitt lymphoma, Kaposi sarcoma, and cervical cancer. B-cell lymphoma is the most frequently diagnosed AIDS-defining malignancy. AIDS-defining malignancies are more common shortly after initiation of active retroviral therapy, particularly among patients with low CD4 counts. Lung, acute myeloid leukemia, and kidney cancer are all non-AIDS defining cancers.

7. *Answer:* A

*Rationale:* cART and antineoplastic agents may have similar toxicity profiles (i.e. diarrhea, hepatotoxicity, pancreatitis, QT prolongation, etc.) and combination therapy may compound the toxicities when utilizing combination therapy for treatment. Therefore, patients should be monitored for overlapping toxicities when undergoing combination therapy. Steroid use increases the risk of inflammatory response (i.e. IRIS) rather than decreasing inflammation. Vaccines should be modified during or after cancer treatment due to continued immune defect, while antineoplastic therapy should continue to be administered in the setting of low CD4+ counts as these counts are a temporary condition.

8. *Answer:* B

*Rationale:* An active EBV infection is present in 44% to 67% of HIV lymphomas. In HIV-related lymphoma, the CD4+ count is typically less than $200/mm^3$, not $400/mm^3$, it lacks the CD20+ marker, and is a late manifestation of HIV infection.

9. *Answer:* C

*Rationale:* Ocular involvement occurs in 20% of patients diagnosed with primary central nervous system lymphoma, and commonly have multifocal lesions. HIV-infected patients do not have extensive bone marrow involvement, nor do they have other organ/tissue involvement. This patient population also has a low CD4+ count and do not generally have concurrent CMV but EBV infection.

10. *Answer:* C

*Rationale:* Immune reconstitution syndrome occurs with severe inflammatory or infectious reactions, as well as with initial cART therapy. Immune reconstitution syndrome has occurred with toxoplasmosis, pneumocystis, other opportunistic infections in HIV disease, and EBV reactivation. Immune reconstitution syndrome has also been linked to rituximab administration. Anaphlaxis to Bactrim would likely occur with the first dose so the patient would not be experiencing symptoms such as altered mental status, fevers, and shortening of breath on Day 2. Superimposing infection or worsening PCP pneumonia would not necessarily be accompanied by altered mental status, so A is incorrect as well.

11. *Answer:* D

*Rationale:* Gastrointestinal lesions or B symptoms (fever, night sweats, unintentional weight loss) shorten the survival in patients diagnosed with Kaposi syndrome. The era of cART has increased survival dramatically, and no decrease in survival rates has been reported. Prior or comorbid major opportunistic infections worsen survival, rather than having no impact. The median survival rate is less than one year, but not less than six months.

12. *Answer:* A

*Rationale:* The nurse should provide education about the use of latex condoms with a water-based lubricant to reduce risk. A water-based lubricant is recommended because petroleum-based lubricants or cosmetic creams weaken the condom, greater increasing the chance of HIV transmission. To decrease the risk of transmission, a latex condom should be used during every episode of vaginal, rectal, or oral intercourse. Personal hygiene items – such as a toothbrush or a razor – should not be shared, so the best method is to avoid sharing altogether. The solution of 1 part household bleach to 10 parts water during cleanup of emesis or other body fluid spills is correct and can be used, but the person cleaning should always wear gloves for protection against the spread of disease.

13. *Answer:* D

*Rationale:* It is correct that studies of antiretroviral adherence reflect low rates of medication adherence among individuals with low health literacy, linking a low health literacy score with adherence to medication. Low health literacy has a large – not a small – impact

**146**

on maintaining regular medical care. In fact, only 17% to 40% of patients who have scored low on health literacy scores have maintained regular medical care. This statistic, though, is greater than the 5% of patients maintaining regular medical care, which is an exaggerated number, making answer C an incorrect response. Finally, low health literacy is associated with English not being the first language, mental health disorder, and lack of understanding of how to access care and support (and interpreters are not readily available in every place where healthcare is being provided).

## CHAPTER 18

1. *Answer:* A

   *Rationale:* Exposure to certain viruses, such as EBV and HTLV-1, is a risk factor for developing ALL. Being of Hispanic descent, not African or Asian, is a risk factor for developing ALLH. Having a genetic condition such as Down syndrome, Li-Fraumeni syndrome, Ataxia telangiectasia, Klinefelter syndrome, and Fanconi Anemia is a risk factor for developing ALL. A diagnosis of measles is not a known risk factor.

2. *Answer:* A

   *Rationale:* Peripheral blast cells are commonly found in a peripheral blood test for a patient newly diagnosed with ALL. Patients often have an elevated BUN/Creatinine at diagnosis. Patients usually have decreased platelet counts at diagnosis, not thrombophilia. Patients often have a change in PT/INR at diagnosis.

3. *Answer:* D

   *Rationale:* Allogeneic HCT is utilized as consolidation therapy after remission is achieved with induction therapy. Pediatric regimen is used for induction therapy in patients with Philadelphia chromosome negative disease and who are less than 65 years of age. Corticosteroids are not used as monotherapy, but in combination with TKI in patients who are less than 65 years of age. Induction therapy for individuals more than 65 years of age with a Philadelphia chromosome typically involves multi agent chemotherapy with a TKI to induce a remission and the patient who would potentially become a candidate for allogeneic HCT.

4. *Answer:* D

   *Rationale:* Midostaurin is the only oral agent listed for FLT3 inhibition. Venetoclax is used for CLL, SLL, and newly diagnosed AML in adults 75 years or older in combination with azacitidine or decitabine or low dose cytarabine. Enasidenib is for relapsed/refractory AML with IDH2 mutations. Ivosidenib is indicated for relapsed/refractory AML with IDH1 mutations.

5. *Answer:* B

   *Rationale:* ATRA + arsenic trioxide + anthracycline is recommended in high-risk disease in the absence of cardiac disease. ATRA + arsenic trioxide is given with or without anthracycline in low-risk disease. Gemtuzumab ozogamicin is used as a single agent in high-risk, relapse, or inability to tolerate arsenic trioxide due to QT prolongation. Intrathecal chemotherapy is used in consolidation therapy for patients with high-risk APL in combination with ATRA + arsenic trioxide + anthracycline.

6. *Answer:* C

   *Rationale:* CLL is a diagnosis that is diagnosed at a median age of 60 years old and less than 15% are diagnosed under the age of 50. CLL is the most frequent form of leukemia. CLL is more frequently seen in a Caucasian population than a Hispanic or Asian population. CLL originates from mature B lymphocytes.

7. *Answer:* A

   *Rationale:* Ibrutinib is used for patients with 17p deletion. There is no known targeted therapy for TP53 mutation. Rituxmiab is used for patients with CD20 antigen. Alemtuzumab is used for patients with CD52 antigen.

8. *Answer:* D

   *Rationale:* Rai stage III, high-risk disease is noted to have anemia Hgb < 11 g/dL and lymphocytosis. The patient may or may not have adenopathy, hepatomegaly, or splenomegaly, and platelets counts are normal. Rai stage I, intermediate-risk disease I noted to have adenopathy and lymphocytosis (no hepatomegaly or splenomegaly, RBC and PLT counts are normal). Rai stage IV, high-risk disease is noted to have thrombocytopenia < 100,00 μL and lymphocytosis (with adenopathy, hepatomegaly and splenomegaly and RBC counts are normal or near normal). Rai stage II, intermediate-risk disease is noted to have splenomegaly and lymphocytosis (may have hepatomegaly, may or may not have adenopathy, and RBC and PLT counts are normal).

9. *Answer:* B

   *Rationale:* One risk factor in developing acute myeloid leukemia (AML) is long-term exposure to benzene. Benzene is a chemical used in heavy industry, including places such as oil refineries, chemical plants, and the gasoline industry. Benzene can also be found in cigarette smoke, and in such common household items such as glue, detergent, and paint. Radiation therapy is not considered a risk factor for AML; however, exposure to high levels of radiation is seen as a risk factor. Those who have been involved in an atomic bomb attack, for instance, or been a survivor of a nuclear accident have an increased risk of developing the disease. Alcohol use and diet are not risk factors, though smoking has been linked to AML. Other risk factors include genetic disorders, such as Fanconi anemia and Down syndrome, family history of AML, as well as treatment of some chemotherapy agents.

10. *Answer:* A

    *Rationale:* Acute lymphocytic leukemia (ALL) is the most common form of leukemia among children and adolescents representing 20% of all cancers among persons less than 20 years representing 3000 new cases annually. The risk declines after 5 years of age until the middle twenties and then rises again after the age of 50. In chronic myelogenous leukemia (CML), the average age at diagnosis is greater than 60 years with half of the total cases being over the age of 65. Chronic lymphocytic leukemia (CLL) is the most frequent form of leukemia

**147**

and originates from mature B lymphocytes. The median age at diagnosis is 60 years, and less than 15% are diagnosed under the age of 50. The lifetime risk of CLL is 1 in 175 and is most commonly diagnosed at 70 years of age. CLL accounts for 25% of all leukemias and is more frequently seen in Caucasians compared with Asians, as well as Hispanics.

11. *Answer:* D

*Rationale:* The Rai staging system for chronic lymphocytic leukemia defines risk or extent of disease as low, intermediate, or high. There is no medium category. Those with lymphocytosis (lymphoid cells > 30%); no lymphadenopathy, splenomegaly, or hepatomegaly are considered low. The intermediate level is defined by lymphocytosis; lymphadenopathy in any site, splenomegaly, or hepatomegaly. In both the low and intermediate levels, red blood cell and platelet counts are near normal. A high level is associated with lymphocytosis; presence of anemia (hemoglobin < 11 g/dL) or thrombocytopenia (platelet count less than $100 \times 10^9$/L) with or without lymphadenopathy, splenomegaly, or hepatomegaly. Mr. M.'s lymphocytes are greater than 6000 which indicates a more than 30% of the total white blood cell count percentage. He has thrombocytopenia, with the platelet count below 100,000. He has two sites of lymphadenopathy, the groin and axilla area, and he is having early satiety, which is likely caused by splenomegaly.

12. *Answer:* A

*Rationale:* Chronic myelogenous leukemia (CML) is a clonal disorder that originates from the Philadelphia chromosome translocation of the BCR-ABL oncogene. The translocation between chromosome 9 and 22 fuses together causing tyrosine kinase activity, which results in initiation of leukemia (Philadelphia chromosome). There are three phases of this disorder, which include chronic, accelerated, and blast crisis phase. Inherited mutations in the ATM (Ataxia Telangiesctasia mutated) gene are associated with increased risk of certain cancers. People who inherit a mutated copy of ATM from one parent are at increased risk of female breast cancer (up to 52% lifetime risk), and possibly pancreatic, prostate, and other cancers. Persons who inherit two copies of the ATM gene develop ataxia–telangiectasia syndrome or Louis-Bar syndrome, which is a rare, neurodegenerative, autosomal recessive disease, which causes severe disability. Persons with inherited (germline) tp53 mutations are at risk for breast, lung, colon, gynecologic, sarcomas, and many other cancers and have a condition known as Li Fraumeni syndrome. Trisomy 21, also known as Down syndrome is a human chromosomal disorder caused by having three copies (trisomy) of chromosome 21.

## CHAPTER 19

1. *Answer:* A

*Rationale:* Pancoast syndrome can result when a superior sulcus, such as lung cancer, destroys lesions of the thoracic inlet and involves the brachial plexus and cervical sympathetic nerves, and is manifested by shoulder pain. Other intrathoracic effects include pleural effusions and superior vena cava syndrome. Lower extremity neuropathy and darkening of the skin are not intrathoracic effects of lung cancer. While hypomagnesia does not have an intrathoracic effect due to lung cancer, it can be associated with hypercalcemia, which is a known oncologic emergency seen in persons with lung cancer.

2. *Answer:* B

*Rationale:* Small cell lung cancer is diagnosed in 0-15% of lung cancers and has a more aggressive, rapidly growing course compared to the other carcinoid types. Since it is a rapidly growing disease, small cell lung cancer is likely to metastasize. Patients with limited disease have a median survival of 15-20 months, and are often treated with chemotherapy in combination with radiation therapy, while patients do not have multiple options for surgery. In fact, surgery is not an option. Small cell lung cancer is associated with a poor prognosis with overall 5-year survival at 5% to 10% and when untreated median survival 2 to 4 months, so it does not have a better prognosis than other forms of lung cancer.

3. *Answer:* C

*Rationale:* Risk of lung cancer increases with the number of years the individual has spent smoking and number of cigarettes smoked per day. To quantify tobacco exposure, the number of packs of cigarettes per day is multiplied by the number of years smoked to obtain pack history. Assessing the age when the patient began smoking, the frequency of smoking, and family history of the patient does not quantify the patient's risk of smoking. Pack years must be calculated to have a more complete risk assessment for developing lung cancer.

4. *Answer:* A

*Rationale:* Current screening guidelines for lung cancer screening are for current or former smokers (> 30 pack-years or quit < 15 years), asymptomatic, age 55 to 74, to have annual screening with low-dose chest CT. The nurse working the local health fair, then, should have provided instructions for answer A. The use of inhaled marijuana and the use of electronic cigarettes have not been established as risk factors in the development of lung cancer.

5. *Answer:* D

*Rationale:* The nurse should advise C.R. on nicotine replacement products. Pharmacologic treatments include nicotine replacement therapy (NRT) such as ibuproprion and Varenicline (Champix), in addition to nicotine patches. Behavioral counseling and cognitive behavioral therapy can be used to focus on thoughts, emotions, and behaviors, and while those types of behavioral therapies are important, they are not known to be as effective as types of NRT. Gestalt therapy focuses on the here and now and isn't related to smoking cessation. Ice chips are frequently used to prevent mucositis in cancer patients, but not in smoking cessation. Vitamin E is not utilized in smoking cessation.

6. *Answer:* B

*Rationale:* The presence of the KRAS mutation is associated with tyrosine kinase inhibitors (TKI) resistance and overall poor survival compared to patients without the KRAS mutation. Having the KRAS mutation and the use of monoclonal antibodies has shown no response in patients who received monoclonal antibodies and in patients who harbored the KRAS mutation, and the use of oral medications alone in therapy has not shown any effect on the KRAS mutation.

7. **Answer:** D

**Rationale:** A VATS (video-assisted thoracic surgery) is a minimally invasive technique often done in conjunction with a wedge resection, where a wedge-shaped piece of lung tissue with a small tumor is removed, and is associated with decreased morbidity. A pneumonectomy is a surgical procedure to remove the entire lung. Overall morbidity is higher for this type of surgery. Sleeve resection is done if the tumor is in the central area of the lung and growing into the bronchus, and this is not a common surgery. A thoracotomy is a major surgical procedure done to access the chest cavity with an incision made through the chest wall. A resuscitative thoracotomy is an emergency procedure done for life-threatening emergencies such as chest hemorrhage.

8. **Answer:** A

**Rationale:** For early-stage NSCLC (stage I or IIa disease), stereotactic body radiation therapy (SBRT) or stereotactic ablative radiotherapy (SABR) is recommended for the patient who is not a surgical candidate or who refuses therapy. Oral chemotherapy is not an indication for treatment for this stage lung cancer. Low energy radiation does not penetrate deeply enough and is used mainly to treat skin cancers, and not NSCLC. Immunotherapy is often used for patients who have failed previous therapies.

9. **Answer:** C

**Rationale:** Pembrolizumab, along with Nivolumab and Atezolimab, are anti-PD-1 human monoclonal antibodies and immune checkpoint inhibitors approved for the first-line treatment of NSCLC. Tyrosine kinase inhibitors are EGRF-targeted therapies that block cancer cells from growing and dividing. Erlotinib is first-line therapy for individuals with advanced, recurrent, or metastatic non-squamous NSCLC. Pemrolizumab does not harbor molecules which break down cancer cells. Immune-checkpoint inhibitors are drugs that block specific proteins involved in downregulation of immune response in cancer cells.

10. **Answer:** A

**Rationale:** Prophylactic cranial radiation therapy is indicated for individuals with complete response to chemotherapy or radiation therapy to reduce the risk of developing brain metastasis. The overall 5-year survival is poor at 5% to 10%. The KRAS oncogene is never mutated in small cell lung cancer but may be seen is non-small cell lung cancers. Surgery is rarely an option for the main treatment of small cell lung cancer, as the cancer has usually spread by the time it is found.

11. **Answer:** B

**Rationale:** Erlotinib is considered first-line therapy for individuals with advanced, recurrent, or metastatic

NSCLC, so that could be an agent used to treat D.J. Molecular-targeted therapy is known to be effective in treating individuals with a genetic mutation and is promising for future developments of targeted therapies for specific pathways of mutation. Bevacizumab is recommended in select patients with advanced NSCLC but in addition to chemotherapy, and not as a single treatment, as misrepresented in the incorrect question.

12. **Answer:** D

**Rationale:** While it is true that more men (14%) will be newly diagnosed with lung cancer than woman (13%) and that 53% of all those diagnosed will be between the ages of 53 and 74, his age and gender are not factors in his diagnosis. His weight is also not a factor, though weight is a factor in many cancer cases especially colon, prostate, and breast cancers. Exposure to paint and paint thinners have been been linked with limited evidence to bladder cancer, however, environmental and occupational factors do increase the risk of developing lung cancer. His potential exposure to asbestos over his long career in home remodeling and demolition could have played a significant role in E.W.'s cancer diagnosis. Those who have been exposed to asbestos have been known to have an increased risk of developing lung cancer. Other potential factors include exposure to radon gas and air pollution.

## CHAPTER 20

1. **Answer:** B

**Rationale:** Early favorable Hodgkin's Lymphoma is a clinical stage I or II without any additional risk factors. The patient has an early favorable stage Hodgkin's Lymphoma, which requires limited amount of chemotherapy (usually two to three cycles) plus involved field radiation therapy. For patients with unfavorable stages, a moderate amount of chemotherapy (four cycles) plus involved field radiation is required. High-dose chemotherapy followed by autologous bone marrow transplant may be required for patients who have relapsed/refractory disease. Combination chemotherapy and radiation is associated with long-term survival in more than 80% of patients. Palliative chemotherapy and radiation therapy are not the correct treatment options for patients who have favorable Hodgkin's Lymphoma.

2. **Answer:** B

**Rationale:** The patient has Stage II diffuse large-B cell lymphoma. Diffuse large-B cell lymphoma is the most common type of non-Hodgkin lymphoma (NHL). Standard treatment options include chemotherapy with or without radiation therapy, and RCHOP. Autologous peripheral blood stem cell transplant is indicated for patients with recurrent NHL. Salvage radiation therapy is not a treatment plan for patients with NHL. Ifosfamide, carboplatin, etoposide (ICE) is a second-line regimen for patients who have relapsed/refractory Hodgkin's Lymphoma.

3. **Answer:** A

**Rationale:** Reed-Sternberg cells on the patient's pathology examination are present with classic Hodgkin's lymphoma. Bone marrow involvement and

**149**

lymphadenopathy with extranodal involvement are typically present in NHL. Metastases to the long bones are not diagnostic of Hodgkin's lymphoma.

4. **Answer:** D

**Rationale:** The Lugano Classification modification of the Ann Arbor Staging system is used to stage lymphoma. Staging is based on the extent of the disease and the presence of systemic symptoms. The Rai staging system is typically used to stage CLL. The Tumor Nodes Metastasis staging is usually used to stage solid cancers; however, the Ann Arbor Staging system is used to stage lymphomas. The Reed-Steenberg pathologic staging system is not a staging system.

5. **Answer:** C

**Rationale:** A risk factor for the development of MALT lymphoma of the stomach is the bacterial infection *Helicobacter pylori* infection (*H.pylori*). Having *H.pylori* does not put a patient at risk for developing breast cancer or cancer of the distal colon, but it does increase the risk of developing gastric cancer and should be treated. A risk factor for development of Burkitt lymphoma is EBV infection.

6. **Answer:** A

**Rationale:** The majority of patients who have a high-grade, localized disease who receive radiation plus chemotherapy or combination chemotherapy alone, have an overall survival at 5 years, which is over 60%. Patients who have aggressive NHL have a cure rate of 50%; however, they can expect to relapse within 2 years after therapy. Those patients with an 80% cure rate are those who are diagnosed with Hodgkin's Lymphoma and who are treated with combination chemotherapy and/or radiation therapy. High-dose chemotherapy (HDCT) followed by an autologous stem cell transplant is sometimes utilized in Hodgkin's Lymphoma or NHL, which is refractory or recurrent, but does not ensure a cure.

7. **Answer:** A

**Rationale:** T.J.'s systemic symptoms - fever, weight loss, fatigue, and night sweats – are considered "B" symptoms of lymphoma. The common clinical presentation of lymphoma is enlarged lymph nodes, spleen, and other immune tissue, with or without the systemic symptoms. Pain in the chest is not a symptom, but some patients do report pain in the nodal site when drinking (though the significance of such pain has not been established). Swelling of the limbs is not symptomatic, and extreme thirst and frequent urination could be signs of many conditions – from dehydration to diabetes – but is not a systemic symptom of lymphoma.

8. **Answer:** A

**Rationale:** To complete staging for non-Hodgkin lymphoma, a computed tomography scan of the chest, abdomen, and pelvis must be completed. In addition, a bilateral bone marrow biopsy and aspirate are done to determine whether bone marrow disease is present. To diagnose lymphoma, a lymph node biopsy is required to determine pathology. If the pathology reveals a CD 20+ tumor, the patient may receive rituximab (Rituxan,

a monoclonal antibody specific for CD 20+ cells, as part of the chemotherapy regimen. The correct answer, then, is A. A 24-hour urine test is not necessary in staging a Hodgkin's Lymphoma.

## CHAPTER 21

1. **Answer:** B

**Rationale:** A known risk factor for developing multiple myeloma is a history of monoclonal gammopathy of undetermined significance (MGUS). Additionally, another risk factor includes exposure to the herbicide and defoliant Agent Orange that was used by the U.S. military during deployment in the Vietnam War during the 1960s and early 1970s. Other risk factors include exposure to ionizing radiation (including low-level radiation, which places radiologists and those working in the nuclear power industry at risk), exposure to certain metals (especially nickel), agricultural chemicals, benzene, and petroleum products, aromatic hydrocarbons, and silicone. Multiple myeloma has also been linked to a family history of the disease, obesity, and immunologic issues (patients with AIDS have been associated with developing multiple myeloma). Finally, ethnicity has been shown as a risk factor, with multiple myeloma with twice the incidence in African Americans than in their Caucasian counterparts. Exposure to EBV is a risk factor for lymphoma but not specific to multiple myeloma. The employment status of a person or female gender are not known risk factors.

2. **Answer:** B

**Rationale:** Multiple myeloma is a B-cell clonal malignancy of the plasma cells that is characterized by monoclonal plasmacytosis in the bone marrow, excessive production of M protein (myeloma-produced immunoglobulin), osteolytic bone lesions, renal disease, anemia, hypercalcemia, and immunodeficiency. Multiple myeloma is most often associated with hypercalcemia versus hypocalcemia and excessive production, and is more likely to present with elevated M protein versus low production of M protein.

3. **Answer:** C

**Rationale:** Bone marrow biopsy is the confirmatory test for establishing the diagnosis of multiple myeloma, which demonstrates the presence of more than 10% clonal plasma cells. Additional tests that might be used to assess the extent of multiple myeloma include serum protein immunoelectrophoresis, urine protein immunoelectrophoresis, serum lactate dehydrogenase, and urinary light chain M proteins (Bence Jones proteins). Multiple myeloma-related organ dysfunction is also evaluated with laboratory assessment for hypercalcemia, renal insufficiency, and anemia, as well as lytic bone lesions. While a bone scan might identify a lytic lesion, it is not diagnostic for multiple myeloma. A renal ultrasound can determine some abnormalities in the kidneys but does not assess for renal insufficiency. A complete blood count will demonstrate anemia, but it is not specific for multiple myeloma.

4. *Answer:* D

*Rationale:* Deletion of chromosome 17p, translocation of chromosomes 14 and 16 and 14 and 20 are features of high-risk multiple myeloma according to Mayo Clinic mSMART Protocol. Standard risk is characterized by trisomies, t (11;14) and t (6;14) translocations, and intermediate risk is characterized by t (4;14) translocation and 1q gain by FISH. Certain characteristics may place patient at standard risk; however, there is no low-risk stratification.

5. *Answer:* D

*Rationale:* Lytic bone lesions are the most common source of pain in persons with multiple myeloma. For this reason, supportive care for persons with multiple myeloma often includes radiation therapy to the lytic lesion as well as the administration of medications such as bisphosphonates. Although there are bone marrow changes that can occur, this is not typically a source of pain. Additionally, neural infiltration of plasma cells and intestinal obstruction are also not common underlying causes of pain in multiple myeloma. Anemia is common in multiple myeloma but symptoms typically include fatigue and possibly shortness of breath, not pain.

6. *Answer:* C

*Rationale:* Shingle prophylaxis is indicated during proteasome inhibitor-based therapy with bortezomib, carfilzomib, or ixazomib secondary to the increased risk during treatment. Shingle prophylaxis includes daily acyclovir or valacyclovir. Although anti-emetics may be administered to patients on this regimen, aprepitant is not routinely used. Although there is a risk for tumor lysis syndrome and hydration is important in the overall care of the patient, they are not standard nursing interventions in caring for persons on this regimen.

7. *Answer:* A

*Rationale:* The correct nursing intervention related to physical, emotional, psychological, social, and spiritual distress is to encourage the patient to verbalize his feelings about the disease and the treatment. While nurses are encouraged to engage the family in coping options, the intervention should be done jointly between the patient and the family, while validating effective mechanisms. The patient should not be referred to pastoral care, unless the patient is requesting to see a pastor, but the nurse should refer the patient to a mental health specialist, community resources, and support groups run by established associations such as the Leukemia and Lymphoma Society, the American Cancer Society, and the International Myeloma Foundation, as needed. Other interventions including teaching the patient and family to identify, manage, and report symptoms, and providing pharmacologic and nonpharmacologic interventions to manage side effects.

8. *Answer:* D

*Rationale:* The diagnostic criteria for active or symptomatic multiple myeloma requiring therapy is calcium elevation in blood, with a calcium level greater than 10.5 ng/L or the upper limit of normal. Seventy percent is the incorrect percentage of clonal bone marrow plasma cells. The correct percentage is 60%. Serum-free light chain ration Kappa: lambda < 100 is incorrect. The correct answer is serum-free light chain ration Kappa: lambda >100. Magnetic resonance imaging (MRI) studies with < 1 focal lesion (>8 mm in size) is also incorrect. The correct answer is magnetic resonance imaging (MRI) studies with >1 focal lesion (>5 mm in size). Other diagnostic criteria include renal insufficiency (with a serum creatinine level greater than 2 mg/dL), anemia (hemoglobin less than 10 g/dL), bone lytic lesions (detected through a metastatic bone survey, MRI, or positron emission tomography/computed tomography (PET/CT) imaging), and bone marrow biopsy demonstrating the presence of more than 10% plasma cells.

9. *Answer:* is B

*Rationale:* Patients who present with hypercalcemia, renal dysfunction, and bone fractures are associated with inferior overall survival. Hypocalcemia is not a presenting symptom for a new diagnosis of multiple myeloma and a normal bone scan would not be indicative of significant disease. Multiple myeloma is a malignancy of the plasma cells; therefore, it would be expected that plasma cells would be present in a new diagnosis.

10. *Answer:* D

*Rationale:* No cure exists for multiple myeloma regardless of trisomy translocations and surgery is not indicated in patients with multiple myeloma for treatment of the disease. Newer therapies have extended the survival of patient with a multiple myeloma diagnosis; however, treatment in this instance is aimed at reduction and control of the disease and a palliative intent.

## CHAPTER 22

1. *Answer:* A

*Rationale:* Pediatric tumors are most often malignant and are diagnosed more often than any other type of cancer in pediatrics except for leukemia.

2. *Answer:* B

*Rationale:* Points of care where neuro-imaging is indicated are pre-operatively, post-operatively, and at follow-up examinations. Preoperatively imaging is used to identify patterns of cerebral edema or location of lesions. Postoperative imaging with CT or MRI is recommended within 24 hours of surgical resection to assess residual tumor volume and establish new baseline to measure treatment effect. Follow-up examinations ordered every 3 to 4 months is the typical standard practice outside of clinical trials, unless clinically indicated otherwise.

3. *Answer:* A

*Rationale:* While corticosteroids may be administered preoperatively, and antiepileptic medications may be given perioperatively, they are to control symptoms of the tumor and are not a primary treatment for the tumor. The most important therapy for a primary brain tumor is maximal surgical resection. Chemotherapy is not effective in many types of brain tumor.

4. *Answer:* C

*Rationale:* Of children and teens diagnosed with a central nervous system tumor, about 75% will be alive

**151**

more than 5 years after the initial diagnosis. This is important for the oncology nurse to anticipate because of the substantial survivorship issues that these children, teens, and parents must endure.

5. *Answer:* A

*Rationale:* The oncology nurse recognizes that a young man with a grade III oligodendroglioma can have a life expectancy of more than 10-15 years with treatment. Thus, while discussing driving, hospice, and outside opinions are of importance at different care points, the most timely education for this young man relative to his chemotherapy treatment is the option of sperm banking PRIOR to starting his chemotherapy treatment.

6. *Answer:* C

*Rationale:* Each of these drug classes may have one or more of these side effects, but corticosteroids are the only one that has all these risks.

7. *Answer:* B

*Rationale:* Of all tumor types, melanoma has the strongest affinity to metastasize to the central nervous system.

8. *Answer:* A

*Rationale:* Of all tumor types, leptomeningeal carcinomatosis is more frequently associated with breast tumors (35%), followed by lung tumors (24%), and then hematologic malignancies (16%).

9. *Answer:* A

*Rationale:* Each of these symptoms may be prevalent in persons with brain cancer, however not with the same frequency or severity as fatigue.

10. *Answer:* C

*Rationale:* While each of these other options may seem plausible, the only correct answer is perioperatively, persons with brain cancer treatment require anti-epileptic medication in the perioperative period. Otherwise, anti-epileptic medication is not indicated unless the person has a known seizure disorder. First-line agents include lamotrigine, levetiracetam, pregabalin, or valproic acid.

11. *Answer:* A

*Rationale:* The AJCC TNM classification system is not used to stage primary central nervous system tumors because two of three indicators are not applicable (there are no nodes and extracranial metastases extraordinarily rare). The World Health Organization (WHO) classification of a central nervous system tumor is universally applicable and prognostically valid. National Comprehensive Cancer Network (NCNN) does not provide staging/classification of disease criteria.

12. *Answer:* D

*Rationale:* The section of the brain responsible for personality is the frontal lobe. The frontal lobe is responsible for not only our personality, but a person's movement, reasoning, behavior, memory, planning, decision-making, judgment, initiative, inhibition, and mood. The occipital lobe accounts for our vision. The temporal lobe accounts for language comprehension, behavior, memory, hearing, and emotions, while the parietal lobe gives us the ability to tell right from left, allows us to do mathematical

calculations, allows to feel sensations, and gives us the power of reading and writing.

13. *Answer:* C

*Rationale:* The most common type of spinal tumor of schwannomas, meningiomas, and ependymomas, comprising 79% of all spinal tumors. Chordomas are the least common of the spinal tumors. The second most common are sarcomas, followed by astrocytomas, and vascular tumors.

14. *Answer:* D

*Rationale:* The section of the brain responsible for coordination and balance is the cerebellum. The cerebellum is also responsible for fine muscle control. The temporal lobe accounts for language comprehension, behavior, memory, hearing, and emotions, while the parietal lobe gives us the ability to tell right from left, allows us to do mathematical calculations, allows to feel sensations, and gives us the power of reading and writing. The pituitary gland controls our hormones, growth, and fertility. The brain stem regulates and controls our breathing, blood pressure, heartbeat, and swallowing functionality.

15. *Answer:* C

Ionizing radiation (IR) is a known extrinsic risk factor. According to various sources, there is a causal relationship between therapeutic irradiation of doses >2500 cGy and development of brain tumors; risk higher for nerve sheath tumors and meningiomas than gliomas. Being immunocompromised, including having a diagnosis of HIV/AIDS, taking immunosuppressive medical therapies, and having a congenital immunodeficiency are all examples of situational risk factors. Exposure to pesticides, vinyl chloride, petrochemicals, electromagnetic fields, inks and solvents, dietary N-nitroso compounds, long-term use of black or brown hair dyes, cell phones, aspartame, and certain viral exposures are unknown risk factors and currently under investigation. Race/ethnicity is an **intrinsic** risk factor. The most at risk are Caucasian with northern European descent, while meningioma is more common in African American populations.

## CHAPTER 23

1. *Answer:* D

*Rationale:* HPV vaccination, Pap testing, HPV screening, and addressing risk factors all encourage prevention, early diagnosis, and early treatment of pre-cancerous or cancerous cervical changes, which decreases the risk of death from cervical cancer. Vaccination for HPV types 16, 18, 31, 33, 45, 52, and 58 is recommended for both males and females starting at age 11 to 12. It can be given as early as age 9. Teenage boys and girls who did not get vaccinated when they were younger should be educated about the vaccine and encouraged to get it. The HPV vaccine is recommended for young women through age 26, and young men through age 21 years. Pre-invasive disease (CIN1-3) may be treated with hysterectomy if fertility sparing is not desired, but more commonly, may

**152**

be treated by fertility sparing modalities such as LEEP, cone biopsy, cauterization, or cryotherapy, followed by surveillance per guidelines. There is not a vaccination for HepC. HIV screening is not routinely done in the general population.

2. *Answer:* B

*Rationale:* Patients with HNPCC/Lynch syndrome have a 60% lifetime risk of endometrial cancer due to genetic susceptibility. Increased estrogen is associated with a higher risk of developing endometrial cancer. Modifiable sources of increased estrogen can come from obesity, a high fat diet, or diabetes. Endometrial cancer is hormonally driven, and tamoxifen can work like estrogen in the uterus and increases the risk of endometrial cancer, similarly to unopposed estrogen therapy. Aromatase inhibitors may actually decrease the risk of developing endometrial cancer. Early menarche and late menopause are risk factors for endometrial cancer as they also extend the period of time the uterus is exposed to hormonal drivers over the course of a female patient's life. Late menarche and early menopause would not be considered risk factors.

3. *Answer:* B

*Rationale:* Most new ovarian cancer diagnoses are in patients over age 55, and hormone therapy replacement is a risk factor, not a protective factor, for ovarian cancer. There is no routine screening test for ovarian cancer, Known risk factors for ovarian cancer include smoking, nulliparity, older age at first birth, hormone replacement therapy (HRT), pelvic inflammation disease (PID), ovarian stimulation for in vitro fertilization (IVF) (in some cases), as well as genetic risk factors. Protective factors include a younger age at first pregnancy, use of OCPs, and breastfeeding. Although most ovarian cancer is not genetic, this patient meets genetic screening criteria because of the history of ovarian in the patient and breast cancer in her sister. Genetic evaluation may help determine if her daughter has hereditary risk for developing breast, ovarian, or other cancers.

4. *Answer:* B

*Rationale:* Chemotherapy is effective with good cure rates and has not been shown to decrease fertility after treatment for GTN. Patients should wait at least 12 months after completing treatment before conceiving, as (1) it is unsafe to conceive while undergoing or immediately after chemotherapy treatment, and (2) most relapses will occur within as 12-month timeframe.

5. *Answer:* A

*Rationale:* Exposure to DES in utero (DES used by the mother, while pregnant) can increase the risk of congenital abnormalities and vaginal cancer in offspring. Breast cancer in a first-degree relative and use of HRT are not known risk factors associated with vaginal, vulvar, or cervical cancer. Asbestos exposure in a parent has not been shown to increase vaginal, vulvar, or cervical cancer risk in offspring.

6. *Answer:* B

*Rationale:* Most testicular cancer occurs in male patients ages 20 to 43, and a painless testicular mass/swelling is a red-flag symptom for testicular cancer, and should be reported by patients to their provider if discovered on self-exam for a full diagnostic evaluation. It is less common in African American or Asian/Pacific Islander men. Other risk factors include a personal or family history of germ cell tumor (GCT), cryptorchidism, testicular dysgenesis, and Kleinfelter's syndrome.

7. *Answer:* B

*Rationale:* Modifiable risk factors for penile cancer include HPV vaccination to prevent HPV infection, prevention of HIV infection, circumcision before puberty, and tobacco cessation The foreskin should be retracted when cleaning the glans to maintain adequate hygiene in uncircumcised patients. Penile cancer is more common in parts of Asia, Africa, and South America than in North America or Europe. It is a rare cancer in the U.S. with usual presentation at 50 to 70 years. HIV/HPV infection (positive in 60%-80% of penile cancers, type 16, 18) is a modifiable risk factor. Other known risk factors include phimosis, balanitis, chronic inflammation, penile trauma, lack of circumcision, lichen sclerosis, tobacco use, and poor hygiene.

8. *Answer:* A

*Rationale:* A rising CA125 is a biochemical sign of relapse or recurrence. Possible signs of ovarian cancer recurrence include abdominal bloating, bowel/bladder changes, weight loss, early satiety, nausea, vomiting, and ascites. Vaginal discharge and bleeding is not a common symptom associated with ovarian cancer.

9. *Answer:* C

*Rationale:* Per National Comprehensive Cancer Network (NCCN) guidelines, the standard of care for endometrial cancer is usually an upfront TH/BSO, which may or may not be followed by adjuvant treatment. Fertility sparing surgery is not usually recommended and is considered as a treatment only in rare cases with genetic counseling, continuous progestin-based suppression, and hysterectomy after childbearing, or on progression of disease. Hormone therapy is generally reserved for patients who are not surgical candidates, and is continued until progression. Assessing for endometrial thickening, or preforming a D&C, is a part of the diagnostic, but not treatment process.

10. *Answer:* C

*Rationale:* Fertility sparing, including conization with cold knife or LEEP procedure, lymph node evaluation if lymphovascular space invasion (LVSI) is present, radical trachelectomy is a treatment for early-stage (IA1–IB1) cervical cancer. Radical hysterectomy and lymph node evaluation is treatment for select IIA1 disease. For IB2, IIA2, or greater nonsurgical candidates, the recommended treatment is definitive chemoradiation (with or without ovarian transposition if premenopausal), and possibly neoadjuvant chemotherapy followed by resection. Primary treatment followed by observation, external beam radiation therapy (EBRT), and/or adjuvant chemotherapy is a treatment for advanced disease.

11. *Answer:* C

*Rationale:* For treatment of metastatic cervical cancer, the recommendation is radiation therapy with or without chemotherapy, palliative systemic agents, and best supportive care. Simple or modified radical hysterectomy with or without lymph node evaluation is a non-fertility sparing option for early-stage disease (IA1–IB1). External beam radiation therapy (EBRT) and neoadjuvant chemotherapy is incorrect. EBRT is used for advanced stage cancers but not in conjunction with neoadjuvant chemotherapy. Neoadjuvant chemotherapy followed by resection, along with definitive chemoradiation (with or without ovarian transposition if premenopausal), is used in IB2, IIA2, or greater nonsurgical candidates: radiation therapy, systemic therapy, local ablation, and surgical resection are treatments for recurrent disease.

12. *Answer:* D

*Rationale:* The stage of testicular cancer that has the best 5-year survival rate in the United States is localized at 99.2%. Distant has a 73.2% 5-year survival rate. Unstaged has a 76.7%, while regional has a 96.1%. The overall survival rate is 95.1%.

13. *Answer:* B

Sperm banking may be done before or after surgery, but ideally before any radiation therapy or chemotherapy since these treatments may have an adverse effect on male fertility.

14. *Answer:* B

Ms. D is perimenopausal. Following surgery, she will be considered menopausal. Surgery and radiation therapy of the abdomen/pelvis and associated pretreatment and posttreatment care, including hypoestrogenism after BSO, which may induce hot flashes, mood, changes, vaginal dryness, pelvic tissue atrophy, osteoporosis, and increased cardiovascular disease (CVD) risk. Alternating constipation and diarrhea as well as change in urinal function are not common complications following a hysterectomy. Risk of cardiovascular disease is increased in postmenopausal women especially those such as Ms. D who are experiencing an early menopause.

## CHAPTER 24

1. *Answer:* A

*Rationale:* The major risk factor for BCC is exposure to the ultraviolet radiation of sunlight, specifically, intermittent exposure early in life. BCCs develop primarily on sun-exposed skin. They are rarely found on palmoplantar surfaces and never appear on the mucosa. Approximately 80% arise on the head and neck area. They tend to be slow growing and arise without precursor lesions. BCCs can be locally invasive tumors. Family history of skin cancer is associated with increased risk but is not the major cause of BCC. Tobacco smoking and young age are not considered risk factors. Risk increases with older age (>65 years).

2. *Answer:* C

*Rationale:* The correct answer is actinic keratoses (AKs). Approximately 60% to 65% of SCCs arise from prior AKs. The presence of atypical nevi and multiple moles are associated with increased risk of melanoma. Skin viral infection is associated with Merkel cell carcinoma; 80% of cases are caused by a common virus (Merkel cell polyomavirus).

3. *Answer:* D

*Rationale:* In a Mohs procedure (called Mohs micrographic surgery), the dermatologist, who has specialized training in this technique, removes tissue in successive thin layers and examines each layer under the microscope to determine the skin depth at which cancer cells are no longer present. In this way, the maximum amount of normal tissue is preserved. The other three types of therapy, cryotherapy with a probe that applies subzero temperature, local chemotherapy injection, and curettage with cautery or electrodessication, are differing techniques used for superficial low-risk skin lesions.

4. *Answer:* B

*Rationale:* Organ transplant is the correct answer. Transplant recipients of solid organs receive immunosuppressive therapies to prevent organ rejection, increasing their risk of Merkel cell carcinoma. Other factors associated with increased risk are male gender, white European ancestry, and age $\geq$ 65 years.

5. *Answer:* C

*Rationale:* A tendency to bleed is the correct answer. Moles that bleed or itch, or demonstrate changes in shape, size, or color are concerning and require specialized evaluation. Normal moles have a symmetrical shape, regular borders, and are uniformly one color. The ABCDE rule can help reinforce characteristics of melanoma. A refers to asymmetry. B refers to border irregularity or faded borders. C refers to color irregularities or having multiple colors. D refers to diameter more than 5 mm. E refers to evolving

6. *Answer:* B

*Rationale:* Immunotherapy is the correct answer. Immunotherapy is considered the standard treatment for metastatic melanoma. Immunotherapy may consist of anti PD-1 monotherapy with pembrolizumab, or nivolumab or combination anti-CTLA-4 + anti-PD-1 with ipilimumab and nivolumab. The other options are not part of standard therapy for metastatic melanoma. Isolated limb perfusion may be used in certain clinical situations, and cranial radiation therapy may be used palliatively for patients with brain metastases.

7. *Answer:* B

*Rationale:* Merkel cell carcinoma (MCC) presents as papules, plaques, and cyst-like structures or pruritic tumors on the lower extremities. MCC most commonly presents as an erythematous or violaceous, tender, dome-shaped nodule on sun-exposed areas on the head or neck of an elderly white male. Develops primarily on sun-exposed skin and rarely found on palmoplantar surfaces and never appears on the mucosa are characteristics of a basal cell carcinoma (BCC). A BCC can also develop at sites of chemical exposure or chronic trauma. Cutaneous squamous cell carcinoma (cuSCC) often presents as a new or enlarging lesion that may bleed, weep, be tender, or be painful.

within 6 hours of the transfusion causing acute respiratory symptoms such as dyspnea, hypoxia, hypotension, fever, and tachycardia. Iron overload is a delayed reaction occurring from frequent RBC transfusions.

5. **Answer:** C

**Rationale:** According to the guidelines, red blood cells are administered when the hemoglobin is less than 7 g/dL or when the patient becomes symptomatic. Platelets are administered if the platelet count is less than 10,000/mm$^3$ with or without bleeding or less than 20,000/mm$^3$ with active bleeding. Neutrophils are administered when an infection is unresponsive to antibiotic therapy and neutrophils less than 500/mm$^3$. Immunoglobulins are administered when immunoglobulin G level is decreased to provide passive immunity.

6. **Answer:** A

**Rationale:** Acetaminophen and diphenhydramine are commonly administered as premedication prior to transfusions especially for a history of a previous reaction. Meperidine is administered for uncontrolled rigors. Hydrocortisone is available for severe reactions and may be added as a premedication for a history of severe transfusion reaction. Diuretica are administered for fluid overload or to reduce intravascular volume.

7. **Answer:** C

**Rationale:** Appropriate filter or blood component set should be attached to the blood product prior to transfusion. Leukocyte reduction filter reduces the number of leukocytes transfused in a unit of red blood cells. Medications or IV fluids should not be added to blood products. Restrict transfusions to those who have clear indications for therapy and only transfuse the minimum number of units necessary. It is recommended to monitor patients for approximately 2 hours after transfusion.

8. **Answer:** C

**Rationale:** Autologous blood is collected from the intended recipient prior to the elective surgery or during surgery by the use of automated "cell saver" device. HLA matched is used for platelet transfusions when alloimmunization has occurred resulting in a poor response to platelet transfusions Blood collected at a blood drive is a homologous blood component from a screened donor. Directly donated blood is collected from a donor and designated to a recipient.

9. **Answer:** D

**Rationale:** Platelets will be transfused with the patient presenting with active bleeding. Guidelines stipulate transfusion of red blood cells when hemoglobin is less than 7 g/dL or symptomatic. Plasma is transfused to correct clotting factor deficiencies or to expand blood volume.

10. **Answer:** B

**Rationale:** Administer iron component therapy for iron deficiency. Use of vitamin supplementation such as folic acid, vitamin B, and vitamin K may be beneficial in decreasing need for blood components. Minimize routine blood testing. Proton pump inhibitors are used to minimize gastrointestinal bleeding, not histimine-2 antagonist. Use pediatric small volume blood collection tubes to minimize blood collected.

11. **Answer:** D

**Rationale:** The initial step in a suspected reaction is to stop the transfusion and keep the intravenous line open with normal saline. The provider should be notified, and orders obtained if standing orders are not available. Diphenhydramine and meperidine could be ordered to control symptoms. Blood bank should be notified of the potential reaction after the transfusion is stopped.

12. **Answer:** D

**Rationale:** The PICC can remain inserted for up to 12 months, however evidence supports longer duration if the device is functioning without complication. PICCs are inserted into a central vein at the antecubital fossa. PICCs are available with single, double, or triple lumens.

13. **Answer:** C

**Rationale:** Chest X-ray, fluoroscopy, or ultrasound (used during placement) can be used to confirm placement of the catheter tip. CT scan is not used to confirm placement. Blood return on aspiration and ease of fluid administration can be used to evaluate the catheter after catheter tip placement is confirmed post initial placement.

14. **Answer:** B

**Rationale:** Bundle care includes frequent hand washing before and after use, optimal catheter site selection, maximal sterile barrier precautions on device insertion, use of alcohol hub decontamination prior to each access, and daily reviewing line necessity with prompt removal if no longer necessary. Incorporating this care has been shown to decrease the risk of line infection. Bundle care does not decrease the risk of bleeding, catheter dislodgement, or catheter migration.

15. **Answer:** C

**Rationale:** The most common cause for a partial occlusion is a fibrin sheath causing a one-way valve effect allowing infusion of IV fluids into the catheter but causing withdrawal occlusion. Deep vein thrombus can cause a partial occlusion with a presentation of edema. Intraluminal blood clot and precipitation are not as common and cause complete obstruction.

16. **Answer:** D

**Rationale:** Elastomeric pumps do not have audible alarms. Peristaltic and syringe pumps are available with audible alarms to alert the patient and/or caregiver of an occlusion, kinked tubing, or pump malfunction. Smart pump is technology equipped in peristaltic and syringe pumps to minimize the risk of incorrect dosing.

17. **Answer:** A

**Rationale:** Intraventricular catheter is implanted directly into the lateral ventricle of the brain providing direct access to the cerebral spinal fluid. Peritoneal catheter provides direct access to the peritoneal cavity. Epidural catheters provide access to the epidural space used for delivery of opioids or anesthetics. Intrapleural catheters give direct access to the pleura cavity.

18. **Answer:** A

**Rationale:** Maintaining a flushing routine and flushing with pulsatile (push-pause) method to cause swirling action in device are preventative measures for occlusion.

**165**

Changing the intrathoracic pressures with a recommendation of having the patient inhale fully and hold his or her breath or exhale fully and hold his or her breath is a restoration of the problem of occlusion. Surgical removal, as indicated, to avoid a fracture, is a restoration of the problem of "pinch-off syndrome." Finally, removing the needle and re-accessing the port using a noncoring needle is an example of restoring the problem of the dislodgement of the port access needle.

19. *Answer:* B

*Rationale:* An example of a restoration of a problem for a mechanical complication of an access device is referring to a physician for repositioning the catheter using fluoroscopy. The physician will need to reposition the catheter due to a complication arising from catheter migration. To prevent catheter migration, the recommendation is to monitor the length of the catheter (tunnel, midline, PICC) to ensure placement is intact. Other recommendations for prevention of catheter migration include protecting the device from potential trauma and anchoring the device appropriately with a securement device. Avoid placing the port at the sites of actual or potential tissue damage (in radiation field) is a recommendation for prevention of erosion of the port through the subcutaneous tissue. High-pressure infusions or flushing with 1 or 3 mL is a prevention technique for complications arising from port-catheter separation.

20. *Answer:* D

*Rationale:* A characteristic of a short-term or intermediate-term peripheral catheter is the capability to infuse fluids, medications, blood products, and peripheral total parenteral nutrition (TPN) and to obtain blood specimens. Short-term or intermediate-term peripheral catheters are single lumen or multi-lumen catheters. Insertion is done peripherally in the forearm or antecubital fossa into the cephalic, basilic, or median cubital vein. Nontunneled catheters are inserted centrally into the jugular vein, subclavian vein, superior vena cava (SVC), or inferior vena cava. Nontunneled venous short-term catheters are available in single or multi-lumen and offer immediate access. Long-term venous catheters are available with a pressure-activated safety valve (PASV) located in the catheter hub and are designed to permit fluid infusion and decrease risk of blood reflux. Also, in long-term venous catheters the tip must be confirmed before initial use by ultrasound (during placement if used), fluoroscopy, or chest X-ray.

21. *Answer:* A

*Rationale:* Blood component therapy (BCT) exposes the patient to components that are foreign to the individual's system and can lead to allergic reactions, as well as the destruction of blood cells (hemolysis). Although fluid volume overload may occur, and the nurse should monitor the patient closely, deep vein thrombosis is not a common reaction. Other coagulation problems are not seen as acute reactions to blood component therapy. Blood components can contain hematopoietic stem cells, and there have been cases of graft-versus-host disease in individuals with impaired immune system function. However, this condition is not seen as an acute reaction. Protocols will indicate when a patient may require irradiated blood products to decrease this risk.

22. *Answer:* D

*Rationale:* Two licensed healthcare professionals must verify that the blood component therapy product is correctly labeled and dated, and that it matches the information on the patient's blood identification band, usually worn as a bracelet. The patient's name must be spelled correctly, and the blood group and blood type must be identified on the both the product and the patient identifiers. Using a gravity flow infusion line is not the priority intervention to maximize patient safety. Gravity infusions, although not the preferred method, may be used if controlled infusion pumps are not available. Slowly adding medications through the Y-port is incorrect. Medications must never be added to blood component therapy (BCT) infusions. Intravenous therapy guidelines recommend larger catheters be used for viscous infusions, such as BCT products. BCT products must be infused within 4 hours, maximum time, to prevent degradation of the components.

23. *Answer:* D

*Rationale:* Although most individuals can be taught to care for commonly used access devices, those who are not good candidates should be considered for an implanted device, as these devices require less self-care. Demonstration of the ability to care for the device is critical for all external devices. The need for chemotherapy infusions and blood samples is a clinical indication for all types of access devices. The patient expressing concerns about the implication is an indication for the nurse to provide additional education.

24. *Answer:* B

*Rationale:* The patient should be able to assess the system to determine that the power is on and the infusion is occurring. The line should be flushed, not with water, but with normal saline. Flushing is unnecessary while infusion is ongoing. Flushing the line with sterile water every 12 hours is incorrect. Normal saline solution would be used, and when the infusion is ongoing, there is no need to flush the line. These systems should be used only for their intended purpose, and only a trained nurse should access the system and determine whether a second line is appropriate. Doses are programmed on the ambulatory infusion pumps with a sequence intended to prevent accidental or uninformed alteration by lay individuals. Changes in dose need to be made by the nurse when an order is changed or when the infusion is complete.

## CHAPTER 31

1. *Answer:* A

*Rationale:* Fever may be the earliest and/or only warning sign of infection in a neutropenic patient. Patients with a single oral temperature of 38.3°C 101°F should be considered to have an infection. The nurse should anticipate orders to obtain cultures and initiate empiric antimicrobial therapy.

2. **Answer:** A

**Rationale:** Ganciclovir is an anti-viral agent that provides coverage for CMV treatment. Levofloxacin and fluconazole do not provide coverage against viruses. Acyclovir is indicated for herpes simplex virus (HSV) and varicella zoster (VZV), not CMV. Valganciclovir is preemptive therapy for CMV.

3. **Answer:** A

**Rationale:** Fever is often the first and only sign of infection in neutropenic patients. Antipyretics, including acetaminophen, aspirin, and non-steroidal anti-inflammatory agents, should be avoided in high-risk individuals as they may mask fever.

4. **Answer:** D

**Rationale:** Vancomycin should not be routinely included in empiric therapy, except in select clinical situations. The routine use of vancomycin can lead to the occurrence of vancomycin-resistant organisms (VRE). Vancomycin is indicated for gram-positive bacterial coverage, and dose adjustments are required to prevent renal toxicity.

5. **Answer:** A

**Rationale:** Amphotericin B adverse effects include nephrotoxicity, electrolyte wasting, and infusion reaction. Pre-hydration and pre-medications are needed to prevent complications.

6. **Answer:** C

**Rationale:** Stewardship tasks performed by the nurse includes reviewing culture results and reporting positive results to the provider in a timely manner. Overuse of antibiotics should be avoided to prevent organism resistance.

7. **Answer:** B

**Rationale:** Influenza is an inactivated virus and safe for patients receiving cancer treatment. Inactivated viruses can be administered two weeks prior to chemotherapy or in between cycles. CD34 markers do not need to be used as a means of timing his vaccination schedule since he is not a stem cell transplant patient.

8. **Answer:** B

**Rationale:** Anti-inflammatory agents work by decreasing the adverse effects of inflammation. Their mechanism of action inhibits cyclooxygenase which leads to decreased prostaglandin production and decreased inflammation. Anti-inflammatory agents should be avoided in individuals at risk for infection and/or neutropenia as they may mask fever which is a side effect. Another side effect is decreased platelet function and increased risk for bleeding.

9. **Answer:** B

**Rationale:** The antiplatelet effects of NSAIDs require that caution be taken when prescribing patients other anticoagulation or antiplatelet medications like clopidogrel. Taking these medications together can increase the risk of adverse reactions and/or potentiate toxicities.

10. **Answer:** D

**Rationale:** Corticosteroids can cause muscle weakness/wasting. The oncology nurse should monitor the patient with cancer's muscle strength, encourage regular exercise, and implement safety measures to prevent fall or injury. Other side effects include hyperglycemia, hypernatremia, hypokalemia, and hypocalcemia, leading to edema, hypertension, diabetes, and osteoporosis.

11. **Answer:** A

**Rationale:** Ondansetron and granisetron are 5-HT3 antagonists, blocking the action of serotonin along nerve pathways. Dopamine is a D2 antagonist. Histamine is a H1 antagonist. Neurokinin is an NK1 antagonist.

12. **Answer:** B

**Rationale:** The general principle of breakthrough chemotherapy-induced nausea and vomiting (CINV) treatment is to introduce one agent from a different drug class to the current regimen. If palonosetron is given prior to chemotherapy, the use of another 5HT3 antagonist is not warranted for the management of breakthrough CINV.

13. **Answer:** B

**Rationale:** Metoclopramide has a black box warning for sudden death related to prolonged QT intervals. This medication should not be administered if QTc is > 500 msec. If the patient experiences shortness of breath or palpitations while receiving this medication, they should immediately notify their healthcare provider. Extrapyramidal side effects may occur.

14. **Answer:** A

**Rationale:** Chronic pain lasts longer than three months and can be a source of background pain for patients with cancer. Chronic pain is commonly associated with breakthrough pain. Analgesic medication management should be prescribed to provide pain control for a 24-hour period. If opioids are used, patients should have long-acting and breakthrough options available when pain is constant. Prophylaxis for constipation with a stool softener and bowel stimulant should be considered for all patients who are started on opioid analgesics, and the regimen should be optimized to assure regular bowel movements. Tolerance occurs in patients who take opioids regularly; that is, they require higher doses to achieve the same amount of analgesia.

15. **Answer:** D

**Rationale:** Abrupt discontinuation of opioids can lead to withdrawal. Symptoms of withdrawal include nausea, vomiting, perspiration, chills, tachycardia, anxiety, and insomnia. Addiction is a psychological sign where the patient craves the drug despite knowing the harm. An assessment for pain and GI is needed to determine adequate pain control and monitor for signs of constipation.

16. **Answer:** A

**Rationale:** Methylphenidate (Ritalin) may be helpful for somnolence or mental clouding from opioids. Metoclopramide is used as an antiemetic. Micafungin is an antifungal agent. Mithramycin is a chemotherapy agent.

17. **Answer:** B

**Rationale:** Opioids can cause nausea and vomiting. Patients should be taught to take medication with food to prevent GI upset.

18. *Answer:* A

*Rationale:* Anxiolytics can be used to reduce anxiety associated with diagnosis and treatment of cancer, to manage anticipatory nausea, reduce pain associated with anxiety, and manage alcohol or narcotic withdrawal.

19. *Answer:* D

*Rationale:* Lexapro is an SSRI. Effects may not be seen for the first 2-4 weeks. To prevent withdrawal, patients should slowly taper off the medication should they experience side effects.

20. *Answer:* C

*Rationale:* Zolpidem (Ambien) is a non-benzodiazepine receptor agonist indicated for sleep latency and mid-night awakenings. Linezolid is used to treat gram-positive bacterial infections. Posaconazole is used to treat fungal infections. Temozolomide is a chemotherapy agent.

21. *Answer:* B

*Rationale:* Antidepressant therapeutic effect can take up to 3 weeks. Patients with major depressive disorder may have suicidal thoughts and should be routinely screened for suicidal ideation or emotional changes until a therapeutic response is achieved. Responses A and C are appropriate assessment questions, but suicide prevention is an important safety issue.

22. *Answer:* D

*Rationale:* Tricyclic antidepressants (TCAs) are associated with anticholinergic effects and have a 4+ toxicity comparison. Fluoxetine, sertraline, and citalopram are SSRIs and do not have anticholinergic toxicities.

23. *Answer:* C

*Rationale:* Carmustine is a chemotherapy drug which has the potential to lower seizure threshold.

24. *Answer:* A

*Rationale:* Somnolence is a side effect associated with levetiracetam. The agent may also be associated with dizziness and rash and occasionally psychosis.

25. *Answer:* A

*Rationale:* Anticonvulsants are enzyme inducers, which causes an increase in metabolism and decreased exposure to the medication. Enzyme inhibitors decrease metabolism, causing exposure of the medication to be increased. A substrate for an enzyme is vulnerable to changes in enzyme activity. If an oncology nurse has concerns about drug-drug interactions while caring for a patient, consider consulting with a pharmacist.

26. *Answer:* B

*Rationale:* Filgrastim is a myeloid growth factor used after autologous stem cell transplant and cord blood transplantation to support neutrophil engraftment.

27. *Answer:* A

*Rationale:* Myeloid growth factors stimulate the proliferation and maturity of neutrophils and macrophages.

28. *Answer:* B

*Rationale:* The oncology nurse should understand the increased risk for thrombotic events when administering erythropoietin. Patients and their families should be taught to monitor for signs of swelling or redness in the lower extremities and to notify their provider should this occur.

29. *Answer:* C

*Rationale:* Splenectomy and functional asplenia may increase the risk of infection where antimicrobials would be warranted. A lobectomy is a surgery to remove one of the lobes of the lungs; an appendectomy removes the appendix and a cholecystectomy is surgery to remove the gallbladder. These surgeries do not impact immune suppression.

30. *Answer:* D

*Rationale:* Serotonin selective reuptake inhibitors (SSRI) may induce anxiety symptoms, not relieve them, early in therapy. SSRIs are started at a low dose, not a high dose, and then increased to an optimal dose. The effect of SSRIs may not be seen for the first 2-4 weeks. Abrupt discontinuation may precipitate withdrawal syndromes.

31. *Answer:* B

*Rationale:* Major depressive disorder is characterized by depressive symptoms lasting most of the day, every day, for at least 2 weeks. Major depressive disorder occurs in about 25% of patients with cancer, leading to poor quality of life and functional status, higher use of healthcare services, and non-adherence with treatment.

32. *Answer D:*

*Rationale:* Dietary modifications to avoid tyramine are critical for patients on monoamine oxidase inhibitors (MAOIs). Tyramine does not impact serotonin selective reuptake inhibitors (SSRIs), serotonin and norepinephrine reuptake inhibitors (SNRIs) or tricyclic antidepressants (TCAs).

33. *Answer:* A

*Rationale:* Therapy should continue for 6 months following improvement in symptoms to avoid relapse of depression. Taking antidepressants as scheduled and allowing the time necessary for a therapeutic response to the medications is required. There is a potential for withdrawal effects with abrupt cessation; therefore, gradually taper of dose should occur at discontinuation.

34. *Answer:* B

*Rationale:* Risk is increased in select patients including: recent surgery or open wounds, prior chemotherapy or radiation therapy, persistent neutropenia, bone marrow involvement of the tumor, liver dysfunction, renal dysfunction, and age greater than 56 years.

35. *Answer:* C

*Rationale:* EPO is associated with an increased risk of venous thromboembolism. Patients who are iron-deficient will not respond to EPO. EPO should not be given in patients with hemoglobin greater than 10 g/dL. EPO decreases, not increases, the number of RBC transfusions required to treat anemia.

36. *Answer:* D

*Rationale:* The cell nadir occurs 7 to 14 days after the chemotherapy treatment. Neutropenia occurs when the absolute neutrophil count (ANC) is less than 500/mm$^3$.

37. *Answer:* A

*Rationale:* Central obesity, moon face, buffalo hump, easy bruising, acne, hirsutism, striae, and skin atrophy occur with use of corticosteroids and would warrant the assessment of the patient's body image and concerns. The oncology nurse should provide the opportunity for the patient with cancer to share concerns and discuss coping strategies, and educate the patient regarding care of skin and safety precautions. NSAIDS: Cox-2 selective agent, salicylates, and aminoglycosides do not cause the degree, if any, body image concerns.

38. *Answer:* B

*Rationale:* The onset of effect for oral Morphine is 30 minutes and Morphine IV is 5-10 minutes. Morphine 10 mg IV has equivalent potency as Morphine 30 mg orally. The peak effect is 10-15 minutes with Morphine IV and 60 minutes for Morphine oral. Morphine IV and oral both have a duration of effect of 3-4 hours.

39. *Answer:* C

*Rationale:* For accurate results, axillary temperature should be avoided. Rectal temperatures should be avoided to prevent potential injury to the rectal mucosa. Temperature threshold for the neutropenic patient should be defined as a sustained oral temperature of 38°C (100.4°F) over 1 hour or a single oral temperature of 38.3°C (101°F).

40. *Answer:* D

*Rationale:* The gold standard for diagnosis in this patient population is to draw one set peripherally and one from central lines when the patient has a central venous catheter. Two peripheral cultures should be drawn if no central venous catheter is in place. Cultures would be obtained before 48 hours, so medication can be administered for symptom relief.

41. *Answer:* A

*Rationale:* Pseudomonas infections are diseases caused by a bacterium from the genus Pseudomonas which is found widely in the environment, such as in soil, water, and plants; this is not a virus. Human immunodeficiency virus (HIV) and respiratory syncytial virus (RSV) are viruses, but only herpes simplex virus (HSV) would routinely warrant antimicrobial prophylaxis.

42. *Answer:* B

*Rationale:* In low-risk patients that are clinically stable with negative cultures and an ANC remaining less than 500, consider discontinuation of antibiotics after a total of 5 to 7 days. Continuing beyond this amount of time may unnecessarily cause additional antimicrobial side effects.

43. *Answer:* D

*Rationale:* Stevens-Johnson syndrome is a severe skin reaction with one of the primary symptoms being the presence of blisters. The infection can spread to the mucous membranes which could cause blisters to form inside the body, making eating and drinking painful. If left untreated, Stevens-Johnson syndrome can spread to other organs. The impact is on dermatologic area, and not the liver, heart, or gastrointestinal.

44. *Answer:* C

*Rationale:* Live virus vaccines use the weakened (attenuated) form of the virus. The measles, mumps, and rubella (MMR) vaccine and the varicella (chickenpox) vaccine are examples. Inactivated vaccines may be administered >2 weeks prior to chemotherapy; live virus vaccines should be given >4 weeks prior to chemotherapy.

45. *Answer:* B

*Rationale:* CD34 is the most commonly used marker for hematopoietic stem/progenitor cells in clinical hematology. Clinicians even use this marker as a quality criterion for the hematopoietic graft. Human leukocyte antigen-DR and vascular endothelial growth factor receptor (VEGFR) are associated markers. A complete blood count (CBC) would not be used alone for timing vaccines.

46. *Answer:* A

*Rationale:* Patients at risk for toxicities with NSAIDs are age 65 or older, history of GI ulcers, renal insufficiency, cardiovascular disease, concurrent aspirin or anticoagulant use, and history of ulcerative colitis. Anticonvulsants, acetaminophen, or corticosteroids would be less toxic with the history presented.

47. *Answer:* D

*Rationale:* Highly emetogenic intravenous chemotherapy would warrant medications such as NK1 RA + 5-HT3 RA + dexamethasone prior to chemotherapy followed by NK1 RA (if needed) and dexamethasone. Agents for breakthrough nausea and vomiting include cannabis (medical marijuana) in addition to dopamine antagonists such as prochlorperazine, droperidol, promethazine, dexamethasone, lorazepam, ondansetron, metoclopramide, and cannabinoids such as dronabinol and nabilone. Legalization of marijuana for medical use is growing in a number of states, but not legal in every state. Cannabis may have long- and short-term side effects, but may still be prescribed for breakthrough nausea and vomiting.

48. *Answer:* B

*Rationale:* Absorption and onset of pain medications vary with patients with any route including buccal, rectal, and subcutaneous. Fat-to-lean body ratio impacts transdermal preparations and is not recommended in cachectic patients and takes a longer time to onset in obese patients.

49. *Answer:* A

*Rationale:* Amphotericin B and fluconazole are antifungals that are indicated for a fungal infection such as *Candida.* Caspofungin (Cancidas) is an antifungal, but ciprofloxacin is an antimicrobial for gram-negative bacteria. Voriconazole (Vfend) is used for *Candida* infection, but imipenem is for gram-positive infections. Cidofovir is an antiviral agent.

50. *Answer:* D

*Rationale:* Doses are based on ideal, not actual, body weight. Ganciclovir, not acyclovir, is the antiviral regarded as being effective preemptive therapy for cytomegalovirus in high-risk patients with cancer. Probenecid is given to patients to prevent renal reabsorption of cidofovir.

51. *Answer:* D

*Rationale:* The serotonin antagonists include ondansetron (Zofran). Prochlorperazine is a D2 antagonist. Aprepitant is an NK-1 antagonist.

52. *Answer:* B

*Rationale:* Major neurotransmitter targets are as follows: serotonin (5HT3 antagonists, e.g., ondansetron),

**169**

neurokinin (NK-1 antagonist, e.g., aprepitant), dopamine (D-2 antagonist, e.g., prochlorperazine), histamine (H-1 antagonist, e.g., promethazine), acetylcholine (muscarinic, e.g., scopolamine), and cannabinoid (cannabinoid agonist, e.g., dronabinol).

53. *Answer:* B

*Rationale:* The pharmacokinetics of fentanyl support B as the correct answer. Fentanyl patch onset is 18 to 24 hours and buccal administration is 5 to 15 minutes.

54. *Answer:* C

*Rationale:* The majority of the serotonin reuptake agents can contribute to sexual dysfunction. The other options – hot flashes, neuropathy, and increased appetite – are not expected side effects.

55. *Answer:* D

*Rationale:* Bone pain is the main side effect of filgrastim. Bone pain occurs as a result of expansion of granulocytic precursors in the patient's bone marrow. Often, a patient's peripheral white blood count will be correspondingly high. Sedation is not a side effect and the other options of liver dysfunction and constipation are not expected side effects.

## CHAPTER 32

1. *Answer:* B

*Rationale:* Complementary and alternative medicine, or CAM, describes the entire domain of therapies that fall outside of conventional medicine. Integrative therapy combines conventional treatment with evidence-based complementary therapy, but integrative therapy is not the domain. Allopathic therapy enhances conventional therapy but is not the domain. Mind body is a complementary therapy but is not the domain.

2. *Answer:* D

*Rationale:* Natural products as well as mind and body practices are the two subgroups defined by the National Center for Complementary and Integrative Health (NCCIH). Massage and acupuncture are therapies within the mind and body group. Tai chi and healing touch are therapies within the mind and body group. Chiropractic and osteopathic manipulation are therapies within the mind and body group.

3. *Answer:* D

*Rationale:* Herbal and botanical medicine can interact with prescribed medication. Herbal/botanical medicine can pose significant risks to the patient due to interactions with conventionally prescribed medications. Herbal/botanical medicine is not FDA approved and is not well-regulated in the U.S. as in other countries. Herbal/botanical medicine safety and efficacy is not guaranteed.

4. *Answer:* A

*Rationale:* Mind body modalities include art and color therapy, music therapy, guided imagery, meditation, yoga, and T'ai chi. Whole medical systems are therapeutic approaches that include chiropractic medicine, homeopathic, and osteopathic medicine. Biologically based therapies use substances found in nature to promote wellness and treat illness, such as biofeedback, hydrotherapy, and energy work. Manipulative and body-based practices include acupuncture, acupressure, dance therapy, and traditional Chinese medicine.

5. *Answer:* C

*Rationale:* Patient values and preferences, which include cultural and religious practices, are part of a comprehensive complementary and alternative medicine (CAM) assessment. Relevant clinical information is incorporated into the assessment and includes items such as comorbidities, allergies, and all medications, including CAM. A comprehensive patient assessment of CAM is done at first visit and ongoing through their cancer care. Biologically based therapies, such as biofeedback, herbal therapy, and energy work, are a part of the CAM assessment.

6. *Answer:* B

*Rationale:* Docetaxel is noted to have interactions with allium sativum, echiacea purpurea, and hypericum perforatum. Adriamycin, Lupron, and Bleomycin are not known to have specific interactions with natural products.

7. *Answer:* C

*Rationale:* Patients with peripheral neuropathy grade 3 or less may receive massage over the affected area. Massage is contraindicated in a patient diagnosed with thrombocytopenia with a platelet count of less than 50,000 due to the risk of bleeding. Patients with suspected or known bone metastasis should not receive pressure or jostling over the affected areas. Patients with severe neutropenia and WBC below 1500 should not receive massage therapy.

8. *Answer:* B

*Rationale:* With the mind-body modality of neuro-linguistic programming (NLP), the patient focuses on positive aspects of his or her life to promote a positive outlook over time. An example of this modality is having a patient record daily entries in a "gratitude journal." The entries focus on recalling positive aspects of his or her life to promote a positive outlook over time. The overriding principle behind NLP is that an individual gets more of whatever that person is focusing on. The modality that has a meditative component that brings harmony to body, mind, and spirit is yoga. Practices within the modality of meditation share characteristics and often involve focused breathing and a relaxed yet alert state that promotes control over thoughts and feelings. Guided imagery is a modality with a structured process that uses live or recorded readings describing different scenarios or detailed images to guide the patient through a certain process.

9. *Answer:* C

*Rationale:* A technique in guided imagery is to lead the patient through progressive muscle relaxation or visualization of a treatment process (e.g., visualization of chemotherapy entering the body and seeking out cancer cells to remove them from the body). Tai chi is a modality that enhances coordination and balance and promotes physical, emotional, and spiritual well-being. Mindfulness-based stress reduction (MBSR) is a technique whereby patients are trained to develop awareness of experiences moment by moment and in the context of all senses. This technique falls under the larger category of meditation. A psychotherapy technique based on the concept that distressing events are associated with specific rapid eye movements is eye movement desensitization and reprocessing (EMDR).

10. *Answer:* D

*Rationale:* The manipulative and body-based practice of acupressure is defined as the use of finger or hand pressure over specific points on the body to relieve symptoms or to influence specific organ function. Acupuncture is an ancient Oriental technique associated with traditional Chinese medicine (TCM), used to restore or promote health and well-being using fine-gauge needles inserted into specific points on the body to stimulate or disperse the flow of energy. The use of manual pressure and strokes on muscle tissue is the definition of massage. Conflicting evidence currently exists as to the effectiveness of massage therapy in patients with cancer. The use of vigorous massage to stimulate flow of lymphatic fluid is the definition of lymphatic therapy.

11. *Answer:* A

*Rationale:* There are currently no standards of practice or processing regulations for aromatherapy since essential oils have a wide range of quality levels. Aromatherapy targets physical imbalances, as well as psychological and spiritual issues. Although individuals can develop an allergy to the transporting vehicle, allergies are not a major safety concern.

12. *Answer:* C

*Rationale:* Feldenkrais refers to a method that teaches movement and manipulation to increase body awareness. Gentle manipulation of the skull to reestablish natural configuration and movement is the definition for cranial osteopathy. Lymphatic therapy is the use of vigorous massage to stimulate flow of lymphatic fluid. The technique that uses movement and touch to restore balance to the body is called the Alexander technique and is not a part of the Feldenkrais method.

13. *Answer:* D

*Rationale:* In Reiki, the practitioner directs the flow of energy by placement of the hands on the body in specific patterns (without applying deep pressure) to redirect or restore energy flow. Therapeutic touch is described in A, while B refers to healing touch, and C describes magnetic therapy.

14. *Answer:* C

*Rationale:* Acupuncture needles applied in one part of the body can affect the pain sensation in another part of the body when impulses stimulate the nerve fibers in the dorsal horn of the spinal cord. Acupuncture treatments could create a placebo effect and could help patients to refocus their concentration, but these are not the primary actions of the therapy. Acupressure, not acupuncture, uses pressure applied to skin surface with the finger and thumb. Acupressure is similar to acupuncture, but without the needles.

## CHAPTER 33

1. *Answer:* D

*Rationale:* A lymph node dissection is related to treatment with surgery and is a treatment-related risk factor for developing lymphedema. An elevated BMI, not a lowered BMI, would be a nonmalignant-related risk factor. Tumor invasion is a cancer diagnosis-related risk factor, not a treatment-related risk factor. Prolonged immobilization is a cancer diagnosis-related risk factor, not a treatment-related risk factor.

2. *Answer:* A

*Rationale:* Treatment of suspected infection by prescribing an antibiotic early will prevent further potentially life-threatening complications including serious bacterial infections of the skin (cellulitis) or an infection of the lymph vessels (lymphangitis). Weight management is important to reduce skin changes and potential infection but occurs over time, not as an urgent, acute management strategy. An exercise program is important but will also be over time, not as acute intervention. Axillary reverse mapping (ARM) facilitates identification and avoidance of arm lymphatics within the axilla during surgery and its use may reduce lymphedema. It is not an urgent priority; it is a prevention strategy

3. *Answer:* D

*Rationale:* Complete decongestive therapy is the standard of care in the management of lymphedema. The use of compression garment is also recommended for practice in persons with lymphedema. Exercise would not be restricted but would be encouraged. The patient should be taught to elevate the affected extremity, not dangle it. Extreme heat may worsen the swelling.

4. *Answer:* C

*Rationale:* Maintenance of healthy weight is encouraged, since obesity is a risk factor for worsening of lymphedema. Loose, not tight, fitting clothes should be worn. The diet should be low sodium and high fiber. Lifelong, not short-term, follow-up will be necessary in persons with lymphedema.

5. *Answer:* B

*Rationale:* Increased capillary permeability can occur with treatment with interleukin-2 or vascular endothelial growth factors. Increased, not decreased, capillary pressure would lead to edema when the volume of blood is expanded or with obstruction. Decreased, not increased, plasma oncotic pressure results in increased fluid in the tissues. When albumin is decreased, fluid leaks into interstitial spaces. Raised, not lowered, hydrostatic pressure drives fluid from the capillaries into the interstitial spaces.

6. *Answer:* D

*Rationale:* Iatrogenic causes of edema occur from plasma expanders, intravenous fluid overload, and blood components. Medications associated with edema may include treatment with hormones, calcium channel blockers, and steroids. An allergic response would be from histamine release. Systemic conditions include diagnoses such as heart failure, nephrotic syndrome, and liver failure.

7. **Answer:** C

**Rationale:** Long distance travel is a known risk factor. Decreased, not increased, mobility is a risk factor. A prior history of edema is a risk factor. Hypertension, not hypotension, is a risk factor.

8. **Answer:** A

**Rationale:** The treatment of the underlying cause of edema is the primary and most effective medical intervention. This includes treatment of congestive heart failure, nephrotic syndrome, liver failure/cirrhosis, thrombophlebitis, lymphedema, and deep vein thrombosis. Beta blockers may be indicated, not restricted, but would be after underlying cause is determined. Dietary sodium intake should be decreased, not increased. Fluid restriction, not increasing fluid intake, is recommended.

9. **Answer:** B

**Rationale:** Mesothelioma is the most common diagnosis associated with malignant pericardial effusion. Melanoma, not basal cell, may be associated with malignant pericardial effusion if metastatic. Brain tumor is not a common cause of malignant pericardial effusion. Amyloidosis is not a common cause of malignant pericardial effusion.

10. **Answer:** D

**Rationale:** Radiation targeted to more than 33% of the heart with more than 300 cGy/day is a risk factor. Fraction doses of 300 cGy/day are tolerated by the heart, however, the iliac crest would not be in field of treatment. Hormones do not cause capillary permeability. Coexisting cardiac disease, lupus, or endocarditis would increase risk. Renal infection is not associated with malignant pericardial effusion.

11. **Answer:** B

**Rationale:** Dyspnea is the most common symptom with malignancy-related pericardial disease. The onset is sudden, not gradual. The cough is nonproductive, not productive. Distention may cause dyspnea but is not related to pericardial disease.

12. **Answer:** A

**Rationale:** Rapidly developing effusions may be symptomatic at 50 to 80 mL. Normal pericardial fluid volume is 15 to 50 mL.

13. **Answer:** B

**Rationale:** Pulse pressure is the difference between systolic and diastolic pressure and "narrowing' if less than 40 mmHg. This occurs with pericardial effusions. There is not sufficient data with vital signs alone to indicate stroke, and the diagnosis needs physical assessment. Widening pulse pressure may be suggestive of valve regurgitation, aortic stenosis, or hyperthyroidism. Pulsus paradoxus refers to a decrease in blood pressure with inspiration and may be associated with a pulmonary embolism or hypovolemic shock.

14. **Answer:** C

**Rationale:** Antimetabolites, such as 5FU, capecitabine, and gemcitabine, can cause coronary artery spasm resulting in angina, arrhythmia, myocardial infarction, cardiac arrest, and sudden death; coronary artery thrombosis and apoptosis of myocardial cells. Alkylating agents, such as cyclophosphamide, can cause, but not limited to, acute myopericarditis, pericardial effusions, and arrhythmias. Anthracyclines, such as doxorubicin, daunorubicin, and epirubicin, can cause toxicity from injury of free radicals that result in myocardial cell loss. Angiogenesis inhibitors, such as thalidomide and lenalidomide, can cause bradycardia, thromboembolism, and hypertension.

15. **Answer:** C

**Rationale:** An acute reaction is reversible. Acute reactions are infrequent, occur within 24 hours of drug administration and usually self-limiting, and cease when the drug is stopped. They may not require discontinuation of the drug.

16. **Answer:** D

**Rationale:** Nurses should document the total cumulative dose of chemotherapy. This is the only nursing intervention and prevention strategy listed. Doxorubicin maximum cumulative dose is $550 \, \text{mg/m}^2$, cumulative dose; mitoxantrone is $160 \, \text{mg/m}^2$ and high-dose cyclophosphamide is 144 mg/kg for 4 days and the nurse should document cumulative dose with each administration and know the maximum cumulative dose. Treating hyperlipidemia is a medical intervention and is used to treat cardiotoxicity, not prevent the complication. Prescription of a beta blocker is a medical intervention and is used to treat cardiotoxicity, not prevent the problem. Prescription of an ACE inhibitor and calcium channel blockers are used to treat hypertension.

17. **Answer:** A

**Rationale:** Risk factors for a thrombotic event include stomach, brain, pancreas, and bladder cancers, advanced stage, lymphadenopathy, infection, renal disease, poor performance status, prolonged immobilization and older age. Risk factors for lymphedema include advanced disease, infection, immobilization, or traumatic injury to an affected extremity. Risk factors for malignant pericardial effusion include mesothelioma direct tumor invasion of the myocardium, obstruction of mediastinal lymph nodes by tumor, infection, and fibrosis secondary to radiation therapy. Risk factors for cardiovascular toxicity include many classes of chemotherapy drugs.

18. **Answer:** B

**Rationale:** Characteristics of an arterial embolus are severe pain in the involved extremity, extremity coolness, pallor, and absent or decreased pulse. Characteristics of venous occlusion would include tenderness over involved vein and unilateral edema of involved extremity. Characteristics of pulmonary embolus would include chest pain, dyspnea, sudden onset of anxiety, and decreased pulse oximetry. Valvular abnormality with S3 or S4 murmurs are characteristic of cardiovascular toxicity, not an embolus.

19. **Answer:** B

**Rationale:** Stage 1 edema is mild, spontaneously reversible, and presents with slight heaviness of the extremity with smooth skin texture with pitting edema. Pain and erythema may be present with stage 1. There is no stage 0; begins with stage 1. Stage 2 characteristics would be moderate, irreversible, with possible tissue fibrosis. The skin is stretched, shiny with non-pitting edema. Characteristics of stage 3 would be severe with lymphostatic elephantiasis, and is irreversible. The skin is discolored, stretched, and firm.

20. *Answer:* C

*Rationale:* In Grade 3 the limb starts to look disfigured, interferes with ADLs and there is more than 30% difference in size at greatest point or mass of limbs. In Grade 1 there is swelling, pitting edema, and a 5-10% difference in size at greatest point of limbs. In Grade 2 there is obvious obstruction, taut skin, and a 10-30% difference in size at greatest point of limbs. Grade 4 often progresses to malignancy is disabling and may need removal of affected extremity.

21. *Answer:* A

*Rationale:* Anthracyclines may cause toxicity from injury of free radicals that result in myocardial cell loss, fibrosis, and loss of contractility resulting in left ventricular dysfunction (LVD), HF, myopericarditis. Agents in this classification include doxorubicin, daunorubicin, epirubicin, idarubicin, mitoxantrone. Alkylating agents are associated with acute myopericarditis, pericardial effusions, arrhythmias, HTN, thromboembolism, and heart failure. An agent in this classification is cyclophosphamide. Angiogenesis inhibitors are associated with bradycardia, thromboembolism, and HTN may be seen, and agents in this classification include thalidomide, lenalidomide, and pomalidomide. Antimetabolites can cause coronary artery spasm resulting in angina, arrhythmia, myocardial infarction, cardiac arrest, and sudden death. Agents in this classification include 5FU, capecitabine, and gemcitabine.

22. *Answer:* D

*Rationale:* Ambulating frequently, and implementing leg exercises, if the patient is bedridden, are techniques that are recommended for oncology nurses to use for the prevention of thrombotic events in high-risk patients. Elevating the patient's foot with their knee flexed is a recommended nursing management technique for prevention. Elevating the patient's foot with their knee extended and elevating the patient's knee with their foot extended are incorrect and not recommended. Finally, employing constant pneumatic compression device is not a recommendation. The recommendation is for the nurse to apply intermittent pressure.

23. *Answer:* D

*Rationale:* Regular measurement of extremities facilitates early recognition of changes. Another action in nursing management for treatment and prevention is the use of elastic sleeves and grading wraps, which serve to facilitate movement of lymph out of the arm. The use of the sterile technique with antineoplastic agents is always indicated and is not specific to patients with lymphedema. It is also important to avoid use of a limb that is at risk for lymphedema. Carefully applied massage therapy has been shown to be beneficial, but vigorous weightlifting with the affected limb is not indicated. Moderate use limits risk, while allowing lymphatic fluid to drain normally.

24. *Answer:* B

*Rationale:* Lymphedema may occur initially years after the surgical procedure has been completed, even if the patient has reported no previous problems. Less invasive breast surgery still requires lymph node dissection for staging. Sentinel node mapping does not eliminate the need for node dissection for biopsy, which can contribute to future lymphedema. Although less extensive node disruption with breast conservation and radiation therapy may well decrease the risk of lymphedema, those treatments do not eliminate the risk.

25. *Answer:* B

*Rationale:* Hypoproteinemia contributes to edema by fluids into the interstitial space. An S2 heart sound is normal. Blood pressure and pulse readings usually increase with edema, while peripheral pulses usually diminish as a result of poor cardiac output.

## CHAPTER 34

1. *Answer:* A

*Rationale:* Cognitive impairment is a functional decline in one or more cognitive domains including executive functioning. Post-traumatic stress is a mental disorder that can occur after a traumatic event. Delirium is associated with a disturbance in the level of an individual's attention and awareness. Decreased confidence is related to belief in one's own abilities.

2. *Answer:* C.

*Rationale:* Cancers, chemotherapy, and immunotherapy treatments can stimulate cytokine dysregulation leading to inflammation and oxidative stress, thus impairing cognition. Surgical removal of central nervous system tumors and/or cranial irradiation may result in structural and functional damage specific to the tumor location. Hormonal therapies impact cognition by altering levels of testosterone or estrogen.

3. *Answer:* D

*Rationale:* Either a CT or an MRI can be ordered to rule out structural abnormalities in patients with focal neurological deficits or who are at high risk for recurrence or metastatic central nervous system disease. A bone scan is more useful to evaluate the presence of an infection, fracture, or bone metastases. Laboratory tests are done to rule out more general causes of cognitive impairment, such as electrolytes for metabolic disturbances, or LFTs for liver dysfunction.

4. *Answer:* A

*Rationale:* Cognitive training is an intervention that is likely to be effective in improving cognitive skills, such as attention or memory. Cognitive training often includes structured repetitive tasks aimed at improving a specific cognitive skill, such as memory or attention. Although the National Comprehensive Cancer Network (NCCN) guidelines suggest that a trial of psychostimulants be considered if non-pharmacological interventions are not effective, effectiveness of acetylcholinesterase inhibitors, N-methyl-D-aspartate receptors, or psychostimulants has not been established for management of cancer treatment-related cognitive impairment. Mindfulness stress reduction is typically utilized to decrease symptoms such as stress, anxiety, or pain.

**173**

5. *Answer:* B

*Rationale:* While changes in other cognitive domains (e.g. motor function, attention/concentration, and memory) may occur, an acute onset of hypervigilance or sedation is the classic symptom of delirium.

6. *Answer:* C

*Rationale:* Treatment toxicities and tumor effects leading to metabolic abnormalities (e.g. calcium, glucose, sodium) may put patients at a higher risk for delirium. Individual characteristics such as advanced age and sensory impairments (e.g. visual, hearing) may contribute to both cognitive impairment and delirium. Dose intensity, cumulative effect, and/or multimodality therapy are risk factors for cognitive impairment. Genetic polymorphisms (e.g. APOE E4 allele) are associated with cancer-related cognitive impairment as well as dementia, but not delirium.

7. *Answer:* A

*Rationale:* The best initial step would be to identify any risk factors for delirium, including medications known to cause delirium or have high anticholinergic potential. A CBC might identify anemia or sepsis, which can contribute to delirium. An MRI of the brain would detect a traumatic brain injury or brain tumor. Lumbar puncture would only be done if etiology is not obvious.

8. *Answer:* B

*Rationale:* Haloperidol, a typical antipsychotic, has the longest track record in treating agitated delirium. Lorazepam is a benzodiazepine, which is a second-line agent, has more paradoxical excitation and respiratory depression than haloperidol. Atypical antipsychotics, such as risperidone and olanzapine, appear to have fewer side effects, but are not as commonly used.

9. *Answer:* D

*Rationale:* Low-dose anti-psychotics may be used to manage severe agitation. Low-dose anti-psychotics may cause drowsiness, but they do not typically affect sleep patterns or treat sleep problems. Metabolic imbalances may be due to dehydration or electrolyte loss and will require hydration and electrolyte replacement. Sensory deficits such as hearing impairment or visual problems should be corrected whenever possible.

10. *Answer:* D

*Rationale:* A nursing management technique for cancer- and cancer treatment-related cognitive impairment is to reinforce cognitive and exercise training plans. Cognitive training and exercise include having the patient participate in structured, repetitive tasks aimed at improving a specific cognitive skill, such as attention or memory. Exercise training may include aerobics, tai chi, or yoga. Avoiding excessive sensory stimulation and/or restraints, incorporating environmental strategies such as having a visible clock or calendar available and keep a room well-lit and surrounded by familiar objects, and providing frequent reorientation and reassurance are all nursing management techniques for patients with delirium.

11. *Answer:* C

*Rationale:* The use of assistive devices, such as eyeglasses or hearing aids, will decrease the distortion of sights and sounds, while decreasing the client's anxiety, and reducing delirium. The remaining choices – removing calendars, not putting-up photos of loved ones, and exposing the patient to environmental noises that might be discomforting and unfamiliar – all serve to increase, and not decrease, the patient's delirium.

## CHAPTER 35

1. *Answer:* D

*Rationale:* Cortisol is the correct answer. Cortisol is a glucocorticoid steroid hormone produced by the adrenal gland. Antidiuretic hormone is produced by the pituitary gland, as is luteinizing hormone. Thyroxine is secreted by the thyroid gland in response to a thyroid stimulating hormone released by the pituitary gland.

2. *Answer:* A

*Rationale:* The presentation of hypothyroidism includes weakness, depression, constipation, and intolerance to cold temperatures. Although weakness and depression may be seen with the other conditions, the presence of cold intolerance differentiates hypothyroidism from the other options. Patients with hyperthyroidism have heat intolerance.

3. *Answer:* A

*Rationale:* Methylprednisolone is the correct answer. Patients being treated with immune checkpoint inhibitors can develop hyperthyroidism. Those who do, and are also at high risk for cardiovascular events, such as patients with a history of coronary artery disease, receive methylprednisolone 1-2 mg/kg daily until thyroid function returns to baseline. Dexamethasone is used as a long-acting glucocorticoid for patients with adrenal insufficiency. Levothyroxine is used as thyroid hormone replacement for hypothyroid patients. Cinacalcet may be used to treat patients with hyperparathyroidism.

4. *Answer:* B

*Rationale:* It takes 4 to 6 weeks for TSH and T4 levels to reach steady state concentration, at which point the levothyroxine dose may be adjusted. Therefore, TSH and T4 levels are monitored every 4 to 6 weeks; after a steady state is reached, TSH and T4 levels are monitored every six months. The other options are inaccurate.

5. *Answer:* C

*Rationale:* Option C, a low calcium, high phosphate diet is the correct answer. Patients with primary hyperparathyroidism have elevated levels of serum calcium (hypercalcemia). They may be advised to avoid calcium-rich foods and to include foods high in phosphorus in their diet. The reason is because calcium and phosphorus levels are regulated in inverse proportion to each other so factors that increase one level will decrease the other. Thiazide diuretics would not be recommended because they can increase the level of calcium in the blood. In addition, dehydration is to be avoided as it aggravates hypercalcemia and fluid intake should be increased. Phosphate binding drugs would not be used because usage of these agents would decrease serum phosphate levels, causing calcium levels to increase.

**6. _Answer:_ D**

_Rationale:_ Serum calcium levels are regulated by parathyroid hormone (PTH) released by the parathyroid glands. When these glands are removed, serum calcium levels decrease to below normal. Calcium replacement is needed at a dose dependent on the level of corrected serum calcium. The other electrolytes - potassium, chloride, and sodium - are not regulated by the parathyroid glands.

**7. _Answer:_ B**

_Rationale:_ Diabetes insipidus is the correct answer. Radiation therapy to the head area has caused pituitary gland dysfunction resulting in hypopituitarism (hypophysitis) and central type 1 diabetes insipidus. The other options are not caused by alterations in pituitary gland function.

**8. _Answer:_ A**

_Rationale:_ The correct answer is A. The patient should wear an alert bracelet indicating steroid stress doses. The alert bracelet should include the patient's condition (adrenal insufficiency) and necessary treatment in the case of an emergency (ie., the need for stress dose steroids). Prior to surgical procedures, the patient may require increased steroid doses rather than decreased. During "minor sick day" periods, such as for a head cold, the patient may need to increase their usual steroid dose two to three times. A five-fold dose increase would be unlikely. Steroid dosing does not change on a weekly basis, but as needed to meet the patient's needs for dose adjustments.

**9. _Answer:_ A**

_Rationale:_ Patients presenting with symptoms of anxiety, agitation, weakness, and heat intolerance, with a physical examination showing the patient has weight loss and hyperactivity, denotes a diagnosis of hyperthyroidism/thyrotoxicosis. Other indications of this condition include tremor, rapid speech, lid lag, hair thinning, tachycardia, an irregular pulse, hyperreflexia, and proximal muscle weakness. A patient presenting with bone pain, fatigue, weakness, and anorexia, with a physical examination revealing hypertension and bradycardia, is showing signs of hyperparthyroidsim. Patients with hypoparathyroidism present with fatigue, anxiety, depression, and irritability. The patient's physical examination might reveal chronic skeletal abnormalities. The patient presenting with visual changes, headache, and myalgias has indications of hypopituitarism and hypophysitis. A physical examination shows the patient has experienced weight loss and is showing signs of hypotension.

## CHAPTER 36

**1. _Answer:_ C.**

_Rationale:_ Elevated rather than lower levels of proinflammatory cytokines, interleukins, and tumor necrosis factor are all underlying mechanisms of fatigue along with 5-hydroxytryptophan dysregulation and circadian rhythm disturbances. Some patients have circadian rhythms that align with morning or evening preference, but no studies suggest this is a risk for cancer-related fatigue.

**2. _Answer:_ C.**

_Rationale:_ All ages and both sexes are susceptible to cancer-related fatigue. Some of the greatest risks include patients receiving opioids during treatment, those with poor performance status, weight loss > 5% in 6 months, and those receiving concurrent chemoradiation. Immobilization, anxiety, pain, and infection are additional risk factors. Therefore, answer c, low performance status is the best answer.

**3. _Answer:_ B**

_Rationale:_ Patient-reported outcomes are those reported directly by the patient. Patient report is considered as the gold standard for fatigue assessment. Onset, intensity, duration, patterns, exacerbating factors, impact on quality of life, and function comprise a comprehensive fatigue assessment. Answer C includes physiologic assessments that are not patient-reported outcomes. Answers A and D include caregiver insight which is not a patient-reported outcome.

**4. _Answer:_ A**

_Rationale:_ Several laboratory analyses can suggest contributing factors of fatigue. These include low thyroid function; electrolyte disturbances; low levels of iron, vitamin B12, folate, and ferritin; low hemoglobin/hematocrit, low hormone levels (e.g. testosterone), and low vitamin D levels. Therefore, answer A is the best choice. SPEP and tumor marker elevations can suggest disease progression, but this may or may not be associated with fatigue as patients can sometimes be asymptomatic. A low platelet count may indicate treatment toxicity or disease but is not always suggestive of fatigue.

**5. _Answer:_ A**

_Rationale:_ Answer A is the best choice, as blood transfusions can correct anemia and improve fatigue. While erythropoiesis-stimulating agents (ESAs) may benefit patients with severe fatigue, benefits should be balanced with risks such as an elevated risk of cardiovascular and thromboembolic complications. ESAs have also been found to shorten overall survival and/or increase the risk of tumor progression or recurrence in patients with breast, non-small cell lung, head and neck, lymphoid, and cervical cancers. Low-dose dexamethasone rather than high dose is sometimes used for severe fatigue. Benzodiazepines often compound the fatigue experience as sedation is a major adverse event.

**6. _Answer:_ D**

_Rationale:_ While answers A, B, and C may improve fatigue, exercise and physical activity have the strongest evidence in the management of cancer-related fatigue. Exercise is shown to be superior to any medical or alternative interventions. The exercise should be tailored according to patient's ability. The type of exercise does not appear to influence fatigue outcomes.

**7. _Answer:_ B**

_Rationale:_ Answer B is the best choice as depression and fatigue can both present with feeling of exhaustion. Screening for depression is important for all patients with cancer, and differentiating between depression and fatigue is essential, although often both may be present. Exercise should be employed as tolerated. No evidence exists that vigorous exercise is more effective in managing fatigue. High-intensity exercise can worsen fatigue if the patient is not ready to tolerate this regimen. Too much stimulation can increase fatigue in some patients; therefore, decreasing environmental stimuli should be considered to alleviate fatigue. While some patients' fatigue resolves over time, fatigue can be long-term in many patients.

8. *Answer:* D

*Rationale:* Fatigue can be caused by a variety of disease-related factors, from fatigue caused by disease-related anemia to fatigue caused by comorbidities and underlying diseases. The correct answer is D. 70% to 80% of patients with cancer report fatigue at some time during the continuum of their disease. Moreover, 29% of all survivors who are in complete remission still report experiencing fatigue. The other percentages are incorrect.

9. *Answer:* B

*Rationale:* Symptoms in patients with cancer that have been known to cluster with fatigue are sleep disturbances, pain, and distress. Anxiety, depression, stress and cognitive changes are not known symptoms to cluster with fatigue in patients with cancer.

## CHAPTER 37

1. *Answer:* A

*Rationale:* During the initiation phase of mucositis, DNA damage occurs, as well as a primary damage response, which includes transcription factors upregulating an innate immune response and activation of gene expression and multiple pathways, leading to production of cytokines and modulators, which are associated with the progression of mucositis. Secondary infection occurs in the ulcerative phase as a result of loss of mucosal integrity, painful lesions, and submucosal breach with bacterial colonization. The development of small nodules due to the absence of angiogenesis and the development of mucositis due to interferons and TNF cell proliferation are not part of the pathogenesis of mucositis.

2. *Answer:* C

*Rationale:* Impaired renal function (high serum creatinine) may increase the risk for mucositis. A BMI of < 18.5 and persistent smoking and alcohol use puts the patient at risk for mucositis. The use of alcohol-based mouth washes does not put the patient at risk for mucositis.

3. *Answer:* D

*Rationale:* Palifermin is a keratinocyte growth factor, and is FDA-approved for patients with hematological malignancies receiving high-dose chemotherapy and total body irradiation followed by autologous HSCT prior to and post-conditioning regimen to reduce the incidence and severity of oral mucositis. Palifermin is not used to alleviate nausea and vomiting or cramping during treatment. Palifermin is also not used to increase blood counts after transplant.

4. *Answer:* A

*Rationale:* Emetogenic chemotherapy damages the gastrointestinal mucosal cells and release serotonin (5HT) from enterochromaffin cells. 5HT binds to and activates 5HT3 receptors on the vagus nerve, initiating emetic signal and acute chemotherapy-induced nausea and vomiting (CINV) during the first 24 hours after chemotherapy. Emetic stimuli cause substance P (SP) binding at neurokin-1 (NK1) receptors in the chemotherapy trigger zone, amplifying the emetic message - particularly during *delayed CINV* that may persist for a few to many days. Small intestine and abdominal contraction do not lead to acute CINV.

5. *Answer:* D

*Rationale:* No or low history of significant alcohol consumption puts the patient at risk for nausea and vomiting. History of smoking, GERD, and use of NSAIDS do not put the patient at risk for chemotherapy-induced nausea and vomiting (CINV). Other risk factors for CINV include being of the female gender, being between the ages 5 and 60 years, a history of motion sickness, and a history of hyperemesis with pregnancy.

6. *Answer:* A

*Rationale:* CINV/RINV standard of care anti-emetics include 5HT3 antagonists, NK1 drugs, a corticosteroid such as dexamethasone, and olanzapine. Dopamine is a rescue antiemetic, and benzodiazapines are typically used for anticipatory nausea/vomiting to decrease anxiety. Anti-secretory drugs are not emetics and are not used for standard of care.

7. *Answer:* C

*Rationale:* Some tumors seed malignant cells within the peritoneal cavity (carcinomatosis), and these are known to increase osmotic pressure leading to malignant ascites. Other causes include cancer cells lining the peritoneum that produce inflammatory cytokines causing large molecules to amass and exert osmotic pressure with subsequent malignant ascites. Another cause is tumor expressed VEGF which induces angiogenesis and alters vascular and peritoneal membrane permeability, leading to increased malignant ascites accumulation. Increased drainage from the malignant tumor and lymphatic cell drainage are not causes of malignant ascites. Too much fluid moving from the intravascular to interstitial space is third-spacing.

8. *Answer:* D

*Rationale:* Paracentesis is safe and well-tolerated with 80-90% of patients stating symptom relief such as decreased abdominal distension and discomfort, dyspnea, nausea, anorexia, fatigue, and mobility. The procedure for paracentesis does not have a risk for bowel obstruction or cardiac effects, but rather there is a low complication risk for bowel perforation. The procedure is done under ultrasound guidance and does not require deep sedation.

9. *Answer:* A

*Rationale:* Metabolic causes, such as dehydration, hyponatremia, hypokalemia, hypercalcemia, hypothyroidism, uremia, and diabetes, may cause constipation. Dietary causes could include insufficient fluid intake. However, the patient's diabetes and uremia make the possibility of metabolic cause more likely. Both kidney stones and a urinary fistula are not the causes of constipation.

10. **Answer:** B

**Rationale:** Rectally administered agents, such as suppositories and enemas, are the preferred method for rapid and predictable evacuation of stool from the rectum and distal colon, such as for patients with fecal impaction. Liquids in enemas do not form fiber and does not soften the stool. Oral stool softeners are ineffective for established constipation and opioid-induced constipation. Oral bulking agent may worsen slow-transit opioid- or anticholinergic-related constipation. Some oral agents are ineffective for established constipation, and are better used as first-line laxatives to prevent constipation. Water taken along with oral medications will not induce cramping and bloating.

11. **Answer:** C

**Rationale:** Drugs that commonly are the cause of diarrhea include 5FU, irinotecan, capecitabine, gemcitabine, methotrexate, cyclophosphamide, cisplatin, oxaliplatin, carboplatin, doxorubicin, paclitaxel, docetaxel, cabazitaxel, and thalidomide. Fecal impaction can lead to overflow diarrhea. Other causes of diarrhea include C-difficile, viral enteritis, and enteral tube feedings.

12. **Answer:** D

**Rationale:** The patient should eat a low-fat, high-potassium diet, with six and eight small meals and snacks per day. The patient should also drink room temperature clear liquids. Dietary modifications to decrease diarrhea include avoiding spicy, fatty, greasy food, as well as those high in fiber (cereals), high in sugar, and stone fruits, such as peaches and nectarines. Beverages that may worsen diarrhea include caffeine, alcohol, fruit juices, lactose-containing dairy products, and hot liquids.

13. **Answer:** B

**Rationale:** Pilocarpine is contraindicated in patients with chronic cardiovascular or pulmonary disease, uncontrolled asthma, narrow-angle glaucoma, or taking β-blockers. Medications that may be considered are cevimeline (Evoxac), Aquoral, Xero-Lube, Biotene Mouthwash, Moi-Stir, NeutraSal, SalivaMAX, and Salivart.

14. **Answer:** C

**Rationale:** The appropriate grading is Grade 3. According to the the National Cancer Institute, Common Terminology Criteria for Adverse Events (NCI-CTCAE) for Gastrointestinal symptoms, tube feeding, TPN, or hospitalization is indicated. For Grade 1, intervention is not indicated. Grade 2 indicates outpatient IV hydration and medical intervention. Grade 4 includes life-threatening complications and treatment is urgent. Grade 5 is death.

15. **Answer:** A

**Rationale:** Oropharyngeal dysphagia (OD) occurs at the start of swallowing and is a symptom of a problem in the mouth or in the pharynx. Usually, this condition causes reflexive coughing and a sense of choking with swallowing. Other possible symptoms include symptoms such as voice change, frequent throat clearing, and earache. Mechanical dysphagia may occur post-surgery from inflammation and edema. The onset of mechanical dysphagia may precede the diagnosis of large (T3–T4) base of tongue, supraglottic, or pharyngeal tumors.

Esophageal dysphagia (ED) is caused by esophageal disease. ED is relatively uncommon, and the patient feels like food is sticking in their neck or upper chest a few seconds after they start to swallow. Radiation therapy is an effective part of treatment for many cancers that arise in the head and neck. However, following radiation for these cancers, some patients develop difficulty swallowing because the radiation caused the muscles and mucosal lining of the mouth, throat, and esophagus to become stiff and deformed. Swallowing becomes effortful and painful.

16. **Answer:** B

**Rationale:** In addition to caffeinated beverage consumption, lifestyle factors include tobacco use, alcohol use, dehydration, heavy snoring, and mouth breathing. Use of an antihistamine and an anticholinergic agent are drug-related causes. Secondary Sjogren syndrome is a disease-related cause.

17. **Answer:** D

**Rationale:** Sialometry is a test to measure saliva flow. The test is performed after an overnight fast or after a 2 hour fast. The patient is sitting upright for the procedure. Results of the test for normal salivary flow rate stimulated is 1.5 to 2.0 mL/min and unstimulated is 0.3 to 0.4 mL/min; less than 0.12 to 0.16 mL/min is abnormal. The evaluation is done at normal bedtime, but upon waking, and the test is also not done after 8 hours of fasting, but 2 hours. The test is not a measure of regurgitation, but of saliva flow.

18. **Answer:** D

**Rationale:** Requesting the patient to make a pretreatment dental examination and providing them with instructions (both written and oral) for implementing an oral hygiene regimen is an example of a preventative nursing management measure. Reminding patients to avoid spicy foods, hot drinks, or foods with too hot temperatures is not a preventative measure but a dietary instruction when the patient is experiencing painful oral mucositis. To ease pain when eating or drinking, patients should eat soft or moistened foods. Instructing patients to use topical protective or coating agents is not a preventative nursing management instruction, but, instead, a tip to provide some temporary relief from oral mucositis pain. Patients can use such agents as benzocaine (Orabase, Oratect Gel, Hurricaine), plus an analgesic such viscous lidocaine. Finally, the instruction to use a solution of normal saline, salt, and baking soda is also not a preventative tip but a way for the patient to reduce pain. The formula for the solution is 0.5 teaspoon each in one cup of warm water.

19. **Answer:** B

**Rationale:** Xerostomia is a drying of the oral mucosa, resulting in a loss of saliva caused by damage that occurs to the salivary glands subsequent to radiation therapy. Dysphagia, mucositis, and trismis do not result in dry mouth. Dysphagia is an inability to swallow or difficulty in swallowing. Mucositis is defined by inflammatory lesions of the mucous membranes and may include the intestine. Trismus is a contraction of the muscles of mastication.

20. *Answer:* B

*Rationale:* Eating popsicles wets the mouth and numbs the mucosa and is an intervention that may provide moisture to the oral mucosa. Decreasing intake of liquids will cause less moisture to be present. The other two answers – encouraging the patient to eat dry and spicy foods and having the patient rinse with a commercial mouthwash - may irritate the mouth and cause excessive burning.

21. *Answer:* B

*Rationale:* Ascites is associated with various tumors, mainly intra-abdominal malignancies. Ovarian cancer accounts for 38% of ascites.

22. *Answer:* C

*Rationale:* Constipation lasting for three days or more is unusual for this patient and suggests a need for immediate relief. At 10 days after chemotherapy, patients are at nadir and susceptible to infection. Rectal medications or treatments should be avoided. Opioids can increase the risk for constipation. Bulk-forming laxatives can take longer to provide relief than oral stimulant laxatives.

23. *Answer:* B

*Rationale:* A low-residue diet will decrease irritation of the gastrointestinal tract. In addition, decreasing spicy, fried, and fatty foods may help. Diet can affect radiation-induced diarrhea; a high-fiber diet will increase irritation of the gastrointestinal tract. The patient should consume solid foods that contain low residue and high protein, while avoiding lactose, if lactose has been a problem.

## CHAPTER 38

1. *Answer:* D

*Rationale:* Stress incontinence is the involuntary loss of urine that occurs with increased abdominal pressure associated with laughing, coughing, sneezing, and other physical activities, such as heavy lifting. Stress incontinence is not associated with psychological distress. It is not caused by neurologic changes that cause urinary sphincter dysfunction or impair reflexes for emptying of the bladder. Urge incontinence is the involuntary loss of urine with an abrupt and strong desire to void. Reflex incontinence is the involuntary loss of urine with no sensation of urge or bladder fullness. Functional incontinence is the state in which an individual experiences incontinence because of difficulty in reaching or inability to reach the toilet before urination. Total incontinence is the continuous loss of urine without distention or awareness of bladder fullness.

2. *Answer:* A

*Rationale:* Treatment-induced bladder inflammation is the correct answer. Radiation therapy to the bladder is associated with an inflammatory reaction within the bladder that increases the risk for urinary incontinence. Reduced size of the bladder tumor is not a risk factor for incontinence. Advanced patient age is not the most likely explanation for urinary incontinence in this patient

whose age is not specified. Radiation to renal structures may lead to permanent fibrosis and atrophy but not kidney stones. Kidney stone development is more likely to be associated with tumor lysis syndrome.

3. *Answer:* A

*Rationale:* Tests to determine the amount of residual urine after voiding provides important information about how completely the bladder empties with voiding. Gathering information about a patient's usual voiding habits and reviewing a patient's bladder diary may be useful but are not diagnostic tests. Colonoscopy is used to visualize changes within the colon.

4. *Answer:* B

*Rationale:* Behavioral techniques, such as voiding at the same time every day, help the patient establish the habit of voiding according to a schedule and gain control of urination. Suggesting that the patient stay shut in the house as much as possible is not therapeutic. Increasing daily fluid intake is more likely to increase uncontrolled loss of urine. Learning bladder self-catheterization is appropriate for patients who are unable to urinate voluntarily.

5. *Answer:* C

*Rationale:* Catheterization of urine will be done every 4 to 6 hours is the correct answer. This type of continent diversion involves creating an internal reservoir for urine from the ileum or large intestine with a stoma brought out to the skin. Urine is removed via catheterization through the stoma several times per day. The other choices are incorrect. A continent diversion does not require an external collection device, and thus is not associated with dribbling of urine, nor with the need to empty a pouch.

6. *Answer:* D

*Rationale:* Emptying the collection pouch when it is half-full is the correct answer. With an ileal conduit, urine collects almost continuously into an external collection pouch, which should be emptied whenever it is one-third to one-half full. The pouch should also be emptied prior to chemotherapy. There are no recommendations to avoid certain foods, such as cruciferous vegetables. The peristomal skin should be cleansed with water rather than alcohol, which causes drying. There is no need to catheterize the stoma because urine is collected externally in the pouch.

7. *Answer:* A

*Rationale:* The presence of renal dysfunction affects many organ systems. Signs and symptoms in the genitourinary system include nocturia, lethargy, and confusion in the neurologic system; and nausea and vomiting in the gastrointestinal system. Prostatic hypertrophy may be associated with nocturia, but not the other signs and symptoms. Disease metastasis to the brain is unlikely to cause nocturia. The signs and symptoms that the patient is experiencing are not indicative of delayed hypersensitivity reaction.

8. *Answer:* B

*Rationale:* Recording daily weights is the order the nurse is most likely to receive and is the correct answer. Daily weights are ordered to provide information about the patient's fluid volume status following medical management with increased hydration and diuretics. Medical management would not include reduction of fluid intake; rather, fluid intake would be increased to maintain adequate hydration and urinary output. Oxygen therapy is unlikely to be ordered for this condition, nor is diphenhydramine, which is an antihistamine drug that can contribute to urinary retention.

9. *Answer:* C

*Rationale:* Hypercalcemia of malignancy is the correct answer. Hypercalcemia of malignancy more commonly occurs in patients with metastatic breast cancer and causes renal dysfunction. When hypercalcemia of malignancy is present, the kidneys become unable to concentrate urine, resulting in diuresis of large amounts of diluted urine. Decreased blood flow to the kidneys would most likely lead to decreased urine output. Breast cancer commonly metastasizes to bone rather than to lymph nodes in the pelvis; obstruction of these lymph nodes would not lead to increased output of urine. Radiation therapy directed to the leg would not cause nephrotoxicity. Radiation therapy is a local treatment and would have no effect on the kidneys if they are not in the radiation treatment field.

10. *Answer:* D

*Rationale:* The nurse realizes that what the patient has been experiencing is most likely urge incontinence. Urge incontinence is when an individual has the involuntary loss of urine, with an abrupt and strong desire to void. Stress incontinence is the involuntary loss of urine during such activities as laughing, coughing, sneezing, or heavy lifting. These activities place increased pressure on abdomen and cause the release of urine. Reflex incontinence is the involuntary loss of urine with no sensation of urge to void or fullness of the bladder. Finally, functional incontinence occurs when a person has a strong desire to void and experiences incontinence because they have difficulty reaching or cannot reach the toilet in enough time before urination occurs.

11. *Answer:* B

*Rationale:* The medical management of renal dysfunction for a patient with cancer as a pharmacologic intervention is treatment of amifostine and sodium thiosulfate for cisplatin nephrotoxicity. Other pharmacologic interventions include saline hydration with appropriate diuretics, and oral or intravenous (IV) sodium bicarbonate to maintain alkaline urine. Other pharmacologic interventions include replacing electrolytes and administering diuretics, as needed. Anticholinergics, tricyclic antidepressants, and potassium channel openers are all examples of medical management for urinary incontinence.

12. *Answer:* D

*Rationale:* Electrostimulation is a medical management treatment for urinary incontinence. Other medical management strategies include anticholinergics, tricyclic antidepressants, potassium channel openers, and a consultation with a urologist. Answers A, B, and C - saline hydration with appropriate diuretic, oral, or intravenous (IV) sodium bicarbonate to maintain alkaline urine, and

replacement of electrolytes – are all examples of pharmacologic interventions for patients with cancer diagnosed with renal dysfunction.

13. *Answer:* A

*Rationale:* A neobladder is a urinary reconstructive procedure in which a surgically constructed bladder is created from the intestine and attached to the urethra. Thus, patients with any intestinal or urethral issues are not appropriate candidates for the surgery. Factors that exclude creation of a neobladder include cancer extending into the urethra, a past history of inflammatory bowel disease, radiation, or short gut syndrome from previous bowel resection. Patients with a history of benign prostatic hypertrophy and urinary incontinence may be appropriate candidates for the surgery.

14. *Answer:* C

*Rationale:* Cisplatin requires aggressive hydration before, during, and after therapy. The other agents do not require aggressive hydration. Daunorubicin can cause the patient with cancer to experience red urine. 5-Flourouracil is not associated with renal toxicity but can cause diarrhea and stomatitis. Flutamide is more commonly associated with side effects of hepatoxicity and gynecomastia.

## CHAPTER 39

1. *Answer:* C.

*Rationale:* Granulocytes are myeloid cells and include monocytes, neutrophils, eosinophils, and basophils. Red blood cells and platelets are myeloid cells but are not granulocytes. Lymphocytes arise from lymphoid progenitor cells.

2. *Answer:* B

*Rationale:* An absolute neutrophil count (ANC) below 1500/mm$^3$ places the patient at increased risk of infection and sepsis. An ANC of 2500/mm$^3$ is within the normal range. A white blood cell count of $4.3 \times 10^9$/L is within the normal range. An increased absolute basophil count can be a sign of chronic inflammation.

3. *Answer:* A

*Rationale:* Febrile neutropenia is present when a patient has a sustained temperature of $\geq 38°C$ (100.4°F) that lasts for more than 1 hour. An ANC $< 1000$/mm$^3$ and a single temperature of $> 38.3°C$ (101°F) also indicates febrile neutropenia. The other options – thrombocytopenia, hypercalcemia, and hemolytic anemia - are not associated with elevated temperatures.

4. *Answer:* D

*Rationale:* One of the most common adverse events associated with G-CSF agents is bone pain. Others are myalgia, arthralgia, and fever. The other options, eye inflammation, acne-like rash, and lung fibrosis, are all associated with use of epidermal growth factor receptor (EGFR) inhibitor agents.

5. *Answer:* A

*Rationale:* Radiation to bone marrow-producing regions, such as the pelvis, ischium, and long bones (eg., femur), can cause prolonged bone marrow suppression. The other options of peripheral neuropathy, wet desquamation, and urinary retention are unlikely to occur.

**179**

6. **Answer:** D

**Rationale:** Fresh flowers are not allowed to be delivered to the room of a patient who is at risk of immunosuppression. The other options are not correct. Recommended interventions include meticulous personal hygiene, including daily baths, and attention to oral and perineal care. So, avoid frequent bathing as it is drying to the skin would be inaccurate. Standing water in pitchers should be changed daily and not every 4 hours. Visits from family members who do not have communicable illness are allowed, so not a visit from every family member would be prohibited.

7. **Answer:** B

**Rationale:** Sore throat can indicate infection. Other signs and symptoms of infection might be the presence of temperature higher than 100.5°F (38.1°C), a productive cough, and painful urination. Therefore, the other options, including the symptoms of a dry mouth, a temperature of 99.8 degrees, and urinary hesitancy, are not correct.

8. **Answer:** C

**Rationale:** Chronic blood loss from the gastrointestinal tract can result in anemia. Iron deficiency, rather than iron overload, can also result in anemia. Alterations in platelet function and estrogen levels are not contributing factors for anemia.

9. **Answer:** A

**Rationale:** Patients with anemia are at an increased risk of fatigue, dyspnea, and tachycardia. These manifestations are not typically seen together in the other conditions of neutropenia, lymphocytopenia, and thrombocytopenia.

10. **Answer:** A

**Rationale:** The target value when transfusing packed red blood cells (PRBCs) is to maintain a hemoglobin level greater than 10 g/dL. The other options, although all are in the normal range, are not taken into consideration when determining the need to transfuse PRBCs.

11. **Answer:** C

**Rationale:** Patients receiving cytotoxic chemotherapy can develop coagulation abnormalities, such as disseminated intravascular coagulation (DIC), a condition in which massive clotting causes platelets (and clotting factors) to be consumed. Results of red blood cell count, and hemoglobin and ferritin levels are not as important as results indicating the presence of thrombocytopenia.

12. **Answer:** A

**Rationale:** Safety measures should be taught to decrease the occurrence of bleeding, which includes fall prevention. Invasive procedures such as enemas are to be avoided, as is shaving with a straight-edge razor. Ice packs are applied to areas of bleeding rather than warm packs.

13. **Answer:** A

**Rationale:** Blood pressure of 86/50 and respiratory rate (RR) of 26 is the correct answer as the presence of hypotension (i.e., 86/50) or tachypnea (RR>24) portend high risk for clinical deterioration. Therefore, a blood pressure of 155/90 (hypertension) and respiratory rate of 20 (normal RR) is not correct. A heart rate of 80 and sleepiness are normal signs. A temperature of 100.1°F is not considered indicative of febrile neutropenia (i.e., a single temperature of 101°F or a sustained temperature of 100.4°F for more than 1 hour), and depression can be a normal response to a cancer diagnosis.

14. **Answer:** C

**Rationale:** Hemorrhage is the correct answer. Signs of hemorrhage include weak or irregular pulse, pale skin, and cold or moist skin. In addition, patients with leukemia, especially nonlymphocytic leukemia, are at increased risk of hemorrhage as a result of a paraneoplastic process. Anemia and thrombocytopenia can result from hemorrhage.

15. **Answer:** B

**Rationale:** Giving the patient tepid sponge baths is the correct answer. Slow cooling of the skin and mucous membranes is recommended for patients experiencing fever and chills. Therefore, heating blankets or immersion in an ice bath are contraindicated. Fluid intake should be increased to prevent dehydration.

16. **Answer:** D

**Rationale:** Dose intensity is a disease and treatment-related risk factor associated with chemotherapy-induced myeloid toxicity. How a patient reacts to a dosage level can affect the risk for myeloid toxicity. Disease-related risk factors include the prevalence of high tumor burden and the bone marrow involvement of a tumor. Decreased immune function is related to the patient and how the host can fend off toxicities, based on treatment, or symptoms of the disease. Recently completed surgery or open wounds is another risk factor associated with the host, as is the example of drug-drug interactions.

17. **Answer:** D

**Rationale:** D is the only correct answer. If the chemotherapy dose is reduced and will not compromise the goal of cancer treatment, growth factor is not recommended. However, if the chemotherapy dose cannot be reduced, growth factor may be prescribed. Colony-stimulating growth factors for neutrophils are not prescribed for anemia or patients with cancer undergoing radiation.

18. **Answer:** B

**Rationale:** Lymphopenia, a reduction in the number of B or T lymphocytes, places the patient at risk for opportunities infections. The other answers are incorrect.

19. **Answer:** C

**Rationale:** Circulating neutrophils are compromised of segmented neutrophils (segs) and bands and are important to fighting infection. If a patient has a decreased number of circulating neutrophils in the blood, the risk of infection is increased. It is important for nurses to know how to calculate an absolute neutrophil count (ANC). The ANC is calculated by taking the % neutrophils (segs 1 bands) multiplied by WBC.

20. **Answer:** C

**Rationale:** Platelets arise from the myeloid stem cells. Lymphoid stem cells produce lymphocytes. Megakaryocyte stem cells are immature platelets. Epithelial stem cells produce skin cells.

21. **Answer:** A

*Rationale:* Granulocytes include basophils, eosinophils, monocytes, and neutrophils.

22. **Answer:** C

*Rationale:* Neutrophils and lymphocytes are part of the white blood cell components and infection. Erythrocytes are red blood cell components. Levels of platelets below 20,000/mm$^3$ increase the patient's risk for severe bleeding.

23. **Answer:** C

*Rationale:* Nadir refers to the lowest point – not the highest point - blood cells reach after a cancer treatment. Nadir occasionally happens after biotherapy administration, but this is not a regular occurrence.

24. **Answer:** A

*Rationale:* When the platelet levels drop below 100,000 mm$^3$, the client has thrombocytopenia.

## CHAPTER 40

1. **Answer:** B

*Rationale:* The subcutaneous tissue is composed of adipose tissue, which serves as an insulator to temperature changes, cushion to trauma, and an energy reservoir. The dermis is highly vascular with afferent sensory nerve receptors, which provides nutritional support to the avascular layer. The epidermis is the avascular outer layer, which serves as a barrier to prevent water loss and renews itself continuously through cell division. The inner connective tissue is the dermis layer.

2. **Answer:** B

*Rationale:* Antihistamines disrupt the action of histamines in the brain which result in drowsiness. Corticosteroids orally can cause an increase in appetite, weight gain, insomnia, fluid retention, and mood changes. Capsaicin topically can cause warmth, stinging or burning at the application site. Calamine lotion side effects include itching, redness, and irritation.

3. **Answer:** A

*Rationale:* Gentle cleansing with tepid water and mild soap and protecting the area with a skin barrier will prevent skin breakdown. Alcohol will dry the skin and create a potential risk for skin breakdown.

4. **Answer:** B

*Rationale:* Graft versus host disease can occur as a reaction to a bone marrow transplant. The donated bone marrow or peripheral blood stem cells view the recipient's body as foreign, and the donated cells/bone marrow attack the body resulting in a serious skin rash. Skin grafting is a surgical procedure that involves removing skin from one area of the body and moving it, or transplanting it, to a different area of the body. A patient would not experience graft versus host disease as a reaction to a skin graft. Melanoma is a tumor of melanin-forming cells, especially a malignant tumor associated with skin cancer. Malnutrition relates to decreased protein stores.

5. **Answer:** D

*Rationale:* Acute radiation dermatitis may occur with all radiation therapy. The mechanism is free radical damage to tissue which can cause erythema, pain, dermal swelling, itching, and necrosis of the skin. Chemotherapy drugs activate immune complexes already circulating due to underlying collagen vascular disease process, causing a circular red scaly rash. This is found in allergic or immune complex reactions. Erythema multiforme rash involves extremities including palms and soles. This is found in allergic or immune complex reactions. Thinning of skin, scarring and contractures, and telanglectasias are associated with chronic radiation dermatitis.

6. **Answer:** B

*Rationale:* A common dermatologic change associated with EGFR inhibitors is an acneiform rash of papules and pustules similar to acne although this rash contains no comedones. This acneiform rash typically involves the face, back, and upper chest. Oncholysis is manifested as a nail lifting from the bed. It is associated with paclitaxel, docetaxel, cyclophosphamide, doxorubicin, 5-fluorouracil (5-FU), and hydroxyurea. Capecitabine is associated with hand and foot syndrome. Cisplatin, hydroxyurea, and bleomycin can be associated with permanent hyperpigmentation of the gums.

7. **Answer:** C

*Rationale:* Photosensitivity makes the patient more sensitive to ultraviolet light. Solar-exposed areas may develop severe sunburn after only limited exposure to the sun. Photo enhancement occurs when the chemotherapy is given several days after sunburn causing the sunburn to reappear in that area. Beah lines appear as transverse lines in nails with bands corresponding to when drug was given. Paronychia is a skin infection around the fingernails or toenails. It usually affects the skin at the cuticle or up the sides of the nail as pain, swelling and redness and can have abscesses.

8. **Answer:** A

*Rationale:* Long-term effects of radiation therapy in port area with thinning of skin, scarring and contractures, telangiectasias, long-term skin sensitivity to irritants and environmental agents is a description of symptoms related to chronic radiation dermatitis. A description of acute radiation dermatitis is the immediate dermatitis occurring in radiated areas with erythema, pain, dermal swelling, itching, and necrosis. Radiation recall dermatitis is defined as occurring in previously irradiated skin within 1-2 weeks after chemotherapy; erythema, edema, superficial ulcerations, and superficial skin sloughing. An allergic response where the drug touches the skin (erythema, local swelling, desquamation, blistering, necrosis possible) is defined as a contact allergy (through activated T cells) and may not develop until 24-36 hours after initial contact with the allergen.

9. **Answer:** B

*Rationale:* A description of symptoms related to Erythema multiforme (antigen–antibody complexes) is a rash with typical target lesions involving extremities, including the palms of the hands and the soles of the feet. This skin reaction can progress to a generalized rash. Itching, redness, and swelling within our hour after the infusion has begun are symptoms of an Immunoglobulin E (IgE) mediated skin reaction. If life threatening, this skin reaction is termed as anaphylaxis and includes decreased blood pressure, decreased level of consciousness, and airway and breathing compromise. Radiation recall dermatitis occurs in previously irradiated skin within 1-2 weeks after chemotherapy. The symptoms include erythema, edema, superficial ulcerations, and superficial skin sloughing. Vasculitis (from antigen-antibody complexes) is a skin reaction that involves generalized vascular inflammation with end organ damage.

10. **Answer:** C

**Rationale:** The skin reaction of Immunoglobulin E (IgE) mediated is known to be caused by treatment through platinum derivatives (cisplatin, carboplatin). Itching, redness, and swelling within our hour after the infusion has begun are symptoms of an Immunoglobulin E (IgE). Acute radiation dermatitis may occur with any or all radiation therapy. The mechanism for the reaction is free radical damage to the tissue. Vasculitis (from antigen-antibody complexes) is caused by methotrexate exposure. Contact allergy skin reactions can from a variety of sources, ranging from chemicals found in poison ivy, oak, and sumac, to materials found in clothing, jewelry, and shoes.

11. **Answer:** D

**Rationale:** J.T.'s skin reaction, which included symptoms of skin blistering, local swelling, and erythemea, is a reaction to a contact allergy. Contact allergies develop after contact – usually with 24 to 48 hours – from a variety of substances, including chemicals found in poison ivy, oak, and sumac, snaps, contact from zippers, and metal-plated objects, contact with neomycin in antibiotic skin ointments, potassium dichromate, a tanning agent, and latex found in gloves and rubberized protective clothing. The source of the allergy most likey came from contact with latex. Food allergies are not a source of contact allergies, as is radiation therapy. A reaction to a medication would result in a systemic response versus a local response.

12. **Answer:** A

**Ratioanle:** Symptoms related to the skin reaction of recall radiation dermatitis occuring in previously irradiated skin within 1-2 weeks after chemotherapy treatnent, and is associated with erythema, edema, superficial ulcerations, and superficial skin sloughing. Chronic radiation dermatitis is associated with the long-term effects of radiation therapy in port area, and is symptomatic of thinning of the skin, scarring and contractures, telangiectasias, and long-term skin sensitivity to irritants and environmental agents. A rash with typical target lesions involving extremities, including palms of the hands and soles of the feet and can progress to generalized rash are symptoms of an immunoglobulin E (IgE) mediated skin reaction. Finally, flulike symptoms, which may progress to life threatening, is a symptom of serum sickness (antigen-antibody complexes).

CHAPTER 41

1. **Answer:** A

**Rationale:** Loss of skeletal muscle mass is the correct answer. Sarcopenia is defined as the subclinical loss of skeletal muscle mass and is commonly observed in patients with malignancy. The other options (bone marrow suppression, joint contractures, and muscle spasticity), even if present, do not fit the definition for sarcopenia.

2. **Answer:** D

**Rationale:** There are many factors that can contribute to the risk of developing musculoskeletal alterations but only option D (increased bed rest) is the correct answer. Complications of increased bed rest can lead to increased bone breakdown associated with diminished weight bearing activities and atrophy of skeletal muscles due to physical inactivity. The use of medical marijuana, enteral tube feedings, and a vegetarian diet are not correct answers.

3. **Answer:** B

**Rationale:** The correct answer is B. Assessment of this patient's functional abilities and signs and symptoms of disease has revealed a KPS of 50. A KPS reading of 50 requires considerable assistance and frequent medical care. The patient is not able to do self-care with effort (KPS of 80), nor is disabled and requires special care (KPS of 40). A patient who shows minor signs or symptoms of disease has a KPS of 90.

4. **Answer:** B

**Rationale:** Gait is the correct answer. Observation of the way a person walks and moves provides useful information about muscle strength and coordination. The other options help provide information about the patient's body build (habitus), personality, or state of mind (cleanliness and body language).

5. **Answer:** C

**Rationale:** The correct option is hypokalemia. Changes in normal levels of serum calcium, magnesium, phosphorus, potassium, and sodium are common after a treatment of chemotherapy and can have a profound effect on skeletal muscle contraction and strength and are generally decreased after cisplatin treatment. Hypokalemia is associated with muscle weakness and muscle cramps. Platelet counts assess the patient's bleeding risk, and it is not likely that a patient would have increased neutrophils two weeks after chemotherapy. Hypermagnesemia is associated with hypotension, respiratory depression, and cardiac arrest.

6. **Answer:** D

**Rationale:** Encouraging a patient to commit to a program of active range of motion exercises every 4 hours is correct. This nursing intervention helps preserve the patient's muscle strength and increase physical function. Active range of motion exercises on unaffected limbs and passive range of motion exercises on affected limbs are recommended at least three or four times per day. The patient's position should be changed every 2 hours rather than every nursing shift. Soft lighting is useful at night to help enhance vision, but not impaired mobility. A restraint vest is unlikely to be ordered for this patient.

7. **Answer:** D

**Rationale:** The Eastern Cooperative Oncology Group (ECOG) Performance Status ranges from sores of 0 to 5. With a score of 3, J.B. is capable of limited self-care, but is restricted to a bed or chair during half of his waking hours. Therefore, the correct answer is D. Patients with a score of 3 have some capacity for self-care but it is limited. For a patient who is completely unable to care for themselves, that is a score of 4, so answer A is incorrect. The patient who is fully active and able to carry on the normal activities that were performed prior to diagnosis rates a score of zero, so B is incorrect as well. The patient who is restricted from strenuous activity but can perform light housework, for example, or sedentary activities scores a 1 on the ECOG Performance Status score.

8. **Answer:** D

**Rationale:** The electrolyte abnormalities might the nurse expect to find in the results is in her sodium levels. Not only does sodium maintain fluid balances but sodium is critical for normal body function and helps regulate nerve function and muscle contraction. Potassium functions to regulate heart function. Calcium stabilizes blood pressure and assists in building strong bones and teeth. Chloride is necessary to maintain a proper balance of bodily fluids.

9. **Answer:** A

**Rationale:** The Eastern Cooperative Oncology Group (ECOG) Performance Status score of 1 means the patient is capable of performing light activities but is restricted in doing any strenuous physical activities. Patients restricted to a bed or chair during half of his waking hours and capable of limited self-care score a rating of 3. Patients who are fully disabled with no means to care for themselves rate a 4 on the scale, while a patient who is dead receives a rating of 5. The ECOG Performance scale ranges from 0 to 5.

10. **Answer:** C

**Rationale:** The electrolyte abnormalities the nurse might expect to find in the results is a change in his potassium levels. Potassium regulates heart function and helps maintain healthy nerves and muscles. Magnesium is another critical mineral and serves much of the same function as potassium. Chloride is important in regulating proper balance of bodily fluids, while calcium stabilizes blood pressure and helps build strong bones and teeth. Finally, phosphates interact closely with calcium.

## CHAPTER 42

1. **Answer:** C

**Rationale:** Individual age under 60 years, and anxiety and depression are not risk factors for neuropathies. Individual risk factors include age greater than 60 years and social issues, including malnutrition and alcohol abuse. Disease-related risk factors include pre-existing neuropathies of diabetes mellitus, HIV infection, and vitamin B complex deficiency, while lumpectomy is not a major risk factor for neuropathies but the incision may be sensitive to the touch.

2. **Answer:** A

**Rationale:** Neuropathies of the central nervous system (CNS) can lead to seizures, encephalopathy, and cerebellar dysfunction. Childhood epilepsy is not a factor in neurologic symptoms in a person with a diagnosis of cancer. Damage to PNS would have symptoms of numbness/tingling not CNS symptoms. Anxiety and depression may be manifested as insomnia, fatigue, trouble concentrating, irritability, and restlessness.

3. **Answer:** C

**Rationale:** Medical management includes the use of mild analgesics and opioids; a fentanyl patch is not mild nor is it appropriate for neuropathic pain. Steroids are not a treatment nor are antianxiety medications. Anticonvulsants neurontin, pregabalin, and depakote are commonly utilized treatments, so the correct answer is C.

4. **Answer:** A

**Rationale:** Nursing management includes to teach patients about hand and foot care (use of massage and lotions). Exercise should be encouraged as should the use of assistive devices to promote safety and assist with mobilization and fine motor skills (not muscle strength). Patients should avoid excess stimulation of the skin.

5. **Answer:** B

**Rationale:** Protecting the patient's hands from cold is important as the neuropathy may prevent the recognition of dangerously cold temperatures. Hand strengthening exercise helps promote independence. Although the prevention of infection is important, hand sanitizer can be drying, leading to small cuts and infection. A three-point can assist with ambulation and would be important for a patient with neuropathy in the feet to promote safety.

6. **Answer:** D

**Rationale:** Proprioception is perception or awareness of the position and movement of the body. A Romberg test can be used to evaluate balance and proprioception: To do the Romberg test, nurses should have the patient stand with their feet together, arms at their side, with the eyes closed and observe the patient's movements. A slight sway is normal. A tuning fork vibration check and assessment of discrimination between sharp and dull shapes provides information about sensory function. Clonus is muscular spasm and it provides information about deep tendon reflexes.

7. **Answer:** B

**Rationale:** Assessing for discrimination between sharp and dull sensations is a procedure for assessing sensory function related to neuropathy. Observing for accurate movement of extremities is an assessment for proprioception, while having patients stand with their feet together, arms at their sides with their eyes closed is part of the Romberg test and is classified as an evaluation for cerebellar and proprioception. Evaluate rapid alternating movement of hands is also classified as an evaluation for cerebellar and proprioception.

8. **Answer:** A

**Rationale:** An intervention to assist patients in improving mobility and self-care is developing an exercise and muscle-strengthening program. Other interventions include collaborating with physical and occupational rehabilitation services and using assistive devices to help with mobilization and fine motor needs. Answers B, C, and D are all examples of nonpharmacologic interventions to manage pain, anxiety, and depression, including offering the patient access to acupressure and acupuncture services, encouraging the patient to implement relaxation techniques, and referring the patient for biofeedback.

9. **Answer:** D

**Rationale:** A nonpharmacologic intervention for symptoms such as pain, depression, and anxiety is to encourage the patient to take-up relaxation techniques. Included are activities such as yoga, meditation, or guided imagery. Teaching the patient about the side effects of cancer and empowering the patient to communicate with her physician and caregivers regarding the severity of her symptoms are interventions to encourage the patient to participate in their own care. Since this patient is already sharing details of her symptoms, this intervention would not be needed. Providing assistive services for the patient in performing daily activities as needed is an intervention to assist with decreased mobility and diminished capacity for self-care.

## CHAPTER 43

1. **Answer:** A

**Rationale:** Confusion may be a sign of electrolyte abnormalities. Patients having complications with nutritional therapy usually have diarrhea, not constipation, and tachycardia and normal respirations, not bradycardia and bradypnea.

2. **Answer:** C

**Rationale:** Cachexia is defined as progressive deterioration with muscle wasting that occurs when protein and calorie requirements are not met, greater than 5% involuntary weight loss has occurred over 6 months, poor quality of life (QOL), impaired functional status, muscle wasting, fatigue, and, ultimately, shortened survival. Malnutrition begins with changes in nutrient levels in the blood and tissues and can progress to organ malfunction. Depression is a risk factor developing cachexia. Anorexia is loss of appetite accompanied by decreased oral intake and is usually accompanied by other symptoms that exacerbate decreased food intake and progressive weight loss, with approximately 80% incidence in patients with cancer from diagnosis to advanced stages.

3. **Answer:** D

**Rationale:** Candies or lozenges will stimulate saliva production to keep the membranes moist and decrease risk of taste alterations. Patients should experiment with flavorings, perform oral hygiene before and after meals, and avoid alcohol.

4. **Answer:** A

**Rationale:** Multi-agent chemotherapy regimens is a risk factor for weight gain especially those regimens that contain steroids. Adjuvant chemotherapy for breast cancer, not lung cancer, is a risk factor for weight gain. Immunotherapy and bisphosphate therapy do not present as an increased risk for weight gain. Hormonal, biologic medications such as interleukin-2 (IL-2), and steroids also lead to weight gain.

5. **Answer:** C

**Rationale:** Patients should consume cold foods to provide comfort, rather than hot foods. Soft and room temperature foods are also associated with improved oral intake. Oral hygiene should be done before and after meals, and pain medications should be given 30-60 minutes prior to eating to provide comfort from pain. Nystatin should be used after meals or at least 30 minutes prior to eating.

6. **Answer:** B

**Rationale:** Dysgeusia is an unpleasant taste sensation, while a decrease in the acuity of taste is hypogeusesthesia, and the loss of taste is ageusia.

7. **Answer:** B

**Rationale:** Participating in preparation of meals can stimulate taste by the aroma of foods. To avoid dry mucous membranes, patients should eliminate the intake of alcohol. Patients should chew gum before eating to change taste and food intake, and consumption of meat should be with gravy and sauces to keep membranes moist.

8. **Answer:** A

**Rationale:** Electrolyte imbalances with hypercalcemia, hypokalemia, hyponatremia, and uremia have been found to be associated with loss of appetite.

9. **Answer:** D

**Rationale:** Enteral feeding is given into the gastrointestinal (GI) tract. The naso-gastric tube is the only tube that is placed in the GI tract. A nephrostomy tube is placed in the kidney to drain urine. A urostomy tube is also placed in the kidney/ureter to drain urine. A tracheostomy tube is placed in the neck to establish a patent airway.

10. **Answer:** C

**Rationale:** Non-Hodgkin's lymphoma is a risk factor for weight loss. Lung cancers and gastrointestinal cancers also put individuals at risk for weight loss. Chemotherapy regimens containing steroids, biologic medications like interleukin-2, and pleural effusions are all risk factors for weight gain.

11. **Answer:** D

**Rationale:** Candidiasis is a known cause of taste alterations. Radiation therapy of the oral cavity can lead to thick saliva which alters taste sensation. Zinc deficiency caused by oncolytic agents which bind and chelate zinc results in loss of taste. Medications associated with taste alterations include cisplatin (Platinol), ironotecan (Camptosar), cyclophosphamide (Cytoxan), dacarbazine (DTIC-Dome), dactinomycin (actinomycin D, Cosmegen), mechlorethamine (nitrogen mustard, Mustargen), methotrexate (Mexate), vincristine (Oncovin), and fluorouracil (5-FU, 5-fluorouracil).

12. **Answer:** A

**Rationale:** A nursing intervention for pneumothorax which is a complication arising from parenteral or nutritional therapy is determining that a chest radiography after insertion of subclavian catheter has been completed to verify placement. Pneumothorax may occur during subclavian catheter insertion, so it is important to observe the patient during insertion for chest pain, dyspnea, and cyanosis. Nurses must assure that a chest radiograph is completed and evaluated after insertion to verify placement. Regulating infusion on a volumetric pump for accuracy is a nursing intervention for fluid overload. For a malpositioned catheter, nurses are recommended to monitor the catheter for migration from the superior vena cava to another vein, while making a notation of patient compliant of pain in the neck and shoulder, as well as swelling in the surrounding area. Checking each bottle or bag before and during infusion for color and clarity of solution is a nursing intervention for a contaminated solution leading to an infection.

13. *Answer:* B

*Rationale:* A nursing intervention for preventing an air embolus which is a complication arising from parenteral or nutritional therapy is securing all IV tubing connections with tape to prevent disconnection. If air emboli are suspected, the nurse is recommended to clamp the tubing immediately and place the patient on left side in the Trendelenburg position. Observing for bright red blood pulsating from catheter is a nursing intervention for an arterial puncture. Infusing 10% dextrose in water solution peripherally or through other lumen of catheter at the same rate as with total parenteral nutrition (TPN) to prevent hypoglycemia is a nursing intervention for a clotted catheter. Finally, Answer D is a nursing intervention for hypoglycemia. If a patient presents with hypoglycemia, a nursing intervention is to administer insulin in TPN, as ordered, monitor capillary blood glucose, monitor serum glucose levels, and observe for signs and symptoms of hypoglycemia. If sudden cessation of TPN occurs, infuse 10% dextrose in water solution peripherally at same rate as TPN. Per physician's order, administer 50 mL of 50% dextrose intravenously.

14. *Answer:* B

*Rationale:* A nursing intervention for preventing contaminated equipment leading to an infection – a complication arising from parenteral or nutritional therapy – is changing all IV tubing per institutional or agency procedure, using aseptic technique, and avoid interrupting TPN for other infusions or blood collecting. Checking each bottle or bag before and during infusion for color and clarity of solution is a nursing assessment for contaminated solution that leads to infection. Infusing 10% dextrose in water solution peripherally or through other lumen of catheter at the same rate as with TPN to prevent hypoglycemia is a nursing intervention for a local infection. Proper dressing changes should also be completed using aseptic technique. Finally, a nursing intervention for hyperglycemia is a recommendation to check a patient's urine for sugar, ketones, and acetone every 6 hours.

15. *Answer:* C

*Rationale:* Giving formula at room temperature is a nursing intervention for the prevention of abdominal distention, and for symptoms such as vomiting and diarrhea. Also, a nursing recommendation is to regulate infusion accurately over 20 minutes. When giving the formula at room temperature, the nurse may need to decrease the volume of the formula given to the patient. Diarrhea may be caused by the formula, by the patient being lactose intolerant, or by bacterial contamination, osmolality, antibiotics, or *Clostridium difficile.* Giving continuous rather than bolus feeding is a nursing intervention for aspiration. Flushing the nasogastric tube with hot water or pulsating motions is a nursing intervention for contaminated equipment or clogged tube. Verifying proper placement via chest radiography and check placement each time using tube is a nursing recommendation for malpositioned tube.

16. *Answer:* B

*Rationale:* Nourishing a patient with cancer may enhance tumor growth, rather than slow it, by improving the supply of nutrients to the body is an example of a controversial stance on long-term nutritional support for patients with cancer. The benefits of nutritional support can be sustained over a long time period is not an example. The controversy surrounds whether or not the beneficial effects are temporary. The psychological impact and the legality of the therapy are not controversial statements.

17. *Answer:* D

*Rationale:* An example of physical assessment is a patient with cancer might undergo as part of an overall nutritional assessment is measuring a patient's weight in comparison with their ideal body weight. Other physical measures include skin turgor, muscle mass as measured by the patient's mid-arm circumference, and fat stores as measured by the thickness of the triceps skinfold. The measure of the patient's daily caloric intake and measures of blood pressure and heart rate are not part of the physical examination and are incorrect. Measures of serum prealbumin, total protein, and serum transferrin to assess protein stores are collected as part of a laboratory assessment of the overall nutritional assessment.

18. *Answer:* D

*Rationale:* An example of laboratory data that could be collected for a patient with cancer as part of an overall nutritional assessment is nitrogen balance. Nitrogen balance levels are collected to assess energy balance. Other aspects of laboratory testing include measuring serum prealbumin, total protein, and serum transferrin to assess protein stores, measuring hemoglobin and hematocrit index, and electrolyte levels. Measuring of allergic reactions to proteins in certain foods is a test to confirm allergies to foods such as peanuts or tree nuts, and not part of an overall nutritional assessment. Skin turgor is part of a physical examination and muscle mass is measured by the circumference of the mid-arm, and another part of the physical exam.

19. *Answer:* C

Protein-calorie malnutrition caused by the metabolic effects of the tumor is a major cause of weight loss in oncology patients. Cancer cell division and growth are associated with increased protein metabolism and calorie use to meet the energy demands of malignant tumors.

**185**

Patients may develop vitamin and mineral deficiencies due to inadequate intake of food. If liver and kidney function are adequate, most pharmacologic agents are metabolized normally. Malignant tumor metabolism is not associated with increased fat metabolism.

20. *Correct answer:* B

*Rationale:* Megestrol acetate and dexamethasone could stimulate a person's appetite. The other drug combinations are incorrect.

## CHAPTER 44

1. *Answer:* B

*Rationale:* The patient is experiencing chronic cancer-related pain. Chronic cancer-related pain can be due to direct tumor involvement, diagnostic/therapeutic procedures, or cancer treatment and lasts longer than 3 months. Answer A is incorrect, because the patient reports it is well-controlled. If the patient's baseline pain becomes uncontrolled and he has acute exacerbations with movement, this would be defined as incident breakthrough pain. Insidious breakthrough pain occurs unpredictably. Answer C is incorrect as the pain is not acute. Acute pain is self-limiting and typically lasts less than six months. Answer D is incorrect. The patient does not show signs of visceral pain.

2. *Answer:* C

*Rationale:* Answer A is incorrect as somatic pain is well-localized and arises from the bone, joint, or connective tissue, and is described as sharp, throbbing, or as pressure. Sympathetically maintained pain is a type of neuropathic cancer pain caused by autonomic dysregulation; therefore, answer B is incorrect. Answer D is another type of neuropathic pain, caused by peripheral nerve injury. The correct answer is C, visceral pain, which is often found in patients with pancreatic, hepatic, and gastrointestinal cancer, leading to distention, compression, and tumor infiltration into the abdominal tissue.

3. *Answer:* D

*Rationale:* The correct answer is D. During modulation, neurons in the brain stem (pons and medulla) descend to the dorsal horn and release neuromediators, which inhibit the transmission of pain impulses at the dorsal horn. Opioids work at the dorsal horn by binding to receptors and preventing transmission of the pain signal to the higher brain centers. Answer A, transduction, is the initiation of the pain process where neurotransmitters are released at the time of injury, generating an action potential to relay the message to the central nervous system. Answer B, transmission, continues to relay the thalmus and other centers in the brain. Answer C, perception, is where the brain finally senses the pain impulse and triggers modulation.

4. *Answer:* C

*Rationale:* The correct answer is C, mucositis. While other pain syndromes can occur with head and neck cancer, almost 100% of patients undergoing combined radiation and chemotherapy develop mucositis and subsequent pain. Answer A, post-surgical head and neck cancer pain,

can occur and increases without consistent mobility and range of motion following surgery. Lymphedema, answer B, is rare with head and neck cancers. Sinusitis, answer D, is not an associated symptom with this therapy.

5. *Answer:* A

*Rationale:* The correct answer is A, post-herpetic neuralgia, which is characterized by burning, aching, and shock-like pain and often occurs as a sequelae to shingles due to immunosuppression from chemotherapy. Answer B is incorrect, as patients are not at increased risk of CIPN when immunosuppressed. Answer C is incorrect because lymphedema, although painful, is due to surgical disruption of the lymph channels not chemotherapy. Answer D, CRPS, is a centrally generated pain syndrome caused by autonomic dysregulation but is not related to immunosuppression.

6. *Answer:* B

*Rationale:* The numeric rating scale, answer B, is the gold standard for pain assessment in all patients who are verbally report pain. School-age children can often conceptualize this scale and provide a perception of their pain. Pain faces, answer A, is often used in children ages 7 or younger. Verbal descriptions, answer C, can be used for patients unable to conceptualize the "0-10" scale. The checklist of nonverbal indicators should only be used when patients are unable to self-report pain.

7. *Answer:* D

*Rationale:* The World Health Organization's analgesic ladder recommends the use of an opioid and possibly an analgesic adjuvant for moderate pain. Answer A, acetaminophen, only contains a nonopioid analgesic. Answer B, morphine, is used for severe pain and is not a good choice because of the metabolites, M3G and M6G, that can accumulate in patients with renal compromise. Answer C, the fentanyl patch, is used for severe pain; additionally, the patient has intermittent pain and does not require around the clock analgesia at this time. The patient may also be opioid naïve, and fentanyl is contraindicated in opioid naïve patients. Answer D is the best answer that incorporates an opioid/acetaminophen combination and is given as needed for intermittent pain.

8. *Answer:* A

*Rationale:* The risk of addiction with opioids is correct; therefore, acknowledging the problem is important. However, nurses should clarify the definition of addiction and reinforce the importance that opioids have on the pain management plan. Answer B is incorrect as addiction can be a concern in some patients. Answer C is incorrect, because an increase in pain is likely due to advanced disease. Tolerance is a physiologic state of adaptation whereby the repeated exposure to a drug results in diminished effect of the drug over time and a possible need to increase the drug dose to achieve the same level of effect. Answer D is incorrect as patients on chronic opioids may experience withdrawal. This is separate from addiction and is a physiological phenomenon.

9. *Answer:* D

*Rationale:* Pain is a complex phenomenon and requires assessment of all domains. Fear of addiction often involves a lack of understanding about the definition of pain. This is a cognitive-psychological concern. Depression is another psychological concern, and the fatigue is a potential physical manifestation of the pain leading to this concern. Lack of mobility is both a physical and social concern as patients may be limited in both their physical and social life. The perception that pain is a punishment is an existential concern; patients have reported feeling that they are punished by God or punished because of their life choices. This concern requires additional assessment and attention.

10. **Answer:** B

**Rationale:** Answer A, mood stabilizers are not a category of antidepressant therapy. The other three categories are different types of antidepressants, which work by blocking the reuptake of neurotransmitters of serotonin, norepinephrine, and/or dopamine at the dorsal horn of the spinal cord. For pain inhibition to occur, the blockage of norepinephrine and/or dopamine is essential. Therefore, SSRIs lack analgesic properties.

11. **Answer:** D

**Rationale:** The correct answer is D. A psychological concern when conducting a comprehensive pain assessment is taking note of a patient's history of mental illness, including such conditions as anxiety and depression. Answer A is incorrect. A patient's financial hardship due to the cost of pain medication is a social concern. The influence of how religion and prayer assist a patient in coping with pain is a spiritual or existential concern; therefore, answer B is incorrect. Answer C is also incorrect. How a patient perceives traditional medicine is also a spiritual or existential concern.

12. **Answer:** C

**Rationale:** The correct answer is C. A social concern when conducting a comprehensive pain assessment is how the family caregiver responds to a patient's pain. Is the caregiver excepting and supportive of the patient's pain, or do they feel the patient is exaggerating? How a caregiver responds to a patient's pain has a strong impact on the level of care. Answer A is incorrect. The patient's experience with coping with pain in the past is a psychological concern as past experience will shape how they react to current or future pain. The patient's willingness to try non-traditional medicine, such as complementary and alternative therapies, is also a psychological concern. Answer B, thus, is incorrect. Answer D is incorrect. The role of a spiritual community in a patient's ability to cope with pain is a spiritual or existential concern.

13. **Answer:** D

**Rationale:** The correct answer is D. The level of cognition, including any signs of confusion or delirium, is a psychological concern when conducting a comprehensive pain assessment. The role of pain in the everyday life of the patient and the amount of support a patient receives, either with family or through the community, are both examples of social concerns. Therefore, answers A and C are incorrect. Answer B is also incorrect. The definition of how patient differentiates pain and suffering is a spiritual or existential concern.

14. **Answer:** D

**Rationale:** Answers A, B, and C – pain, position, and proximity – are all incorrect and not part of the acronym for the pain assessment known as PQRST. The correct answer is D. The "P" stands for Provocation/Palliation. Provocation refers to what caused the pain and palliation refers to what relieves the pain. The rest of the acronym is as follows. "Q" stands for quality of pain. How does the pain feel? The "R" in the acronym stands for region or radiation. In this case, the patient is asked where the pain is located and if the pain radiates. The "S" stands for severity. Patients are asked to rate their pain on a scale of 0 to 10. Finally, the "T" is timing. Is the pain constant or intermittent?

15. **Answer:** D

**Rationale:** Answers A and B are incorrect. The terms "region" and "radiation" refer to the "R" in the PQRST pain assessment. Answer C is an incorrect response. The correct answer is D. The "R" in the OLDCART pain assessment refers to factors in relieving the patient's pain. The rest of the acronym is as follows. The "O" refers to the onset of the patient's pain. "L" stands for the location, and if the pain is limited to a single place on the body. The "D" stands for duration. Patients are asked how long the pain lasts and whether it is constant or intermittent. The "C" is for characteristics. Patients are asked about the intensity of the pain and how they might describe the nature pf the pain. The "A" is for aggravating factors and what makes the pain feel worse. Finally, the "T" in OLDCART is for treatment. The patient is asked to list the treatments they have already tried and how they are working to relieve the pain.

## CHAPTER 45

1. **Answer:** B

**Rationale:** Compression of the tracheobronchial tree may occur from bronchospasm, laryngeal swelling from hypersensitivity reactions related to chemotherapy, and/or biotherapy treatments or superior vena cava syndrome. Abnormal fluid accumulation of fluid within the lung is due to the development of a pneumothorax, hemothorax, hydrothorax, or empyema. An aveolar hemorrhage is most often as the result of an autoimmune disorder and is not a hypersensitivity symptom. Bronchitis is an inflammation of the lungs and is not a hypersensitivity reaction.

2. **Answer:** D

**Rationale:** Risk factors for respiratory problems include exposure to irritants such as pollution, pesticides, chemicals, and irritants. Hair stylists are exposed to hair-coloring agents, hair spray, and hair-straightening products which contains formaldehyde, a known carcinogen, and causes eye, nose, throat, and lung irritant. History of receiving radiation therapy to the right breast, recent upper respiratory disease, and lymph node dissection do not put the patient at risk for development of respiratory problems.

3. **Answer:** A

**Rationale:** The inability to perform activities of daily living, including shortness of breath while showering, is a sign of respiratory problems. Acute anxiety within two to three weeks, and chronic anxiety greater than two months is a sign of a potential respiratory problems. A one-time episode of anxiety, five years ago, is not a risk factor. Two pillows used to sleep is an average amount. Clear, thin sputum production is not a risk factor. However, thick, colored sputum production or hemoptysis may be a sign of a respiratory problems.

4. *Answer:* B

*Rationale:* A PET scan or positron emission tomography is done to delineate anatomic extent of involvement. It is a nuclear medicine functional imaging technique used to observe metabolic processes in the body as an aid to the diagnosis of a disease. A pulmonary function test (PFT) is often performed to quantify air flow limitation. A dexascan is a test done to determine amounts of minerals and calcium to measure bone density. A test to measure vital capacity measures the amount of air a person can expel from their lungs.

5. *Answer:* D

*Rationale:* To maximize safety, the patient should be encouraged to use supplemental oxygen and assistive devices such as a cane or a walker as needed with ambulation to prevent hypoxia. Keeping the temperature warm may cause dehydration, which could lead to difficulty breathing. Cool temperatures and drinking plenty of fluids are encouraged. The patient should keep active. This may improve quality of life, and may lower fatigue and depression, as well as improve muscle strength.

6. *Answer:* D

*Rationale:* An inflammation process affects the interstitial lung parenchyma, which can cause an infectious and non-infectious lung injury. The release of hormones and signaling an antigen response are not causes of immunotherapy-induced pulmonary toxicity. Proportionate amounts of drugs and the volume of the drug administered do not contribute to immunotherapy-induced pulmonary toxicity.

7. *Answer:* C

*Rationale:* Dyspnea is the cardinal sign of pneumonitis. Pneumonitis is an inflammation of the lung tissue. Other symptoms include nonproductive cough, malaise, fatigue, and fever. Dyspnea may develop over weeks to months, but may also develop quickly, within a few hours, and may also occur years following drug exposure. An elevated heart rate and the development of crepitus are not signs of pneumonitis.

8. *Answer:* B

*Rationale:* The chemotherapy agent may be discontinued, or the dose may be reduced for prompt resolution. While rest is desirable, strict bedrest is not required. Physical activity and breathing exercises should be those that promote oxygenation throughout the lungs. Monitoring of EKG's and ECHO are required to monitor for cardiac toxicity. An ABG may be required if the patient is hypoxic, however, serial ABGs are not required.

9. *Answer:* A

*Rationale:* Cerebral metastasis, which affects the respiratory center or stimulates the central and peripheral

chemoreceptors, can cause dyspnea. Co-existing pulmonary, cardiac, or neuromuscular disease puts the patient at risk due to compromised lung expansion or blood flow to the lungs. Advancing age, comorbidities associated with Crohn's disease, and 200 mL total amount of IV fluids of patient received over a 24-hour period do not put the patient at risk of dyspnea.

10. *Answer:* C

*Rationale:* On assessment, clubbing of the fingers due to chronic hypoxemia, cyanosis, pallor, jugular vein distention, upper extremity swelling, and venous congestion in the chest may be found in patients with dyspnea. Palpation of a carotid artery on assessment is normal. A perfusion index (PI) is normally monitored with a pulse oximeter. A PI of 0.2% indicates a very weak pulse, whereas a perfusion index of 20% indicates an extremely strong pulse. A ventilation rate (respiratory rate) of 20 is normal.

11. *Answer:* D

*Rationale:* Immediate-release and parenteral opioids decrease central respiratory drive by reducing ventilator demand and is recommended for practice. In dyspnea, hyperventilation reduces carbon dioxide producing deep sighs. Histamines are typically released during an immune response to foreign pathogens, for example during an allergic reaction, which leads to high levels of histamines. Opioids do not increase physical and psychological demand to increase oxygen.

12. *Answer:* A

*Rationale:* Benign and malignant pleural effusions may be caused by increased negative pressure in the pleural space, or atelectasis. Spontaneous hemopericardium is the rupture of blood into the pericardial sac. Inflammation of the pleural space is due to pleurisy. The formation of pustules is not a cause of pleural effusion.

13. *Answer:* C

*Rationale:* On auscultation, egophony caused by lung consolidation and fibrosis is often found in persons with a pleural effusion. Egophony is an increased resonance of voice sounds heard within auscultating the lungs. Diminished or absent breath sounds will be found, rather than rhonchi and rales, which are typically heard with pneumonia. A tracheal shift is common in pneumothorax. Dullness to percussion is typically found in pleural effusion.

14. *Answer:* D

*Rationale:* Therapeutic aspiration using an intrapleural chemical agent such as talc is the most efficacious, evidence-based treatment. Indwelling pleural catheters are used to manage pleural effusions, not peritoneal catheters. A VATS (video-assisted thoracoscopic surgery) is also a form of pleural effusion management. Both chemotherapy and radiation therapy may be effective in tumors that responsive such as lymphoma or small cell lung cancer (SCLC).

15. *Answer:* C

*Rationale:* The patient's subjective responses, such as pain and dyspnea, and rate of re-accumulation of fluid should be monitored. The type of fluid drained is pleural fluid and this type of fluid does not need to be monitored continually. Fluid buildup does not typically occur around the insertion site. The potential for hypoproteinemia may occur after the procedure. Magnesium levels do not need to be monitored.

16. *Answer:* D

*Rationale:* Bevacizumab is associated with the pulmonary and radiologic abnormalities of bilateral ground-glass opacities and consolidation with the pattern of lung involvement classified as hemoptysis. Bortezomib is linked to bronchiolitis, which is associated with hyperinflation and air trapping. Alpha-interferon is associated with bronchiolitis, and includes air flow obstruction, airway hyperreactivity, and hyperinflation. Erlotinib is associated with interstitial pneumonitis and is categorized as diffuse, patchy, and ground-glass opacities.

17. *Answer:* A

*Rationale:* Sorafenib is associated with pulmonary and radiologic abnormalities associated with acute pneumonitis. Indications of acute pneumonitis includes diffuse patchy ground-glass opacities, and diffuse reticular pattern. Other agents associated with acute pneumonitis is bortezomib, cetuximab, dasatinib, erlotinib, everolimus, gefitinib, gemcitabine, idealisib, imatinib, irinotecan, pemetrexed, piritrexim, procarbazine, rituximab, sunitinib, temozolomide, and temsirolimus. Busulfan is associated with bronchiolitis and is indicated by hyperinflation and air trapping. Isolated acute chest pain is associated with etoposide, as is doxorubicin.

18. *Answer:* B

*Rationale:* L-asparaginase is associated with pulmonary and radiologic abnormalities associated with hypersensitivity reactions. Hypersensitivity reactions are indicated by air flow obstruction, airway hyperreactivity, and hyperinflation. Other agents associated with hypersensitivity include alpha-interferon, cetuximab, etoposide, gemcitabine, obinutuzumab, panitumumab, rituximab, taxanes, and vinca alkaloids. Sorafenib is associated with pulmonary and radiologic abnormalities associated with acute pneumonitis. Carmustine is associated with pneumothorax. Thalidomide is associated with pulmonary embolus (PE).

19. *Answer:* B

*Rationale:* A pneumothorax is caused by air in the pleural space. An empyema is an abnormal accumulation of inflected fluid collecting in the pleural space. A general term for a lung disorder that affects the deeper aspects of the lung tissue is defined as diffuse parenchymal lung disease. A pleural effusion is a collection of abnormal amounts of fluid in the pleural space.

20. *Answer:* B

*Rationale:* An empyema is an abnormal accumulation of infected fluid or pus in the pleural space and is generally treated with systemic antibiotics. Radiation therapy is done to reduce obstructions caused by lung tumors. Epinephrine is used to treat anaphylaxis, while oxygen is used to treat anaphylaxis or the patient who is hypoxemic.

21. *Answer:* C

*Rationale:* Bleomycin in combination with radiation therapy places a patient at high risk for pneumonitis. Answers in A, B, and D present options that are not associated with this patient's therapy regimen.

22. *Answer:* B

*Rationale:* Glucocorticoids decrease local inflammation. Bronchodilators serve to relax airway constriction, thus increasing the flow of air to the lungs. Antibiotics are used to treat sensitive infections, which may have a component of pulmonary inflammation. However, the target of the antibiotic treatment is not the pulmonary inflammation itself, but the bacteria causing the infection. Diuretics decrease fluid overload.

## CHAPTER 46

1. *Answer:* B

*Rationale:* The definition of a sleep-wake disturbance is an actual or perceived disturbance in night sleep with resulting daytime impairment. Sleep-wake disturbances can include insomnia, sleep-related breathing problems, circadian rhythm disorders, and excessive sleepiness. These issues often occur in combination with fatigue, anxiety, and depression. An active biobehavioral process is the definition of sleep, while a transient inability to initiate or maintain sleep describes insomnia. Circadian rhythm disorders are included as part of sleep-wake disturbances.

2. *Answer:* A

*Rationale:* Antihistamines can be used to help patients fall asleep. They may be preferred if concerned about cross-dependence. Antihistamines should be used with caution for older adults. Antipsychotics have a sedating effect but should be considered as a last course of treatment due to the drug's serious side effect profile. Alpha adrenergic receptor blockers relax muscles, but do not help patients fall asleep. Antidepressants are effective if used for insomnia, associated with depression.

3. *Answer:* D

*Rationale:* Patients should try to avoid caffeine after 12 o'clock pm, when possible, due to caffeine's stimulating effect. Patients should develop a routine of only going to bed when sleepy at about the same time each night and waking at the same time each day. Patients should be encouraged to make their bedrooms restful, free of distractions like televisions, tablets, and cell phones, and should try to keep their rooms cool and dark.

4. *Answer:* D

*Rationale:* By waking up at the same time each morning, limiting use of caffeine to the morning hours, and exercising each day, the individual is making a routine conducive to sleep. Enjoying an afternoon nap may impact his ability to fall asleep and stay asleep. Risk factors for sleep-wake disturbances include daytime naps, use of caffeine and or nicotine close to bedtime, lack of daily exercise, and lack of a regular bedtime routine.

5. *Answer:* C

*Rationale:* The sleep-wake cycle consists of two phases. The two cycles are Rapid Eye Movement (the active phase) and Non-Rapid Eye Movement (quiet or restful phase). These phases repeat with each cycle lasting approximately 90 minutes. Four to six cycles occur during a 7- to 8-hour sleep period. There is not an awakening phase.

6. *Answer:* D

*Rationale:* Although it is important to check a patient's sleep cycle at each of the time points given, D is the best answer, as sleep assessments should be done throughout the patient's entire duration of treatment and should coincide with any changes in health status. Sleep should not only be checked at the initial assessment or after their first cycle of chemotherapy and at the end.

7. *Answer:* D

*Rationale:* Concern over losing his job, feeling anxious and afraid of what the future holds all describe psychological stressors. Pain in the patient's hip describes a physical stressor. Physical stressors can play a role in sleep-wake disturbances and should be assessed and treated appropriately to minimize their effect on the sleep-wake cycle.

8. *Answer:* B

Polysomnography is a diagnostic tool to diagnose sleep-wake disturbances such as sleep-related breathing disorders and limb movement disorders. An EEG assesses electrical energy in the brain and is often helpful when evaluating seizure activity. The NCCN distress thermometer looks at distress. Lack of sleep can lead to a higher level of distress, but it is not a diagnostic test. Assessment of the characterization of sleep, including bedtime routine, time to sleep and sleep duration, should be assessed but they are not part of a diagnostic test.

## CHAPTER 47

1. *Answer:* B

*Rationale:* Body image is based upon how a person feels about their body's actual or perceived appearance and/or change in function. While others' perceptions – including friends, family, and strangers - might influence the patient's perception of physical change, the patient's perception is the sole focus of the concept of body image.

2. *Answer:* C

*Rationale:* Patients' self-identification of coping strategies provides buy in for success, and nurses' support with self-compassion has been shown to be effective in improved perceptions and adjusting to changes in body image. Grief has no time frame and can vary greatly from individual to individual. Body image is not affected by contact with long-lost relatives. Education and knowledge in family members does not necessarily facilitate personal acceptance of a body image change in the patient. It is important to educate patients about treatment and potential body image changes so they can anticipate and prepare for changes as much as possible.

3. *Answer:* D

*Rationale:* The nurse's role to assist in reintegration is to focus on positive coping strategies of role-play and problem solving. Role playing and practicing how to respond to various situations can facilitate reintegration and make the patient more confident about reintegration. Telling the patient not to worry and to get back to work demonstrates a lack of empathy on the part of the nurse. Taking additional time off when the patient is capable of returning to work encourages avoidance. Going to the workplace and discussing patient treatment information without the consent of the patient is an example of improper disclosure.

4. *Answer:* A

*Rationale:* Hair loss is total and includes eyelashes, nose hair, and pubic hair. Hair loss typically starts 2 weeks after chemotherapy treatment, may occur over a day to weeks, and occurs later when the patient is treated with low dose of chemotherapy. Hair regrowth usually starts 6 to 8 weeks after completion of treatment. Hair may come back slowly, thinner, or take up to a year to regrow.

5. *Answer:* B

*Rationale:* Social support decreases body image distress. Altered body image issues are a concern for both males and females. Young individuals may be at higher risk for altered body image than older adults. Body image satisfaction is not dependent on time since diagnosis.

6. *Answer:* C

*Rationale:* Actively serving as a volunteer represents actual, rather than a plan for adaptation, and represents reintegration with a constructive objective. Planning to return to work does not fully represent health adaptation – because it may not be actualized. Being able to state body image changes and why they occurred is a demonstration of knowledge not necessarily adaptation. Knowing emergency resources demonstrates attention to safety but not necessarily adaptation.

7. *Answer:* C

*Rationale:* The mother and daughter should talk about the illness and be encouraged to do so. The mother should speak with the daughter so they can both share feelings and concerns. When another family member or individual discusses the issue, instead of with the mother, it implies that the mother cannot or is unwilling to help or communicate with the daughter. The communication should be open and age-appropriate, not necessarily limited or structured. The communication should be ongoing and not just when the disease outcome in known.

8. *Answer:* D

*Rationale:* Letting the patient know that the nurse understands that what she is going through is a huge adjustment as she gets accustomed to her new body shape is an example of an empathic approach to communication. Empathic communication is a preferred approach. The nurse's statement of "don't worry, you look great" is a typical approach and is classified as a premature reassurance. Asking the patient what she sees in the mirror and if she has discussed her feelings with her husband are exploratory approaches, which are also preferred.

9. *Answer:* C

*Rationale:* The nurse telling the patient that if he doesn't get the bag, he will die of his cancer is an example of a typical response. Specifically, the statement is

blood disorder characterized by the formation of thromboses in small blood vessels of the body that can possibly lead to organ damage. DIC is caused by extensive intravascular thrombi causing end organ damage and hemorrhage due to the consumption of platelets and coagulation factors. Sepsis can be a life-threatening organ dysfunction caused by impaired regulation of the patient's response to infection, involving pro- and anti-inflammatory responses. Neither sepsis nor DIC is caused by the release of chemical mediators from mast cells and basophils.

16. **Answer:** A

**Rationale:** Currently, first-line therapy pharmacologic for anaphylaxis is epinephrine. Additional helpful pharmacologic treatments can include inhaled beta agonists, IV fluids, corticosteroids, and H1 receptor antagonists.

17. **Answer:** D

**Rationale:** Ms. A. is at increased risk for infection leading to sepsis because she is older than age 65, has cancer, and has a compromised immune system related to the presence of neutropenia resulting from her chemotherapy treatments. Neutropenic fever, defined as a temperature >100.4 F, may be an early sign of sepsis. Sepsis is life-threatening organ dysfunction caused by impaired regulation of the patient's response to infection, involving pro- and anti-inflammatory responses. Septic shock is a subset of sepsis causing profound metabolic, cellular, and circulatory compromise leading to hypotension that requires vasopressors to maintain mean arterial pressure Septic shock has a greater potential for mortality than sepsis with a rate greater than 40%. Confusion may also be present as sepsis progresses and in septic shock.

18. **Answer:** A

**Rationale:** A white blood cell count with a left shift can be one abnormal lab value of a patient who is experiencing sepsis. Additionally, abnormal laboratory values include a suspected or documented infection. Leukocytosis or leukopenia may be present. There may be a prolonged PT or aPTT. Arterial hypoxemia, decreased platelets, decreased fibrinogen, hyperglycemia, increased lactic acid, positive blood cultures, and elevated creatinine >0.5 mg/dL are also sometimes present in sepsis. Abnormal laboratory values indicative of septic shock (in addition) include elevated liver functions, elevated lactate, urine output <0.5 mL/kg per hour for at least 2 hours without hypovolemia, Increased creatinine >2.0 mg/dL, anemia, thrombocytopenia <100,000 cells/μ, and hypoglycemia.

19. **Answer:** C

**Rationale:** Tumor lysis syndrome (TLS) is an oncologic emergency in which large amounts of tumor cells are rapidly destroyed spilling their cellular contents into the systemic circulation, potentially resulting in serious complications which can manifest as electrolyte abnormalities including hyperuricemia, hyperkalemia, hyperphosphatemia, and hypocalcemia. TLS can occur within 6 hours of cancer therapy initiation. Newer targeted treatments for cancer may also cause TLS.

20. **Answer:** A

**Rationale:** Management of tumor lysis syndrome (TLS) will likely include administering IV hydration 24-48 hours prior to treatment initiation for high-risk patients to facilitate renal perfusion and increase urine output minimizing the risk of uric acid and calcium phosphate deposition in the renal tubules. Prior to their initial cytotoxic treatment, patients at risk of TLS receive medication prophylaxis with uric acid lowering agents, such as allopurinol and rasburicase. Rapid lysis of massive amounts of malignant cells results in the release of the intracellular contents into the circulation causing electrolyte disturbances (i.e., hyperkalemia, hyperphosphatemia, and hyperuricemia), which need to be managed. Oncology nurses need to identify and report symptoms of TLS as soon as possible. Assessment includes high acuity monitoring including ECG changes, intake and output, daily weights, and indications for the need for kidney dialysis. Restriction of potassium rich foods and educating patients and their significant others concerning TLS and TLS interventions..

21. **Answer:** C

**Rationale:** Hypercalcemia of malignancy is an abnormally high level of calcium corrected for albumin (> 10.5 mg/dL) and is the most common oncologic emergency occurring in 20% to 30% of all cancer patients. Tumor lysis syndrome (TLS) is an oncologic emergency in which large amounts of tumor cells are rapidly destroyed spilling their cellular contents into the systemic circulation potentially resulting in serious complications which can manifest as electrolyte abnormalities. TLS can occur within 6 hours of cancer therapy initiation. Newer targeted treatments for cancer exhibit TLS. Syndrome of inappropriate antidiuretic hormone (SIADH) is a condition in which antidiuretic hormone (ADH), in activated form called arginine vasopressin (AVP), is inappropriately triggered despite the presence of normal or increased fluid balance. This results in hyponatremia and hypoosmolality. In the oncology setting, ADH can be inappropriately produced by cancer. Disseminated intravascular coagulation (DIC) is a systemic disorder of coagulation. Within DIC extensive intravascular thrombi cause end organ damage and hemorrhage due to the consumption of platelets and coagulation factors

22. **Answer:** A

**Rationale:** Tumors associated with hypercalcemia of malignancy include breast, lung, prostate, multiple myeloma, lymphoma, and hematologic malignancies. Other risk factors include hyperparathyroidism, vitamin D intoxication, chronic granulomatous disorders, and some medications including diuretics and lithium

23. **Answer:** B

**Rationale:** Symptoms of hypercalcemia depend on the severity. Gastrointestinal symptoms include anorexia, abdominal cramping, loss of appetite, nausea, vomiting, pancreatitis, and peptic ulcer. Neurologic symptoms include restlessness, difficulty concentrating, lethargy, confusion, seizures, and coma. Muscular symptoms include fatigue and generalized weakness, ataxia and pathologic fractures. Renal symptoms include frequent urination, nocturia, polydipsia, and renal failure. Cardiovascular symptoms include orthostatic hypotension, shortened QT, ventricular arrhythmia, and ST segment elevation.

24. *Answer:* C

*Rationale:* Denosumab is a monoclonal antibody that decreases bone resorption. It is utilized in patients unable to receive bisphosphonates. Denosumab is not excreted through kidneys, therefore, may be used in patients with renal insufficiency. This agent is also used in patients who are refractory to bisphosphonate therapy. Bevacizumab is used to treat metastatic cancer. Infliximab (Remicade) is used to treat rheumatoid arthritis, ankylosing spondylitis, psoriatic arthritis, psoriasis, Crohn's disease, and ulcerative colitis. Pembrolizumab is used to treat melanoma and other cancers.

25. *Answer:* A

*Rationale:* Hypercalcemia is demonstrated by an elevated calcium level. Patients with a diagnosis of lung cancer and breast cancer comprise about 80% of all patients in whom hypercalcemia develops. Mental status changes are one of the signs and symptoms of hypercalcemia.

26. *Answer:* A

*Rationale:* In treating patients with hypercalcemia, the aim is to release serum calcium absorption, increase urinary calcium excretion, and decrease intestinal calcium absorption. Initially, the patient is given 0.9% saline intravenously to increase the circulating volume. Calcitonin then works to reduce the serum calcium level. A loop diuretic is often instituted to reduce fluid overload, but it does not work to reduce serum calcium. After rehydrating the patient, bisphosphonates are administered. Vasopressor drugs are not normally used in the treatment of hypercalcemia.

27. *Answer:* B

*Rationale:* Signs and symptoms of anaphylaxis include urticaria and angioedema. Pain or itching around intravenous insertion sites describes a localized hypersensitivity reaction. Feelings of fatigue are common in patients with cancer, but are not indicative of anaphylaxis.

## CHAPTER 53

1. *Answer:* B

*Rationale:* The cranium is a rigid, non-expandable chamber that contains brain tissue, blood and cerebrospinal fluid (CSF) that are maintained within a narrow range of intracranial pressure (ICP). Any increase in the volume of one of these components causes the ICP to increase. An increase of ICP >20 mmHg in adults is considered pathologic. Increased intracranial pressure in this patient with breast cancer results from metastatic tumor deposits that increase the volume of brain tissue and occupy space in the intracranial cavity. Neurologic changes resulting from increased ICP may range from subtle to severe. It is possible that head injury could lead to increased intracranial pressure, but in this patient, it is more likely that the presence of brain metastases that occupy space within the cranium is the cause of the increased intracranial pressure.

Vitamin deficiency and increased hormone production are not associated with increased intracranial pressure.

2. *Answer:* C

*Rationale:* Treatment with high-dose cytosine arabinoside increases the risk for developing increased intracranial pressure. A history of cervical spine surgery does not put the patient at risk for developing increased intracranial pressure. The patient's diagnosis of multiple myeloma does not put the patient at risk. However, a diagnosis of leukemia or lymphoma is a risk factor. The patient's history of degenerative disc disease is also not a risk factor.

3. *Answer:* D

*Rationale:* Patients with lung cancer have increased risk for metastases to the brain. The entire brain may be irradiated prophylactically to destroy any metastatic cells that may be present and are too small to be seen on imaging. Brain irradiation increases the risk of developing increased intracranial pressure. Early signs and symptoms of intracranial pressure may be subtle and may include headache that is worse in the mornings, and are aggravated when bending over, or during Valsalva maneuvers. The patient may also experience nausea, vomiting, and weakness. The presence of dehydration may be associated with weakness, but headache in the mornings or with bending or during Valsalva maneuvers are unlikely. The signs and symptoms the patient is experiencing are not indicative of seizures or dementia.

4. *Answer:* D

*Rationale:* ICP monitoring via intraventricular, intra-parenchymal, subarachnoid, or epidural site is the most reliable method to diagnose ICP, with the goal being to keep ICP less than 20 mmHg, and cerebral perfusion between 60 and 75 mmHg. While PET with CT scan is a method of diagnosing ICP, it is not reliable. Bone marrow biopsy is not a test used to diagnose ICP. Labs for glucose and protein do not diagnose ICP; however, CSF examination is used if leptomeningeal metastasis or meningitis is suspected.

5. *Answer:* C

*Rationale:* The most effective method to rapidly decrease ICP is hyperventilation, which causes vasoconstriction and decreased cerebral blood volume and ICP. Ms. C would need to be sedated and intubated and ventilated to a partial pressure of carbon dioxide (PCO2) between 26 and 30 mmHg. The effects of hyperventilation are short-lived. While radiation therapy to the head may be used to shrink metastatic tumor in the brain in some patients, this treatment would be contraindicated for Ms. C. because brain RT is the causative factor of her increased intracranial pressure. Systemic biotherapy administration is not an effective method to rapidly reduce ICP. Administration of chemotherapy or targeted agents intrathecally is a treatment; however, it is not a rapid means of reducing ICP. Injection of steroids into the cervical spine is not a method to reduce ICP.

6. *Answer:* A

*Rationale:* The nurse should monitor the patient for any changes indicating decreasing cardiac output, such as decreased urinary output, changes in vital signs, and changes in mentation. Patients should avoid the prone position or activities that exert pressure on the abdomen. The patient's head of bed should be elevated to about 30 degrees. Endotracheal suctioning should be minimized.

7. *Answer:* C

*Rationale:* The spinal cord is compressed by the collapse of vertebral bone involved with tumor. Hypertrophy of vertebral bone due to disease involvement is not sufficient to compress the spinal cord. Regeneration of bone marrow cells in the vertebrae is not a cause of spinal cord compression. Improvement in the size of the tumor resulting in misalignment of the vertebrae is also not a cause of spinal cord compression.

8. *Answer:* D

*Rationale:* The diagnostic procedure of choice for evaluating spinal cord compression is an MRI of the entire spine as multiple sites of metastasis may exist. Positron emission tomography is both sensitive and specific but less available than MRI and is not recommended to be used alone for diagnosis or treatment guidance. Diagnostic radiology films of the thoracic spine may show bone abnormalities and soft tissue masses in that area, but miss the rest of the spine and are not used to diagnose or rule out spinal metastasis. Computerized tomography of the spine is used as an alternative when MRI unavailable or contraindicated but is less sensitive than MRI.

9. *Answer:* B

*Rationale:* Patient and family should be instructed to assess for signs of compromised feelings or sensations. Patient should report any changes in sensory or motor function, as well as sexual dysfunction, which may indicate sensory deficits. Mobility should be based on findings of stable or unstable spine and patient should maintain a safe level of independents with the limits of the SCC. The nurse should monitor for progression of motor or sensory deficits, including bowel patterns and frequency. Incontinence of stool may indicate autonomic dysfunction. Palpation for bladder diction should be done if the interval between voiding increases. Long periods without voiding may indicate autonomic dysfunction.

10. *Answer:* C

*Rationale:* When obstruction of the superior vena cava (SVC) occurs, there is decreased venous return to the heart from the head, neck, thorax, and upper extremities, and hemodynamic compromise occurs from mass effect on the heart. SVC occurs because of compression or obstruction of the vessel such as by tumor, lymph nodes, or thrombus. Thrombosis may concomitantly occur but is not the cause of superior vena cava syndrome (SVCS). Myocardial infarction is not a cause of SVCS.

11. *Answer:* D

*Rationale:* The presence of non-small lung cancer, especially in the right lung, accounts for the most cases of SVCS. When obstruction of the superior vena cava occurs, venous blood return to the heart from the head, neck, thorax, and upper extremities is compromised and characteristic symptoms of SVCS develop. Symptoms include dyspnea, sensation of head fullness, headache, blurred vision, nasal stuffiness, hoarseness, dysphagia, nonproductive cough, chest pain, and orthopnea (the need to sleep in an upright position). Symptoms are more pronounced in the morning and improve after being in an upright position after a few hours. Sinusitis and pneumonia may have similar symptoms; however, symptoms usually do not improve. Churg-Strauss syndrome is a rare disorder caused by blood vessel inflammation.

12. *Answer:* B

*Rationale:* The signs of orange-brown, malodorous feculent emesis are signs of a distal small intestine obstruction or colonic obstruction. Rapid-onset, bitter, bile-stained emesis that may be projectile would be a sign of a proximal small intestine obstruction. Signs of a small bowel obstruction include more severe nausea and vomiting. Non-bile colored, sour emesis with undigested food would be a sign of gastric outlet obstruction.

13. *Answer:* C

*Rationale:* Fluid accumulation in the pericardial sac may occur secondary to increased permeability of cardiac capillaries caused by chemotherapy or biotherapy. Coronary artery disease and leakage of fluid into the chest from pneumothorax do not cause fluid to accumulate in the pericardial sac. Inaccurate insertion of a central line may puncture the pericardial sac and cause fluid accumulation in the pericardial sac.

14. *Answer:* A

*Rationale:* Surgical management includes colectomy with primary anastomosis with or without ostomy. Hyperosmolar agents and methylnaltrexone are treatments for constipation. Insertion of a biliary stent is not a surgical procedure to treat bowel obstruction.

15. *Answer:* D

*Rationale:* Checkpoint inhibitor immunotherapy is associated with increased risk of pneumonitis. Pneumonitis may be an adverse event of several of the checkpoint inhibitor agents including PD-1/PD-L1 inhibitors, as well as many other biotherapy agents. Systemic hyperthermia is an alternative treatment for cancer and is not a risk factor for a patient developing pneumonitis. Issels immunotherapy vaccine and dendritic cell treatment are the same and are not factors for developing pneumonitis. Another major risk factor for pneumonitis is radiation therapy to the chest.

16. *Answer:* C

*Rationale:* The patient's symptoms most likely indicate bowel perforation. Patients may be able to pinpoint the precise time of bowel perforation, noting a sudden relief of pain, followed by more severe pain. In addition, the patient's recent abdominal surgery increases the risk of bowel perforation. A post-surgical ileus is not considered a risk factor for bowel perforation. Patients receiving pain medication short term to manage postoperative pain will not become addicted to pain medication.

17. *Answer:* A

*Rationale:* Having a history of vertebral compression fractures puts a patient at risk for spinal cord compression. A history of chronic myelogenous leukemia is not a

**201**

precursor to patients developing SCC. Cancers that typically metastasize to the bone, including breast, lung, and prostrate cancers, as well as multiple myeloma, which develops in the bone marrow, account for the greatest percentage of cases of SCC. Osteomyelitis is an inflammation of the bone and does not put a patient a risk for SCC. History of childhood scoliosis is not a risk factor.

18. *Answer:* C

*Rationale:* While radiation therapy is the primary treatment for SVCS for patients with SCLC, the urgency of this patient's admission makes percutaneous intravascular stent placement the most effective treatment to restore blood flow and resolve symptoms. Chemotherapy is also a treatment; however, it should follow the patient's initial urgent treatment. Surgical resection is rarely used due to the effectiveness of stent placement.

19. *Answer:* D

*Rationale:* Pneumonitis is the correct answer. Pneumonitis due to chest radiotherapy may occur between 4 and 12 weeks after completion of radiation therapy. Factors that may contribute to risk of pneumonitis include undergoing combination therapy, as well as immunotherapeutic agents such as rituximab for treatment of her lymphoma. Symptoms may include low grade fever and hypoxia. Myocardial effusion and cardiac tamponade are not correct because patients do not typically present with a low grade fever. While patients with superior vena cava syndrome often present with dyspnea, the other symptoms of chest pain and low grade fever are not common.

20. *Answer:* B

*Rationale:* The patient is at risk for developing cardiac tamponade due to his history of cardiovascular disease, diagnosis of mesothelioma, and treatment with Doxorubicin (which may cause cardiotoxicity), and more than 4000 cGy of radiation to the chest. While the patient's diagnosis of mesothelioma and complaints of dyspnea may put the patient at risk for SVCS, symptoms of SVCS are usually more pronounced in the morning and improve or disappear after being upright for several hours. Radiation recall, which is a severe skin reaction that occurs in the radiation treatment field when certain chemotherapy drugs are administered during or soon after radiation therapy to the involved area, is not accurate. The patient is not at risk for developing cardiomyopathy based on the data provided.

21. *Answer:* A

*Rationale:* The most common cause of cardiac tamponade is malignant disease that causes a pericardial effusion. The severity of the cardiac tamponade depends on the amount of fluid in the pericardium, rate of accumulation, and degree of compromise. Cardiac tamponade is a life-threatening situation of excessive accumulation of fluid in the pericardial sac exerting extrinsic pressure on the cardiac chambers, resulting in impaired intracardiac filling, decreased cardiac output, and compromised cardiac function. Patients particularly at risk include patients with primary tumors of the heart, including mesothelioma and sarcomas (including Kaposi sarcoma), and patients with metastatic tumors to the pericardium—lung, breast,

GI tract, leukemia, Hodgkin or non-Hodgkin lymphoma, sarcoma, melanoma. Other patients at risk include those with who have received more than 4000 cGy of radiation to a field in which the heart is included. Patients receiving chemotherapy or biotherapy associated with increased capillary permeability (e.g., anthracyclines, interferon, interleukin, granulocyte-macrophage colony-stimulating factor) are also at increased risk.

22. *Correct answer:* C

Superior vena cava syndrome (SVCS) results from compromised venous drainage of the head, neck, upper extremities, and thorax through the superior vena cava (SVC) because of compression or obstruction of the vessel such as by tumor, lymph nodes, or thrombus. The SVC is a thin-walled major vessel that carries venous drainage from the head, neck, upper extremities, and upper thorax to the heart. The SVC is located in the mediastinum; surrounded by structures of the sternum, trachea, vertebrae, aorta, right bronchus, lymph nodes, and pulmonary artery. The SVC is a low-pressure vessel easily compressed; compression (acute or gradual) can occur from multiple causes. Right-sided lung cancers responsible for most cases of SVCS. When obstruction of the SVC occurs, venous return to the heart from the head, neck, thorax, and upper extremities is impaired

23. *Correct answer:* A

The biggest risk factor for SVCS is the presence of chest malignancy, most often non–small cell lung cancer (NSCLC) and SCLC, followed by lymphoma. Other malignancies can cause SVC syndrome but not as frequently. Other risk factors include the presence of central venous catheters and pacemakers, previous radiation therapy to the mediastinum resulting in vascular fibrosis, associated conditions (e.g. fungal infection, benign tumors, aortic aneurysm), and underlying cardiovascular disease

24. *Answer:* C

*Rationale:* Patients with a chest malignancy, especially lung cancer, have an increased risk of developing superior vena cava syndrome (SVCS). The SVC is an easily compressed low-pressure vessel that is located in the mediastinum surrounded by several fairly rigid structures. SVCS may occur because of compression or obstruction of the SVC by tumor mass, enlarged mediastinal lymph nodes, or thrombus formation. The presence of a right-sided lung tumor accounts for the most cases of SVCS. Plaque deposition in the carotid artery, pulmonary embolism, and myocardial infarction are not associated with the development of SVCS.

25. *Answer:* C

*Rationale:* The leptomeninges are the two inner-most layers of the meninges. Cerebrospinal fluid (CSF) circulates between these layers. Leptomeningeal metastases are often seen in acute leukemias and are a result of metastatic spread of malignant cells through the CSF spaces. Lymph node metastases are also seen with leukemias. The spleen and the liver can be involved, but this is less common.

**26. *Answer:* A**

*Rationale:* Patients with increased intracranial pressure (ICP) can display a variety of neurological symptoms, including headaches, blurred vision, lethargy, and changes in level of consciousness. Some of the most emergent late signs and symptoms comprise Cushing's triad and include bradycardia, respiratory depression, and hypertension. Answers B and C describe digestive and neurologic symptoms. A variety of urinary symptoms are related to ICP, depending on the cause. Urinary frequency is more often found than decreased urination.

**27. *Answer:* C**

*Rationale:* The most common presenting symptom of spinal cord compression (SCC) is neck and back pain. Pain can occur before the actual compression of the spinal cord and before the development of any neurologic symptoms. The common progression of symptoms in SCC is pain, motor weakness, sensory loss, motor loss, and autonomous dysfunction.

**28. *Answer:* C**

*Rationale:* Obstruction of the superior vena cava causes jugular vein distention and edema of the face, neck, upper thorax, breasts, and upper extremities. Abdominal distension and fever are not associated with superior vena cava syndrome (SVCS). Tachycardia, not bradycardia, usually occurs with SVCS. Cheyne Stokes respirations are not indicative of SVCS.

## CHAPTER 54

**1. *Answer:* B**

*Rationale:* The Oncology Nursing Society *Scope and Standards of Practice* describe the expectations for oncology nursing practice across various care settings. For each standard, criteria for demonstrating competence are provided at the RN level that apply to all nurses who provide care to patients with cancer or practice in an oncology setting. Additional standards that apply to graduate-level prepared nurses and advanced practice registered nurses are included for some standards. The *Standards of Oncology Nursing Education* were developed to guide educators in the oncology nursing setting and schools of nursing about preparing nurses to care for cancer survivors across many settings. The ASCO/ONS Chemotherapy Administration Safety Standards are interprofessional standards outlining best practices for reducing errors related to chemotherapy processes. The nurse recruiter represents the institution's job specification not origin of professional standards.

**2. *Answer:* B**

*Rationale:* Nursing standards of practice and professional performance (NSPPP) set expectations for competent nursing practice and serve as powerful guides for ensuring evidence-based, quality nursing care and provide direction to nurses and their employers related to expectations and development of competence. As a nurse educator, the nurse is focused on policy and development for the entire staff, not individual professional growth. Staff may or may not agree with a policy, but such policies should be based on standards and evidence-based practice. The nurse educator may also be responsible for continuing education of the staff but when working on a policy she is looking at NSPPP and promoting evidence-based practice.

**3. *Answer:* C**

*Rationale:* The ASCO/ONS Chemotherapy Administration Safety Standards are interprofessional standards that outline best practices to reduce the risk of error during the process of chemotherapy provision. They are not tiered but interprofessional. These standards address appropriate staff and policies, planning, consent and education for patients and caregivers, ordering, preparing, administering by parenteral and oral routes and documentation and monitoring adherence, side effects, and complications. They do not include information for locating clinical trials or information for patients/public to understand efficacy/side effects of chemotherapy.

**4. *Answer:* B**

*Rationale:* Clinical practice guidelines recommendations utilized to optimize patient care and are based on a systematic review of evidence and an assessment of the benefits and harms of alternative care options. The ONS Symptom Interventions are written by teams of oncology nurse scientists and summarize and synthesize available evidence on the management of symptoms commonly encountered in oncology nursing practice. Oncology nurses can access this information to guide clinical practice. Standards for professional nursing practice are statements that define the duties that all nurses, regardless of role, are expected to perform competently. Standards and clinical guidelines are not the same and are differentiated by expectations of compliance. There is an expectation of compliance with standards. There are standards specific to oncology nursing such as *Oncology Nursing Scope and Standards of Practice* and standards specific to oncology professionals such as the ASCO/ONS Chemotherapy Administration Safety Standards. An evidence-based protocol might be adopted by an institution based on a review of practice and literature.

**5. *Answer:* D**

*Rationale:* ONS *Nursing Documentation Standards for Cancer Treatment* describe nursing documentation requirements for persons with a diagnosis of cancer undergoing cancer treatment and requiring supportive care and reflect the minimal elements to include documentation about people undergoing treatment for cancer. They address chemotherapy and biotherapy administration, radiation therapy, blood and marrow transplantation, oncologic surgery, central venous access devices, blood product transfusion, and extravasation management. A side by side comparison of current documentation practices with the standards for documentation can identify gaps and potential areas for improvement. Ease of locating policies will not necessarily result in appropriate documentation. A consultant could review policies but without a side by side comparison it is not clear if the documentation is appropriate and meets the requirements of the standard. The compliance department may be more concerned with coding and reimbursement.

6. *Answer:* B
   *Rationale:* *Standards of Oncology Practice* include the following components: assessment, diagnosis, outcomes identification, planning, implementation, coordination of care, health teaching and health promotion, and evaluation. Standards of Oncology Professional Performance include the following components: ethics, culturally congruent care, collaboration, communication, leadership, education, evidence-based practice and research, quality of practice, professional practice evaluation, resource utilization, and environmental health.

7. *Answer:* C
   *Rationale:* The full definition for standards for professional nursing practice, as stated by the American Nurses Association (ANA), is an "authoritative statements of the duties that all registered nurses [RNs], regardless of role, population, or specialty, are expected to perform competently" (ANA, 2015a, p. 3). According to the Institutes of Medicine (IOM), clinical practice guidelines are defined as "statements that include recommendations intended to optimize patient care that are informed by a systematic review of evidence and an assessment of the benefits and harms of alternative care options" (IOM, 2011, p. 15). Therefore, any statement with a recommendation is not defined as a standard. Finally, the standards of professional nursing are meant for all nurses, including, and not limited to, subspecialties.

8. *Answer:* B
   *Rationale:* The definition for the education component in the Standards of Professional Performance is the oncology nurse seeks and expands personal knowledge and competence that reflect the current evidence-based state of cancer care and oncology nursing and contributes to the professional development of peers, assistive personnel, and interprofessional colleagues. Collaboration is defined as the oncology nurse partners with the patient and family, the interprofessional team, and communityresources to optimize cancer care. The definition of evidence-based practice and research is the oncology nurse integrates relevant research into clinical practice and identifies clinical dilemmas and problems appropriate for study while supporting research efforts. Finally, resource utilization is defined as the oncology nurse considers factors related to safety, efficiency, effectiveness, and cost in planning and delivering care to patients.

## CHAPTER 55

1. *Answer:* D
   *Rationale:* A nonpayment for complications model exists when EBP is not followed which supports pay for performance. EBP has not been implemented throughout the United States or globally consistently. EBP supports pay for performance initiatives. Evolution of evidence is not limited, but instead evolves on a continual basis.

2. *Answer:* A.
   *Rationale:* P = Patient population of interest. I = is not Improvement, but Intervention or issue of interest. O = is not Opportunity, but Outcomes. T = is not Theory, but Time Frame. C = Comparison Intervention or Control Group

3. *Answer:* A
   *Rationale:* Level 1 is the highest level of evidence on which to base practice change. Level 1 is a systematic review of randomized control trials (RCTs). Level 2 is single-site RCT studies. Level 5 is a systematic review of descriptive or qualitative studies. Level 7 is the lowest level of evidence on which to base practice change; it is an expert opinion.

4. *Answer:* C
   *Rationale:* Practice changes should first be implemented or piloted in one or two practice areas to ensure feasibility, sustainability and outcomes. Incorporation into a policy may take place after the pilot. Publishing may take place after the pilot. Review by the IRB would take place before research starts if patients are involved.

5. *Answer:* B
   *Rationale:* EBP is most valuable when clinical practice changes and the impact of the practice on patient outcomes is communicated effectively and adopted. Information about outcomes should be disseminated such as through grand rounds, professional journals and national conferences, but impact on clinical practice and patient outcomes are most important and valuable components of EBP.

6. *Answer:* D
   *Rationale:* Qualitative research is used to describe or explore phenomena or gain understanding into some aspect of the patient/provider care experience. Characteristics of qualitative research are that it is process-focused, subjective, and not generalizable. Types of qualitative research include descriptive, survey, phenomenology, and content analysis. Quantitative research to describe relationships between variables, examine cause and effect, and identify facts. Characteristics of quantitative research are that it is outcome-focused, objective, and may be generalizable. Types of quantitative research include quasi-experimental, experimental, and correlational.

7. *Answer:* D
   *Rationale:* A systemic review of randomized control studies (RCT) studies is the highest level of evidence on which to base practice change. Single-site randomized control studies (RCT) studies are considered at a level 2 of evidence. A single descriptive study or qualitative study is a level 6, while a case or cohort study is a level 4. Other levels include quasi-experimental studies (level 3), systematic review of descriptive or qualitative studies (level 5), and expert opinion (level 7) and the lowest level on which to base practice change.

8. *Answer:* D
   *Rationale:* Starting journal clubs, ongoing evidence-based practice (EBP) education, and access to key databases is an example of creating a sense of inquiry and create an EBP culture, which is also the first step in the multistep process of using evidence to support clinical practice. Identifying a problem or trigger is a second step in the process, which can be either problem-focused or knowledge-focused. Searching and critiquing the literature for relevant studies, and identifying of information and stakeholders needed to solve the problem are steps later in the process.

## CHAPTER 56

1. **Answer:** D

   **Rationale:** Focus groups are used for community assessment before the development of targeted patient education programs and materials. Individual assessment would involve specific questions for that exact person to understand specific educational needs of that individual person. Caregiver assessment would involve specific questions related to care delivery or the needs of the caregiver. Survivors would be an individual assessment with specific questions for the survivor.

2. **Answer:** B

   **Rationale:** M = Measurable. S = Specific. A = Attainable. R = Realistic. T = Timely

3. **Answer:** D

   **Rationale:** List four vegetables with high fiber content includes specific outcome criteria. It is specific about what (vegetables with high fiber content) and specific about the number (four). This outcome is measurable. Understand nutritional impact on body is vague, not an objective outcome. It is not clear what constitutes understanding and nutritional impact. Prepare low fat foods is vague, not an objective outcome, as it does not identify what prepare means (once, twice, without assistance etc.). Maintain adequate sodium intake is vague, not an objective outcome, as it is not specific as to what constitutes adequate sodium intake and it is not clear what maintain means (1 week, 1 month, 6 months, etc.)

4. **Answer:** A

   **Rationale:** Diagnostic methods are routinely used in testing nurses' and other staff members' competency and knowledge base in specific areas. Patients are assessed using specific questions related to the needs of the patient. Caregivers are assessed using specific questions related to their needs or the needs of the recipient of their care. The community is assessed using specific methods, such as a survey, checklist, or interviewing a focus group.

5. **Answer:** C

   **Rationale:** Performance analysis of information from quality improvement, incident reports, and other data, such as infection control data, are used in the evaluation phase. Development of the teaching plan uses principles of adult learning elements. Determination of teaching objectives is stating the goals of education. Content identification is within the teaching plan development phase.

6. **Answer:** A

   **Rationale:** Social learning theory encompasses learning by watching and imitating others. Cognitive learning theory is an internal process that requires attention, thought, and reasoning. Behavioral learning theory is based on observable behaviors that are reinforced to increase the strength of the behavior. Humanistic learning theory encompasses the uniqueness of all individuals and is a learner-directed approach.

7. **Answer:** C

   **Rationale:** Adult learning theory is described as someone who is self-directed, independent, and problem-centered which includes the internet search example. Operant conditioning is also known as behavioral learning and is based on observable behaviors that are reinforced to increase the strength of the behavior. Motivational theory is focused on how human behavior is activated. Pedagogy (teaching children) is the opposite of andragogy (adult learning).

8. **Answer:** C

   **Rationale:** Motivational learning is activated through internal and external cues. The foundation of motivational learning is studying the processes that explain the "why" and the "how" human behavior is activated and directed through external and internal cues. An internal cue could be an inner drive to stop smoking for a person's health or to "be there for my family." An external cue could be the cost of cigarettes or having to work around a nonsmoking policy in a person's workplace. Social learning theory revolves around watching and learning from the behavior of others. Cognitive learning is an internal process that requires attention, repetition, and ultimately, retention. Humanistic learning theory is a learner-directed approach, with a foundation based upon the theory that everyone is unique and learn in different ways.

## CHAPTER 57

1. **Answer:** C

   **Rationale:** State Boards of Nursing (BoN) provide oversight of nursing practice by enforcing the state nurse practice act to protect the health, welfare, and safety of the public. The National Council of State Boards of Nursing (NCSBN) develops the National Council Licensure for Registered Nurses (NCLEX) examination. The NCSBN also encourages and facilitates consistency among state boards of nursing. Nurse practice acts define nursing role, titles and scopes of practice. The NCLEX is the licensing examination not a regulating body. The NCLEX is a standardized exam that each state board of nursing uses to determine whether or not a candidate is prepared for entry-level nursing practice

2. **Answer:** B

   **Rationale:** The Affordable Care Act (ACA) provides coverage to Americans with pre-existing conditions (cancer is a pre-existing condition). The ACA also mandates insurers to offer dependent coverage for children to age 26 regardless of if they are in college. The ACA prohibits annual and lifetime limits on coverage. The ACA prohibits arbitrary withdrawals of insurance coverage, mandates essential health services (such as screening examinations or vaccination), and allows four tiers of benefit coverage from low to high monthly premiums and out-of-pocket costs.

3. **Answer:** D

   **Rationale:** Oncology specific accreditation and certification agencies and programs include the Oncology Nursing Certification Corporation (ONCC), American College of Surgeons – Commission on Cancer (ACS-COC) and the Quality Oncology Practice Initiative (QOPI). The QOPI, which is associated with the American Society of Clinical Oncology is a quality program designed for outpatient-oncology practices to promote self-assessment and improvement. The QOPI uses over 190 evidence-based quality measures and generates individual performance scores by practice, site, and provider, as well as bench-marked scores comparing all participating practices. The Joint Commission accredits and certifies healthcare organizations and programs for meeting specific performance and quality standards. The NIH is a federally funded bio-medical research agency. CMS administers the Medicare program and works in partnership with state governments to administer Medicaid and other related programs.

4. *Answer:* C

*Rationale:* Approximately 3% of cancer survivors file for bankruptcy which requires legal consultation. Insurance and prescription coverage would be insurance company issues and social workers, navigators and patient advocates can often assist with obtaining coverage and reimbursement. Many cancer survivors face employment discrimination which would require legal services; a promotion is not employment discrimination.

5. *Answer:* B

*Rationale:* Breach of duty is defined as a failure to meet an acceptable standard of care. Malpractice is a deviation from a professional standard of care. Negligence is a deviation from the acceptable standard of care that a reasonable person would use in a specific situation. Proximate cause is a cause that directly produces an event and without which the event would not have occurred.

6. *Answer:* D

*Rationale:* Common causes of litigation against nurses include issues associated with lack of informed consent, improper operation of a medical device, not following standards of care, failure to communicate appropriately, inadequate or inappropriate patient assessment, inadequate teaching, lack of patient advocacy, medication errors, inappropriate delegation or supervision, inadequate documentation, and working while impaired. Following standard of care is not a litigation risk. Communicating effectively/appropriately is not a litigation risk factor nor is advocating for patients.

7. *Answer:* D

*Rationale:* Communicating clearly when educating patients and families is an example of the development of interpersonal communication, while fostering positive relationships with patients and their families can minimize risk of malpractice. When a nurse has clearly explained and educated a patient on, for example, treatments, their potential side effects, and how to effectively manage those side effects, the nurse improves the level of patient care, but also lessens her chances for malpractice or disciplinary risk later in the patient's journey, since the patient has been well-educated and informed. Attending continuing education programs, obtaining specialty certifications, and becoming involved in patient advocacy programs are examples of maintaining knowledge and skills, another strategy in minimizing personal risk for nurses.

8. *Answer:* B

*Rationale:* The correct answer is negligence. Negligence is the deviation from the acceptable standard of care that a reasonable person would use in a specific situation. Malpractice, on the other hand, is a deviation from a professional standard of care. The two terms are often confused and the line between them is thin, but distinct. Defamation involves harming the reputation of someone by making false statements to a third person. Breach of duty, unlike malpractice and negligence, is the failure to meet an accepted standard of care.

9. *Answer:* C

*Rationale:* Malpractice is the deviation from a professional standard of care. Examples of medical malpractice include a misdiagnosis or a failure to diagnosis. Negligence is the deviation from the acceptable standard of practice. An example of negligence in nursing is misusing equipment or perhaps taking a personal phone call in the middle of a patient's treatment. Slander is defined as making a defamatory statement expressed in a transitory form, especially speech. Duty is a care relationship between a patient and provider.

## CHAPTER 58

1. *Answer:* A

*Rationale:* Increased technology and availability of life support measures increases the likelihood of aggressive care longer, contributing to concerns of overtreatment. Effective collaboration between the physician and nurse about treatment and a request by the patient to continue treatment would not cause moral distress in the nurse. Helping the patient complete an advance directive would not cause moral distress. Nurses who lack knowledge and time to help the patient make an autonomous decision might put the nurse at risk for moral distress.

2. *Answer:* C

*Rationale:* Informed consent ensures the patient has adequate understanding of the risks, benefits, alternatives, and consequences of treatment. Completing the entire treatment plan, and guaranteeing cure of his disease are not provisions of the informed consent. The informed consent consists of risks and benefits. Therefore, there may be risks of treatment that may cause harm to the patient. The informed consent process ensures the patient has an adequate understanding of risks, benefits, alternatives, and consequences of treatment and supports autonomy and human dignity. Informed consent touches on issues of beneficence, justice, and veracity.

3. *Answer:* A

*Rationale:* Advocating for patients is of the provision of promoting, advocating, and protecting the rights, health, and safety of the patient. The other answers are part of the provisions are of the code that establishes boundaries of duty and loyalty, delineating nursing's responsibilities toward social justice, health policy and advancement of nursing as a science and profession.

4. *Answer:* C

*Rationale:* Deontology is the theory that argues that an action's goodness is derived from intention and certain actions are intrinsically right or wrong. Utilitarianism is the theory that what is good is what will result in the most benefit for most people. Ethical egoism is the theory that it is always good to promote one's own good, and divisability is not any ethical principle.

5. *Answer:* B

*Rationale:* In Shared Decision-Making, the patient chooses treatment options in conjunction and with guidance from the physician. Informed consent ensures the risks and benefits of treatment, and supports an autonomous decision. Power of Attorney involves allowing another person to make decisions, and combined decision-making is not a type of decision-making.

6. *Answer:* D

*Rationale:* The ethical principle that is defined by the duty to not harm others is nonmaleficence. Nonmaleficence, in nursing terms, can mean ensuring that the benefits of treatment outweigh the potential harm. Beneficence is doing good or do what is of benefit. However, this term is often shaded in grey, for what is good or one person may not be of benefit to another person, so trying to act with beneficence may prove ethically challenging for some nurses. Autonomy is showing respect to an individual for their right to choose or their right to self-determination. Autonomy in nursing, according to the American Nurses Association, stems from a core value of giving a patient their dignity. Justice, as it relates to medical and nursing care, is allowing each patient, no matter what their life circumstances or morality, access to the same resources.

7. *Answer:* D

*Rationale:* Justice is allocating the same resources to each patient, no matter their socioeconomic status, race, religion, or moral standing. In nursing care, that means making available the same level of care or treatment to the rich and the poor, the morally just and those who have committed crimes. It is the same resources for all. Ensuring the benefits of a patient's treatment outweighs the harm is an example of nonmaleficence. Showing compassion toward a patient in a nurse's care is an example of beneficence, while respect for a person's right to choose their own destiny, or, in medical terms, their own plan of care, is an example of autonomy.

8. *Answer:* C

*Rationale:* Step 3 in identifying ethical concerns is to analyze the problem using ethical theories or approaches. In this step, nurses are to discuss what principles, codes, laws, or perspectives are relevant. Exploring practical alternatives is the fourth step. Nurses are to discuss possible courses of action, with the goal of an action that is ethically reasonable and most likely to achieve the desired outcome with the least harm. Gathering the information and obtaining the facts is the first step in the process towards identifying ethical concerns. Finally, the last step in the process (Step 5) is evaluating the process and outcome. Debriefing sessions with those involved are critical for exploring whether the problem was adequately resolved, and for discussing implications for future similar situations. In Step 1, the nurse gathers information from key participants and obtains the facts to understand the multiple complex perspectives of the ethical problem. In Step 2, the nurse identifies the type of ethical problem that exists.

## CHAPTER 59

1. *Answer:* B

*Rationale:* Barriers to building a collaborative relationship include a lack of clearly defined, distinct domain of influence, a lack of understanding regarding scope of practice, overlapping and changing domains of practice that produce competition, lack of recognition of knowledge and expertise of a profession, and legal responsibilities. Interdisciplinary team meetings provide an opportunity for collaboration and team building among professionals. Developing and initiating change of shift reporting practices promotes nurse to nurse collaboration.

2. *Answer:* D

*Rationale:* Existential advocacy is defined as acknowledging that various experiences in healthcare such as the definition of health versus illness, pain versus suffering, and the experience of dying are highly personal. Human advocacy is a personal extension of self, such as disclosing one's own views on health issues and life as a means to connect more deeply with the patient. Paternalistic advocacy is defined as doing something for or to another without that person's consent on the premise that it serves the person's own good. Simplistic advocacy occurs when one person pleads the cause of another.

3. *Answer:* C

*Rationale:* Certification helps assure the public that the certified nurse has the knowledge and qualifications needed to practice in his or her clinical area of nursing. It is not a guarantee of increased pay although some employers do acknowledge the value of certification with increased pay or promotion. It is not mandated for relicensure or by the BRN.

4. *Answer:* C

*Rationale:* The Plan-Do-Study-Act (PDSA) model is used in quality improvement studies. It typically seeks to answer three fundamental questions, which include identification of the goal, determining how a change will be recognized as an improvement, and what changes will result in improvement. It typically occurs in settings and situations where everyday care occurs. The PICOT question format is a consistent approach and strategy for developing answerable, researchable questions. **P: stands for** Population/patient; **I: stands for** Intervention/indicator (Variable of Interest). **C: stands for** Comparison/control. **O:** stands for Outcome and **T: stands for** Time it takes for the intervention to achieve an outcome or how long participants are observed

5. *Answer:* B

*Rationale:* The Institute of Medicine (IOM) provides a national focus on knowledge regarding safety and setting national safety goals and tracking their progress. Institutions should develop and implement safety systems and development of a "culture of safety" where safety is an explicit organizational goal. Recognizing and removing faulty equipment helps promote safety. Certification helps assure that the nurse has knowledge and qualification for practice in a specific area but it does not assure that medical errors will not occur. Sitting on an evidence-based care committee may increase awareness of potential problems but does not necessarily prevent individual medical errors. Reading nursing journals may increase knowledge about nursing practice but the specific content may not be at reducing medical errors.

6. *Answer:* D

*Rationale:* Paternalistic advocacy is defined by doing something for or to another without that person's consent on the premise that it serves the person's own good. An example of that type of advocacy could be paying for someone's transportation to a medical appointment or even raising funds to help with medical costs, without their knowledge. Simplistic advocacy is personally pleading a case on someone's behalf. Consumer advocacy is ensuring that patients have adequate information

Human advocacy is the extension of self and involves disclosing a person's own beliefs on issues related to healthcare, such as advocating for equal access to health or reducing costs for certain treatments.

7. *Answer:* D

*Rationale:* The Individual Mandate as part of the Affordable Care Act requires individuals to sign-up for health insurance or face a tax penalty. The Individual Mandate was repealed in 2017 as part of an effort to repeal and replace the Affordable Care Act. The other options – annual health screenings, wellness programs, and prevention education – are all false.

## CHAPTER 60

1. *Answer:* B

*Rationale:* Compassion fatigue is a state of physical and emotional distress, or apathy which results from caring for those experiencing pain or is a result of the constant demands of caring for other. For example, those patients seen on an inpatient oncology unit or in a busy infusion area are populations with constant demanding care needs. Exhaustion, cynicism, and inefficacy from chronic job stress are symptoms of burnout. Compassion fatigue is often correlated with burnout, but there are differences. C and D are not syndromes relating to any problem.

2. *Answer:* C

*Rationale:* Caring for high acuity patients and working under high levels of stress with a large caseload on an inpatient unit such as those on a bone marrow transplant unit over a long period of time can cause compassion fatigue. Other risk factors include nurses who are young and single with less than 10 years of experience in the nursing. Overconfidence is not a risk factor; having a high level of self-judgment imposed by either the nurse or the employer puts the nurse at risk for developing compassion fatigue.

3. *Answer:* B

*Rationale:* Scheduling a day at a spa is a way of managing compassion fatigue because the nurse is doing something for herself and exhibits self-care. Other self-care activities include good nutrition and sleep. Staying out late and binge drinking are not ways of managing self-care. This may be a behavioral sign of compassion fatigue. Adequate sleep is recommended; however, lying in bed for weeks at a time is not. Getting the adequate amount of sleep along with exercise is a better way of taking care of one's self. Verbalizing feelings to friends, family, and coworkers may offer support. Speaking to facility social workers or chaplains may also provide counseling and support.

4. *Answer:* C

*Rationale:* Burnout occurs over a prolonged period of time and is due to chronic job stressors. Individuals with burnout may experience cognitive, emotional, or physical exhaustion, feelings of detachment and distancing from work, including social interactions. They may also have feelings of incompetence and being overwhelmed. Compassion fatigue is emotional and physical distress due to the prolonged demands of caring for high acuity individuals or those in pain. Chronic fatigue syndrome is an unexplained medical disorder. Cognitive disorders are related to cognitive disabilities and may include confusion and poor judgment.

5. *Answer:* C

*Rationale:* While the Maslach Burnout inventory is an assessment tool used for diagnosing compassion fatigue, the Professional Quality of Life Scale (ProQOL) uses subscales including assessing for secondary stress disorder, burnout, and compassion satisfaction. The tool is easy to use and score and is the most commonly used. The secondary scales provide more extensive assessment data. The Mental Status exam and Montreal Cognitive Assessment scale are frequently used to assess cognitive changes in individuals.

6. *Answer:* D

*Rationale:* Making time for prayer and meditation is an example of a self-reflection exercise that a nurse can try as part of self-care management. Spending time in prayer or in mediation is a good way to center thoughts and allow for self-reflection. Indulging in a massage, spending time exercise (recommend three to four times weekly for 20-30 minutes), and enjoying a hobby, listening to music, humor, and enjoying nature are all activities that emphasize self-care.

7. *Answer:* C

*Rationale:* An example of managing self-care through grief counseling and support are through activities that focus a person's attention on the present experience, becoming more aware of one's physical, mental, and emotional condition, in a way that is nonjudgmental. Mindfulness has been shown to be effective at reducing stress. The interventions can be offered individually or in a group setting. Establishing good nutrition and eating well, as well as scheduling preventive and medical care appointments, are examples of emphasizing self-care. Sending cards to the family, reminiscing about time spent with patients, sometimes attending the funeral of patients with whom there has been a close bond, is a self-reflective exercise.